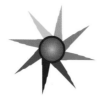

Perspective Press

THE

PHARMACY TECHNICIAN

SECOND EDITION

MORTON PUBLISHING COMPANY

www.morton-pub.com

Morton Publishing

Second Edition
Copyright © 1999, 2004 by Morton Publishing Company

Printed in the United States of America.

Morton Publishing Company
925 West Kenyon Avenue, Unit 12
Englewood, CO 80110
phone: 1-303-761-4805
fax: 1-303-762-9923

International Standard Book Number
0-89582-650-X

10 9 8 7 6 5 4 3 2

NOTICE

To the best of the Publisher's knowledge, the information presented in this book follows general practice as well as federal and state regulations and guidelines. However, please note that you are responsible for following your employer's and your state's policies and guidelines.

The job description for pharmacy technicians varies by institution and state. Your employer and state can provide you with the most recent regulations, guidelines, and practices that apply to your work.

The Publisher of this book disclaims any responsibility whatsoever for any injuries, damages, or other conditions that result from your practice of the skills described in this book for any reason whatsoever.

THE PHARMACY TECHNICIAN

SECOND EDITION

TABLE OF CONTENTS

TABLE OF CONTENTS

TABLE OF CONTENTS

ACKNOWLEDGEMENTS

CONTRIBUTORS

I'd like to thank the following people for their continuing contributions to this book. Aside from developing and revising their specific chapter(s), they have been a great help with the whole book from making suggestions to providing general, and often frequent, assistance.

Robert P. Shrewsbury, Ph.D., R.Ph., Associate Professor of Pharmaceutics, University of North Carolina-Chapel Hill.
> *Bob developed the material for chapters 4, 7, 8, 9, 10, and 11. His involvement in this book has been invaluable.*

Brenda Hanneson Vondereau, B.Sc. (Pharm.), Clinical Services Pharmacist, Catalyst Rx, A HealthExtras Company
> *Brenda developed the chapter on Prescriptions.*

Mary F. Powers, Ph.D., R.Ph., Associate Professor, University of Toledo College of Pharmacy
> *Mary developed the Financial Issues chapter, did an extensive revision of the Calculations chapter, prepared most of the end of chapter multiple choice questions, and is revising the workbook accompanying this text.*

Cindy Johnson, R.Ph., M.S.W., Pharmacist, Colorado Mental Health Institute
> *Cindy developed the Information chapter.*

Betsy A. Gilman, Pharm.D., Director, Singac Pharmacy
> *Betsy developed the material on Community Pharmacy and helped in getting valuable photography that has been transformed into art in this book.*

Pamela Nicoski, Pharm.D., Clinical Pharmacist, Loyola University Medical Center
> *Pamela developed the Institutional Pharmacy chapter.*

In addition I would like to thank the following reviewers who provided feedback on the first edition and suggestions for the second:

> James Austin, R.N., B.S.N., CPhT, Program Chair, Pharmacy Technology Program, Weatherford College, Weatherford, Texas

> Marisa Fetzer, Institute of Technology, Clovis, CA.

> Claudia Johnson, M.S.N., R.N.C., A.P.N., Allied Health Instructor, Pharmacy Technician Program, Polytech Adult Education

> Mary Anna Marshall, CPhT, Richmond Apothecaries; Virginia Institute for Pharmacy Technicians, J. Sargeant Reynolds Community College, Virginia Pharmacist Association

> Peter Vondereau, R.Ph., Pharmacy Manager, Scolan's Pharmacy

> Walgreen Co.

I would also like to thank two great artists for their assistance: Tammy Newnam and Anna Veltfort. Dona Mendoza and Chrissy Morton at Morton Publishers were always helpful and pleasant, even when having to ask about deadlines. I would like to especially thank Dennis Hogan for giving me the opportunity to work on this book. And, finally, I'd like to thank my husband Ned, without whom I do not know what I would do; Malcolm and James, who had to share their dad a little more than usual; Peggy, who helped on several fronts; and my son Beckett, who stayed many extra hours at day care while "mommy was working on her book."

Alison Reeves

HOW TO USE THIS BOOK

This book has been specially designed and developed to make learning easier and more productive. Besides the extensive use of illustrations to both provide information and reinforce text discussion, the text uses a distinctive facing page design that makes it easier to identify important points and to make connections between concepts. Illustrations are never a page or two away from the text. Topics are presented in perspective. Information is easy to find and understand. Some of the other key features of this design are:

➡ A **running glossary** represented by the symbol at right is presented throughout the text to emphasize important vocabulary.

➡ We have used the **Rx symbol** to indicate points of emphasis and suggestion because these are a recipe for success.

➡ End of chapter **Reviews** that provide:

✔ a checklist of the **Key Concepts** in the chapter;

✔ a **Match the Terms** section that tests knowledge of the terminology;

✔ **Multiple Choice** questions in the *choose the best answer* format.

CHANGES IN THE SECOND EDITION

The book has been revised extensively throughout from updating and clarifying to adding new material on important topics, as well as revisions to the pedagogical material. Some revisions are:

➡ Information on pharmacy technician trends, training, education and certification in chapter 1 and especially in chapter 2 has been updated significantly based on data in *"The White Paper on Pharmacy Technicians 2002"*.

➡ New material on the *Health Insurance Portability and Accountability Act* has been added wherever relevant, especially in chapters 2, 3, 5, and 15.

➡ Chapter 5 has an expanded section on prescriptions to labels, and a major section on HIPAA.

➡ Chapter 6 on Calculations has been revised and expanded significantly, including new material on fractions, decimals, significant figures, and calculations for business.

➡ Chapters 7 through 11 have been thoroughly updated and revised, with many new illustrations.

➡ Information sources and descriptions have all been updated in chapter 12; the chapter also includes a new section on Personal Digital Assistants (PDAs).

➡ Chapter 13 includes new information on automated dispensing systems.

➡ The description of Medicare in chapter 14 reflects the new laws passed in 2003.

➡ Chapters 14 and 15 include new material on Disease State Management Services.

➡ Chapter 16 on Institutional Pharmacy has been greatly updated, expanded and reorganized, including new sections on Organization of Medications, Order Processing, and Safety.

➡ Chapter 17 includes a new discussion on On-Line Drugstores.

➡ The number of multiple choice questions per chapter has increased from about 4 to about 25.

➡ The Classifications Appendix has been revised and reorganized for greater clarity.

We think you'll find this book a useful guide to understanding the principles, career concepts, and pharmacy skills you'll need to be a successful pharmacy technician. We also hope that you find this to be one of the best texts you will use.

Dear Student or Instructor,

The American Pharmacists Association (APhA), the national professional society of pharmacists in the United States, and Morton Publishing Company, a publisher of educational texts and training materials in healthcare, are pleased to present this outstanding textbook, *The Pharmacy Technician, second edition*. It is one of a series of distinctive texts and training materials for basic pharmacy and pharmacology training published under this banner: *American Pharmacists Association Basic Pharmacy and Pharmacology Series*.

Each book in the series is oriented toward developing an understanding of fundamental concepts. In addition, each text presents applied and practical information on the skills necessary to function effectively in positions such as technicians and medical assistants who work with medications below the prescriber level and whose role in healthcare is increasingly important. Each of the books in the series uses a visual design to enhance understanding and ease of use and is accompanied by various instructional support materials. We think you will find them valuable training tools.

The American Pharmacists Association and Morton Publishing thank you for using this book and invite you to look at other titles in this series, which are listed below.

John A. Gans, Pharm.D.
Executive Vice President
American Pharmacists Association

Douglas N. Morton
President
Morton Publishing Company

TITLES IN THIS SERIES:

The Pharmacy Technician, second edition
Pharmacy Technician Workbook and Certification Review, second edition
Basic Pharmacology
Drug Card Workbook

THE
PHARMACY TECHNICIAN
Second Edition

ORIGINS

In earliest times, medicine was based in magic and religion.

Like many ancient peoples, Sumerians living between the Tigris and Euphrates rivers around 4,000 B.C. believed that demons were the cause of illness. They studied the stars and the intestines of animals for clues to the supernatural causes of man's condition and fate. In many cultures, physicians were priests, and sometimes considered gods or demi-gods. The Egyptian Imhotep, for example, born around 3,000 B.C., was a priest and adviser to pharaohs and was the first physician known by name. After his death, he was named a demi-god and eventually a god: the Egyptian god of medicine.

The supernatural approach to treating illness gradually gave way to a more scientific approach, based on observation and experimentation.

Around 400 B.C., the Greek physician Hippocrates developed a more scientific approach which has guided Western medicine for much of the time since. He promoted the idea of diagnosing illness based on careful observation of the patient's condition, not supernatural or other external elements. He also wrote the oath which physicians recited for centuries and still honor today: the Hippocratic Oath. From Hippocrates and others following in his footsteps, an approach to medicine in which natural causes were examined scientifically gradually grew to become the dominant approach to treating human illness.

 synthetic with chemicals, combining simpler chemicals into more complex compounds, creating a new chemical not found in nature as a result.

The Greek god of Medicine

The ancient Greek Aesculapius was said to have been such an extraordinary physician that he could keep his patients from dying and even raise the dead. This skill angered Pluto, the god of the underworld, because it reduced the number of his subjects. At Pluto's request, Zeus killed Aesculapius with a lightning bolt, then named him the God of medicine. Aesculapius's daughter, Panacea, became the goddess of medicinal herbs.

MEDICAL MYTH

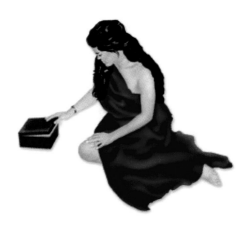

Pandora's Box

As punishment for Prometheus's theft of fire for mankind, the Greek God Zeus created Pandora and had her collect "gifts" for man from the gods. These gifts were really punishments that included disease and pestilence. They were released upon the world when Pandora opened her box.

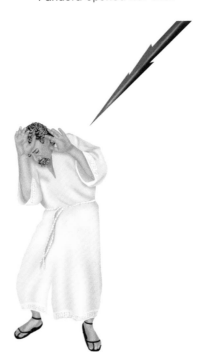

NATURE'S MEDICINE

A Treatment for Malaria

Malaria had long been one of the most deadly diseases in world history, until medicine made from the bark of a Peruvian tree, the Cinchona, was discovered. The medicine was **quinine,** popularly called "Jesuit's powder" for the Spanish priests that sent it to Europe from the New World. Its use along with preventive measures aimed at eradicating the cause of malaria brought the deadly disease under control.

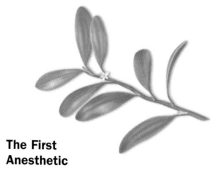

The First Anesthetic

Long before Spanish explorers noticed it, the Indians of the Andes chewed coca leaves for their medicinal effects, which included increased endurance. The active ingredient in the leaves was **cocaine,** which in 1884 was shown to be the first effective local anesthetic by Carl Koller, a Viennese surgeon. This discovery revolutionized surgery and dentistry, since previously anesthesia was administered on a general basis— that is, to the whole body. Eventually, because of its harmful properties when abused, a man-made substitute was developed, called **procaine** or **Novocain®.**

Besides looking to the supernatural, ancient man also looked to the natural world for medical answers.

Early man understood that plants and other natural materials had the power to treat or relieve illness. The ancient Sumerians used about 250 natural medicines derived from plants, many of which are still used today. Around 3000 B.C., the Chinese Emperor Shen Nung is said to have begun eating plants and other natural materials to determine which were poisonous and which were beneficial. One of the first known practitioners of "trial and error" drug testing, he is believed to have established 365 "herbs" that could be used in health treatments. Over the centuries, this number was gradually expanded by various Chinese physicians into the thousands. Herbal medicine remains a major component of Chinese medicine today.

Through the ages, people have used drugs to treat illnesses and other physical conditions.

Ancient cultures around the world used medicines made from natural sources, many of which contained drugs that we still use today. Over the past two centuries, however, science found ways to create *synthetic* drugs, which often have advantages in cost, effect, and availability. Some of these man-made drugs replaced natural drugs and others were for entirely new uses. Today, while we still rely on many drugs derived from natural sources, we use more than twice as many synthetically produced drugs as naturally produced ones. As a result, the number of illnesses and physical conditions that can be treated with drugs is constantly increasing.

Nature's Aspirin

The ancient Greek physicians Hippocrates and Dioscorides both wrote about the pain relieving ability of the bark of a white willow tree that grew in the Mediterranean. In the 1800's, more than 2,000 years after Hippocrates' time, the active ingredient in the willow bark, **salicylic acid**, was derived by chemists. However, because of difficulties in taking salicylic acid internally, **acetylsalicylic acid**, popularly known as **aspirin**, was developed and it eventually became the most widely used drug in the world.

MEDICINE THROUGH THE AGES — A TIMELINE —

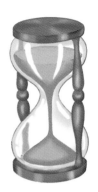

4000 B.C.

Ancient **Sumerians** studied the stars and animal intestines to divine man's fate and physical condition.

3000 B.C.

The **Egyptian Imhotep,** born around 3,000 B.C., was a priest and adviser to pharaohs and the first physician known by name. After his death, he was named a demi-god and eventually a god: the Egyptian god of medicine.

500 B.C.

The **Greek Alcmaeon,** a student of Pythagorus, saw diseases as a result of a loss of the body's natural equilibrium, rather than the work of the gods.

```
4000 B.C.    3000 B.C.    2000 B.C.    1000 B.C.    500 B.C.    250 B.C.
```

3000 B.C.

The **Chinese Emperor Shen Nung** is said to have begun tasting plants and other natural materials to determine which were poisonous and which were beneficial. One of the first known practitioners of "trial and error" drug testing, he is credited with establishing hundreds of herbal medicines.

1500 B.C.

The most complete record of ancient Egyptian medicine and pharmacology, called the **Papyrus Ebers,** dates back to 1500 B.C. This 1100 page scroll document includes about 800 prescriptions using 700 drugs, mostly derived from plants.

600 B.C.

A cult following **Aesculapius, the Greek god of Medicine,** established centers where medicine was practiced. These early clinics became training grounds for the great Greek physicians of later years.

400 B.C.

A number of medical documents are written by different Greek physicians under the name **Hippocrates.** The works avoid the supernatural and religious and represent an approach to medicine that is grounded in scientific reasoning and close observation of the patient. They contain writings about the conduct of physicians, including the famous Hippocratic oath.

pharmacology the study of drugs—their properties, uses, application, and effects (from the Greek *pharmakon:* drug, and *logos:* word or thought).

pharmacognosy derived from the Greek words "pharmakon" or drug and "gnosis" or knowledge; the study of physical, chemical, biochemical and biological properties of drugs as well as the search for new drugs from natural sources.

materia medica generally pharmacology, but also refers to the drugs in use (from the Latin materia, matter, and medica, medical).

100 B.C.

King Mithridates of Pontos practiced an early form of immunization by taking small amounts of poisons so that he could build his tolerance of them. It is said that he was so successful at this that when he eventually decided to kill himself through poisoning, he was unable to, and had to be killed by someone else. The potion Mithridates developed, Mithridaticum, was believed to be good at promoting health and was used for fifteen hundred years.

77 B.C.

Dioscorides, a Greek physician working in the Roman Legion, wrote the **De Materia Medica**, five books that described over 600 plants and their healing properties. His work was the main influence for Western pharmaceutics for over sixteen hundred years. One of the remedies he described was made from the bark of a type of willow tree, the active ingredient of which was salicylic acid, the natural drug on which acetylsalicylic acid (aspirin) is based. He also described how to get opium from poppies.

162 A.D.

The Greek physician **Galen** went to Rome and became the greatest name in Western medicine since Hippocrates both through his practice and extensive writings, nearly 100 of which survive. He believed there were four "humours" in man which needed to be in balance for good health, and he advocated "bleeding" to assist that balance. He also believed in the vigorous application of a scientific approach to medicine and his emphasis on education, observation, and logic formed the cornerstone for Western medicine.

200 B.C.   100 B.C.   1 A.D.   100 A.D.   200 A.D.

200 B.C.

The first official Chinese "herbal," the **Shen Nung Pen Tsao**, listing 365 herbs for use in health treatments, is believed to have been published. This can be considered an early Chinese forerunner to the FDA approved drug list.

100 A.D.

The **Indian physician Charaka** wrote the **Charaka Samhita**, the first great book of Indian medicine, which among other things described over 500 herbal drugs that had been known and used in India for many centuries.

 Note: since the use of drugs goes so far back in history, we use many terms based on Greek or Latin words.

 pharmacopeia an authoritative listing of drugs and issues related to their use.

pharmaceutical of or about drugs; also, a drug product.

panacea a cure-all (from the Greek *panakeia*, same meaning).

MEDICINE THROUGH THE AGES

— A Timeline —

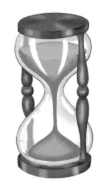

900 A.D.

The **Persian Rhazes** wrote one of the most popular textbooks of medicine in the Middle Ages, the **Book of Medicine Dedicated to Mansur**. A man of science, Rhazes was also an **alchemist** who believed he could turn lesser metal into gold. When he failed to do this, the Caliph ordered him beaten over the head with his own chemistry book until either his head or the book broke. Apparently, it was a tie. Rhazes lost sight in one eye but lived to continue his work.

1500 A.D.

When the Spanish found them, the **Indians of Mexico** had a well established pharmacology that included more than 1,200 drugs and was clearly the result of many hundreds of years of medical practice. One plant, the sarsaparilla, became very popular in Europe for its use on kidney and bladder ailments and can be found to this day in many medicinal teas.

1580 A.D.

In China, **Li Shi Zhen** completed the **Pen Tsao Kang Mu**, a compilation of nearly 2,000 drugs for use in treating illness and other conditions.

1630 A.D.

Jesuits sent **quinine** back to Europe in the early sixteen hundreds. Also called Jesuit's powder, it was the first drug to be used successfully in the treatment of the dreaded disease malaria.

---

750   1000   1250   1500   1750

1000 A.D.

Perhaps the greatest Islamic physician was **Avicenna**. His writings dominated medical thinking in Europe for centuries. He wrote a five volume encyclopedia, one of which was devoted to natural medications and another to compounding drugs from individual medications.

1500 A.D.

In the early fifteen hundreds, a Swiss alchemist who went by the name of **Paracelsus** rejected the "humoural" philosophy of Galen and all previous medical teaching other than Hippocrates. Though he had many critics, he is generally credited with firmly establishing the use of chemistry to create medicinal drugs. Included in his work is the first published recipe for the addictive drug laudanum, which became a popular though tragically abused drug for the next three hundred years.

1721 A.D.

A smallpox epidemic strikes Boston and **Dr. Zabdiel Boylston** (who had already contracted the disease as a child during an earlier epidemic) becomes the first Westerner known to administer a **smallpox vaccine**. The first people he inoculated were his six year old son and two slaves, all of whom developed only a mild case of the disease and then recovered. Even though the inoculation was successful, much of the Boston population was at first extremely suspicious. After several months, 249 people were eventually inoculated, six of whom died, compared with 844 of the 5980 people who contracted the disease naturally.

1796

Edward Jenner successfully uses a vaccine from the milder cowpox disease to inoculate against smallpox.

ABCD *antitoxin* a substance that acts against a toxin in the body; also, a vaccine containing antitoxins, used to fight disease.

antibiotic a substance which harms or kills microorganisms like bacteria and fungi.

hormone chemicals produced by the body that regulate body functions and processes.

human genome the complete set of genetic material contained in a human cell.

1785 A.D.

The **British Physician, William Withering**, publishes his study of the **foxglove** plant and the drug it contained, **digitalis**, which became widely used in treating heart disease. Foxglove had been used since ancient times in various remedies but Withering described a process for creating the drug from the dried leaves of the plant and established a dosage approach.

1803

The German pharmacist **Frederich Serturner** extracts morphine from opium.

1846

In Boston, the first publicized operation using **general anesthesia** is performed. Ether is the anaesthetic.

1899

Acetylsalicylic acid, popularly known as **aspirin,** is developed because of difficulties in using salicylic acid, a drug contained in certain willow trees that had long been used in the external treatment of various conditions.

1921

In Toronto, Canada, **Frederick Banting** and **Charles Best** show that an extract of the hormone, **insulin,** will lower blood sugar in dogs and so may be useful in the treatment of the terrible disease diabetes. The biochemist James B. Collip then develops an extract of insulin pure enough to test on humans. The first human trial in January, 1922 proves successful and dramatically changes the prospects for all diabetics.

1957

Albert Sabin develops an **oral polio vaccine** using a weakened live virus that could be taken orally rather than by injection. However, because of risk of an associated disease from the live virus, only the injectable form of the vaccine is used to inoculate children after January 2000.

1960

The **birth control pill** is introduced.

1981

First documented cases of **AIDS.**

1987

AZT becomes the first drug approved by the FDA for AIDS treatment.

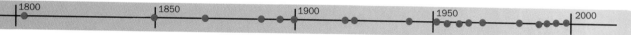

1864

Louis Pasteur's experiments show that microorganisms cause food spoilage, and that heat can be used to kill them and preserve the food. Though others had proposed principles of **"germ theory"** previously, Pasteur's work is instrumental in it becoming widely accepted.

1884

In 1884, **Carl Koller,** a Viennese surgeon, discovers that cocaine, the active ingredient in coca leaves, was useful as a local anesthetic in eye surgery, and cocaine is established as the **first local anesthetic**.

1890

Effective **antitoxins** are developed for diptheria and tetanus, giving a major boost to the development of medicines that fight infectious disease.

1928

In Britain, **Alexander Fleming** discovers a fungus which produces a chemical that kills bacteria. He names the chemical, **penicillin.** It is the first antibiotic drug.

1943

Russell Marker is able to create the **hormone progesterone,** the first reliable birth control drug, from a species of Mexican yam.

1951

James Watson and **Francis Crick** identify the structure of **DNA**, the basic component within the cell that contains the organism's genetic code.

1955

Dr. Jonas Salk succeeds in developing a refined **injectable polio vaccine** from killed polio virus. (In 1954 polio had killed more than 13,000 and crippled more than 18,000 Americans.)

1988

The **Human Genome Project** is begun with the goal of mapping the entire DNA sequence in the human genome. This information will provide a better understanding of hereditary diseases and allow the development of new treatments for them.

1989

Amgen, a **biotechnology** company that develops products based on advances in cellular and molecular biology, introduces its first product, Epogen, an anemia treatment for dialysis patients.

1996

HAART (Highly Active Anti-Retroviral Therapy) is introduced for AIDS treatment. Made up of a combination of one protease inhibitor and usually two antiretroviral drugs, it proves extremely effective in slowing HIV progress and is partially responsible for a 47% decrease in the AIDS death rate in 1997.

THE 20TH CENTURY

The average life span in the United States increased by over twenty years in the Twentieth Century.

In 1900, the average American lived only into their early fifties. By 2000, the average life expectancy at birth in the United States had risen to 77 years. Similar changes were seen throughout the industrialized world and to a lesser extent in developing countries. The growth of hospitals, advances in the treatment of disease, improved medical technology, better understanding of nutrition and health, and the rapid increase in the number of effective drugs and vaccines have all contributed to this profound change in improved life experience.

A major factor in the increased health and life expectancy seen in this century was the dramatic growth in pharmaceutical medicine.

Since the eighteenth century, there was a growing interest and success in creating man-made or synthetic medicines. The creation of aspirin in 1899 was followed by more pharmaceutical research and discoveries that spurred the growth of a worldwide industry committed to creating medicines for virtually every illness and condition. The discovery of the antibiotic penicillin was followed shortly by a World War in which its mass production was seen as critical to Allied success. This and other war related drug needs stimulated the U.S. pharmaceutical industry to dramatically boost its capacity and production. Ever since, pharmaceutical research and development in the U.S. has grown substantially and continually, making it the world's leading producer of medical pharmaceuticals with more than $100 billion in annual worldwide sales.

LIVING LONGER

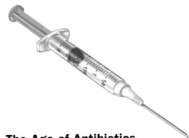

The Age of Antibiotics

In World War I, more soldiers died from infections than the wounds themselves. Although penicillin was discovered as an antibiotic in 1928, it was difficult to produce and for years not much was made of the discovery. With the start of World War II, however, British scientists looked again at penicillin and established that it was effective in fighting infections. Already under attack from Germany and unable to develop mass production methods for penicillin, the British sought help in the United States. In 1942, the Pfizer pharmaceutical company was able to develop a method for mass production of the drug, and by D-Day the Allied army was well stocked with it. Its use saved many thousands of lives during the war and revolutionized the pharmaceutical industry. A period of intense research and discovery in the field of antibiotics began, and many new antibiotics were developed which have dramatically contributed to improved health and increased life expectancy.

Living Longer

Improved pharmaceutical products have had a major effect on the life span of Americans and others in the twentieth century. In the U.S., the life span increased about 64% % in the last century, with much of the increase due to the discovery and use of disease fighting drugs.

source: National Center of Health Statistics

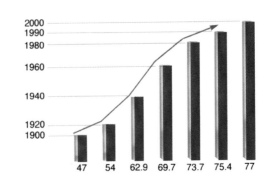

47	54	62.9	69.7	73.7	75.4	77

THE DRUG INDUSTRY

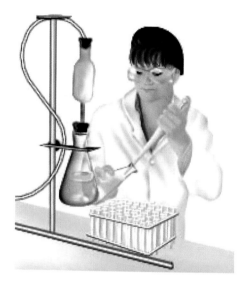

With the increasing availability of powerful drugs, their regulation became more important than ever.

Leaders and governments have long sought to regulate the use of medicinal drugs because of their effect on the population's health. The explosive growth of pharmaceuticals in the twentieth century made governments throughout the world keenly aware of the importance of setting and maintaining standards for their distribution and use.

In the United States, drug regulation is performed by the Food and Drug Administration.

FDA activity is a major factor in the nation's public health and safety. Before a drug can be marketed, it must be shown through testing that it is safe and effective for its intended use. Once marketed, the FDA monitors drugs to make sure they work as intended, and that there are no serious negative (adverse) effects from their use. If drugs that are marketed are found to have significant adverse effects, the FDA can recall them (take them off the market).

The discovery of new drugs requires a major investment of time, research, and development.

The pharmaceutical industry employs thousands of scientists and devotes about one-sixth of its income to research and development. Bringing a new drug to market is a long and difficult process in which the vast majority of research does not produce a successful drug. Thousands of chemical combinations must be tried in order to find one that might work as hoped. Once a potentially useful drug is created, it must undergo an extensive testing and approval process before it can be made available to the public. In the United States, the length of time from the beginning of development through testing and to ultimate FDA approval is often more than ten years.

Patenting Discoveries

As with other scientific and technological areas, patenting new discoveries is an important part of the pharmaceutical development process since it protects against illegal copying of the discovery. The company holding the patent is then able to control the marketing of the product and use this as a way to recover their original investment. Since patenting generally occurs long before a drug is approved, however, a company generally has only about ten years of patent protection left in which to market their product without competition from direct copies called "generic" versions. For more information, see the section on New Drug Approval and Marketed Drugs in chapter 3.

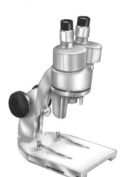

It's in the Genes

One of the most exciting areas of pharmaceutical research is performed by molecular biologists studying human genes. While antibiotics are the answer for many infectious diseases, many other diseases which seemed based on heredity are effectively untreatable. The study of the human genome has shown that many diseases are related to genetic defects. This has led to the creation of new drugs that can successfully treat many diseases previously considered untreatable. As a result, the field of biotechnology has become the most dynamic area of pharmaceutical research and development.

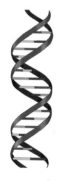

PHARMACY TODAY

A "prescription" drug is one that has been ordered or "prescribed" by a physician or other licensed prescriber to treat a patient. Though physicians occasionally give patients the actual medication, in most cases the individual who dispenses the prescribed medication to the patient is a pharmacist. Pharmacists at the more than 50,000 community pharmacies account for approximately half of the distribution of prescription drugs in the United States. The rest reach consumers primarily through hospitals, mass merchandisers, food stores, mail order pharmacies, clinics, and nursing homes-- all of which employ pharmacists for the dispensing of medications.

The pharmacist has consistently been rated as one of the most highly trusted professionals in the U.S.

The sheer number of available drugs, their different names and costs, multiple prescriptions from different physicians, and the involvement of third-party insurers are among the many factors which make using prescription drugs a complex area for consumers. As a result, they rely on pharmacists to provide information and advice on prescription and over-the-counter medications in easy to understand language. They also routinely ask the pharmacist to make recommendations about less expensive generic substitutes for a prescribed drug.

In 1990, the U.S. Congress required pharmacists to provide counseling services to Medicaid patients in the Omnibus Budget Reconciliation Act (OBRA).

Since then, a number of states have begun requiring this for all patients, and it is generally considered a fundamental service for pharmacists to provide.

The number of prescriptions filled increased between 44 and 54% from 1990 to 1999.

At the same time, the number of active pharmacists increased by only 5%. Between 1999 and 2004 the number of new prescriptions filled is expected to increase by 36% while the number of pharmacists will increase by only 4.5%.

To help with this increasingly complex environment, pharmacists use powerful computerized tools and specially trained assistants.

Computers put customer profiles, product, inventory, pricing, and other essential information within easy access. **Pharmacy technicians** perform many tasks that pharmacists once performed.

THE PHARMACIST

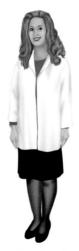

A Trusted Profession

Pharmacists consistently rank as one of the mostly highly trusted and ethical professions in the United States, according to Gallup Polls. In 2003, the top five professions were:

1. nurses
2. medical doctors
3. veterinarians
4. pharmacists
5. dentists

Education

To become a pharmacist, an individual must have earned a Doctor of Pharmacy degree from an accredited college of pharmacy (of which there are about 80 in the U.S.), pass a state licensing exam (in some states), and perform an internship working under a licensed pharmacist. Once licensed, the pharmacist must receive continuing education to maintain their license. Pharmacists seeking to teach, do research, or work in hospitals often must have postdoctoral training in the form of residency and fellowship training. Three out of five pharmacists work in community pharmacies; one out of four in hospitals.

PHARMACY SETTINGS

Most pharmacists and pharmacy technicians work in either a community pharmacy or hospital setting, with community pharmacy being the area of greatest employment (about half of all pharmacists and technicians). However, there are a number of other environments where significant employment can be found. The primary environments for pharmacist and technician employment are:

➡ **community pharmacies:** the area of greatest employment

➡ **hospitals:** the next greatest area of employment

➡ **mail order operations:** pharmacy businesses that provide drugs by mail to patients—a fast growing area.

➡ **long-term care:** residence facilities that provide care on a long-term rather than acute or short-term basis.

➡ **managed care:** care that is managed by an insurer, such as Kaiser Permanente.

➡ **home care:** care provided to patients in their home, often by a hospital or by a home care agency working with a home care pharmacy.

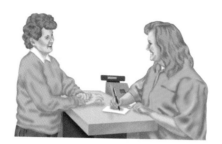
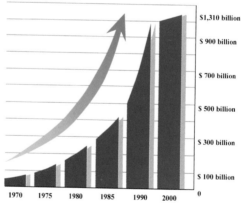

ECONOMIC TRENDS

From 1970 to 2000, the cost of health care in the United States rose over 1,500 percent! Preliminary data from the Department of Health and Human Services for 2003 shows that costs increased an additional 18% between 2000 and 2003, to a total of $1.55 trillion; the increase between 2002 and 2003 was the largest in eleven years.*

As a result of these escalating costs, there have been increasing efforts by government, industry, and consumers to find ways to control the costs of care. Though drugs represent only a small fraction of overall health care expenses, they have also been included in these efforts.

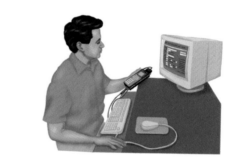

➡ A result of the **managed care** movement is that the majority of prescriptions are now paid by private third parties such as HMO's and other insurance companies, instead of directly by consumers.

➡ Along with this is a trend toward the use of closed "formularies," lists of drugs which are approved for use. These lists rely substantially on substituting generic drugs in place of more expensive brands that may be prescribed by the physician.

➡ Another cost cutting trend is the increasing use of "therapeutic substitution" in which a chemically different drug that performs a similar function is substituted, usually because it is less expensive.

*as reported by The New York Times, *Friday, January 9, 2004, p. A1*
source for illustration: U.S. Statistical Abstract

COMPUTERS IN PHARMACY

Pharmacies use powerful computerized tools that help productivity.

Computerized pharmacy management systems put customer profiles, product, inventory, pricing, and other essential information within easy access. They also automate elements like label printing, inventory management, stock reordering, and billing. As a result, pharmacies and pharmacists dispense more prescriptions and information than ever before.

Pharmacy computer systems may be developed by the user to meet specific needs, purchased ready-made, or provided by a drug wholesaler.

Wholesalers provide inventory management systems to their customers as part of their service. The wholesaler actually owns the system. It is primarily designed for placing orders with the wholesaler, though it may also contain various other elements. Large pharmacy chains have the business volume to justify the expense of developing comprehensive systems that are tailored to their needs. Smaller operations usually buy a commercially available system. Whatever the operation, a computerized pharmacy management system is an indispensable productivity tool.

Although each pharmacy computer system has its own specific features, many general principles of computer usage apply to all systems.

The most important element is stated in the classic computer axiom: garbage in, garbage out. That is, the information produced by the computer is only as good as the information that is entered into it. This means special care has to be taken when entering information (generally called data) to make sure it is correct. A simple mistake in data entry can result in the wrong medication being given to the wrong patient or in any number of other serious problems.

 keyboard skills: Considering how much data entry is required, being able to type at least forty five words per minute is an important skill.

computer knowledge: Many systems use personal computers or similar custom hardware, so familiarity with using computers is important.

A SAMPLE COMPUTER SYSTEM

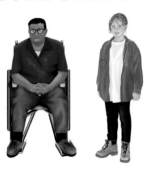

Patient Profile

Allows complete information about patients, including prescribers, insurer, and medication history, and medical history, including allergies; identifies drug interactions for patients taking multiple medications.

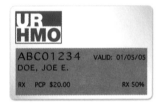

Billing

Checks policies of third parties such as HMOs and insurers; authorizes third party transactions and credit cards electronically.

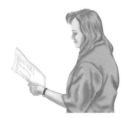

Management Reporting
Forecasting, financial analysis.

data information that is entered into and stored in a computer system.

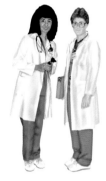

Prescriber Profile

Includes state identification numbers and affiliations with facilities and insurers.

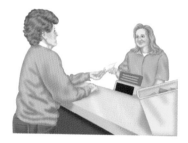

Education/Counseling

Patient information about drugs, usage, interactions, allergies, etc.

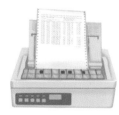

Product Selection

Locates items by various means–brand name, generic name, product code, category, supplier, etc. Gives updates of prices and other product information.

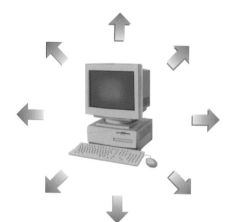

Pharmacy computer systems generally offer most or all of these features, as well as a number of others.

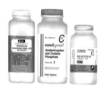

Inventory

Adjusts inventory as prescriptions are filled; analyzes turnover; produces status reports; automatically re-orders based on inventory levels, generates purchase orders.

Pricing

Provides prices for medications and possible substitutes; automatically updates prices; scans prices from bar codes.

Security

Password protection restricts access to authorized users for different features.

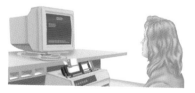

Labeling

Creates label, receipt, customer information and usage instructions.

REVIEW

KEY CONCEPTS

ORIGINS

- ✔ People have used drugs derived from plants to treat illnesses and other physical conditions for thousands of years.
- ✔ The ancient Greeks used the bark of a white willow tree to relieve pain. The bark contained salicylic acid, the natural forerunner of the active ingredient in aspirin.
- ✔ Cocaine was the first effective local anesthetic.

MEDICINE THROUGH THE AGES

- ✔ The foxglove plant contains the drug digitalis, which has been widely used in treating heart disease.
- ✔ Louis Pasteur's experiments show that microorganisms cause food spoilage, and that heat can be used to kill them and preserve the food.
- ✔ Frederick Banting and Charles Best showed that an extract of the hormone, insulin, lowered blood sugar in dogs and might be useful in the treatment of diabetes.
- ✔ Alexander Fleming discovered the antibiotic chemical, penicillin.
- ✔ The Human Genome Project is an attempt to map the entire DNA sequence in the human genome. This information will provide a better understanding of hereditary diseases and how to treat them.

THE 20TH CENTURY

- ✔ The average life span in the United States increased by over twenty years in the Twentieth Century.
- ✔ In World War I, more soldiers died from infections than the wounds themselves.

PHARMACY TODAY

- ✔ To become a pharmacist in the United States, an individual must graduate from an accredited college of pharmacy, pass a state licensing exam, and perform an internship working under a licensed pharmacist.
- ✔ Once licensed, the pharmacist must receive continuing education to maintain their license.
- ✔ Increasing costs of health care have brought increased efforts to control the cost of prescription drugs, one aspect of which is the use of closed "formularies" that rely substantially on substituting generic drugs in place of more expensive brands.

COMPUTERS IN PHARMACY

- ✔ Computerized pharmacy management systems put customer profiles, product, inventory, pricing, and other essential information within easy access. One result has been that pharmacies and pharmacists dispense more prescriptions and information than ever before.

SELF TEST

MATCH THE TERMS.

answers can be checked in the glossary

antibiotic

antitoxin

hormone

human genome

materia medica

panacea

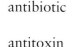pharmaceutical

pharmacology

pharmacopeia

synthetic

- combining simpler chemicals into more complex ones, creating a new chemical not found in nature.

- an authoritative listing of drugs and issues related to their use.

- of or about drugs; also, a drug product.

- a cure-all.

- the study of drugs—their properties, uses, application, and effects.

- generally pharmacology, but also refers to the drugs in use.

- a substance that acts against a toxin in the body

- a substance which harms or kills microorganisms like bacteria and fungi.

- chemicals produced by the body that regulate body functions and processes.

- the complete set of genetic material contained in a human cell.

CHOOSE THE BEST ANSWER.

the answer key begins on page 347

1. The ancient Greek goddess of Medicinal Herbs was
   a. Pandora.
   b. Panacea.
   c. Hippocrates.
   d. Euphrates.

2. The Egyptian god of Medicine was
   a. Imhotep.
   b. Aesculapius.
   c. Plato.
   d. Pandora.

3. An authoritative listing of drugs and issues related to their use is a(an)___
   a. pharmaceutical.
   b. pharmacology.
   c. pharmacopeia.
   d. panacea.

4. Derived from the bark of the Peruvian tree, "Jesuit's Powder," used along with preventive measures, helps keep this disease under control.
   a. smallpox
   b. malaria
   c. polio
   d. tuberculosis

REVIEW

5. Aspirin is made from salicylic acid from the bark of the _____ tree.
   a. willow
   b. cinchona
   c. tea
   d. fig

6. _____ was the first effective local anesthetic.
   a. Quinine
   b. Cocaine
   c. Heroin
   d. Morphine

7. _____ showed that heat can be used to kill microorganisms associated with food spoilage.
   a. Pasteur
   b. Banting and Best
   c. Watson and Crick
   d. Fleming

8. _____ discovered penicillin could kill some bacteria.
   a. Banting and Best
   b. Watson and Crick
   c. Fleming
   d. Marker

9. _____ are substances produced by the body to regulate body functions and processes.
   a. Hormones
   b. Antitoxins
   c. Antibiotics
   d. Genomes

10. _____ identified the structure of DNA.
    a. Watson and Crick
    b. Banting and Best
    c. Serturner
    d. Koller

11. The pharmaceutical manufacturing industry devotes about _____ of its income to research and development.
    a. 1/10
    b. 1/6
    c. 1/3
    d. 1/2

12. _____ protect(s) against illegal copying of new discoveries
    a. Generics
    b. Brand names
    c. Patenting
    d. The FDA

13. The FDA is required to
    a. ensure that a drug is safe and effective for its intended use.
    b. to monitor a drug after it is marketed to ensure it works as intended.
    c. to monitor a drug for any adverse effects.
    d. all of the above.

14. The length of time from the beginning of development of a new drug to FDA approval is often more than _____ years.
    a. two
    b. five
    c. ten
    d. twenty

15. In most cases the individual who dispenses the prescribed medication to the patient is the
    a. prescribing physician.
    b. nurse.
    c. medical office assistant.
    d. pharmacist.

16. The Omnibus Budget Reconciliation Act (OBRA) requires that pharmacists provide
    a. counseling services to all patients.
    b. mail order medication to Medicaid patients.
    c. counseling services to Medicaid patients.
    d. HMO coverage to all patients.

17. To become a pharmacist in the United States:
    a. an individual must graduate from an accredited college of pharmacy, pass a state licensing exam, and perform an internship working under a licensed pharmacist.
    b. an individual must graduate from a non-accredited college of pharmacy and pass a state licensing exam.
    c. no internship experience is required unless the pharmacist intends to practice in community pharmacy.
    d. an individual must graduate from an accredited college of pharmacy, and perform an internship working under a licensed pharmacist, however, no examination is required.

18. The area of greatest employment for pharmacists is
    a. hospitals.
    b. mail order operations.
    c. community pharmacies.
    d. managed care.

19. As for employment opportunities, the Pharmacy Technician may find the greatest opportunity in
    a. the hospital setting.
    b. the community setting.
    c. home health care.
    d. mail order operations.

20. In managed care, care is managed by a(an)
    a. patient.
    b. physician.
    c. pharmacist.
    d. insurer.

21. Lists of drugs approved for use by managed care organizations are called
    a. OBRA.
    b. mail order operations.
    c. HMOs.
    d. formularies.

22. Information that is entered and stored into a computer, such as a patient's name, is called
    a. product.
    b. inventory.
    c. data.
    d. billing.

PHARMACY TECHNICIAN

In health care, "technicians" are individuals who are given a basic level of training designed to help them perform specific tasks.

This training often is provided at community and technical colleges or even on the job. By comparison, health care "professionals" such as physicians and pharmacists receive more extensive and advanced levels of education.

To perform their duties, pharmacists today rely upon the assistance of trained support staff called pharmacy technicians.

Technicians perform essential tasks that do not require the pharmacist's skill or expertise. They work under the direct supervision of a licensed pharmacist who is legally responsible for their performance.

Pharmacy technicians perform such tasks as filling prescriptions, packaging doses, performing inventory control, and keeping records.

Having technicians perform these tasks gives the pharmacist more time for activities which require a greater level of expertise, such as counseling patients. As the job of the pharmacist has become more complex, the need for pharmacy technicians has increased. As a result, pharmacy technician is a rapidly growing occupation offering many opportunities. There are currently about 250,000 pharmacy technicians in the United States and it is estimated this number will grow by at least 36% by 2010.

Like pharmacists, most pharmacy technicians are employed in community pharmacies and hospitals.

However, they are also employed by or in clinics, home care, long term care, mail order prescription pharmacies, nuclear pharmacies, internet pharmacies, pharmaceutical wholesalers, the Federal Government and various other settings. Depending upon the specific setting and job, they may perform at different levels of specialization and skill. An introductory level technician job at a pharmacy requires general skills. In various hospital and other environments, there are specialized technician jobs which require more advanced skills developed from additional education, training and experience. Compensation for these specialized positions is greater than it is for entry level positions.

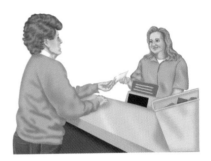
receiving prescriptions

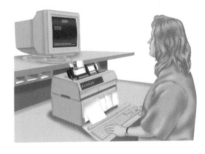
using computers

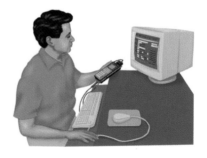
inventory control

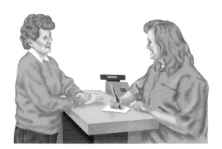

taking patient information

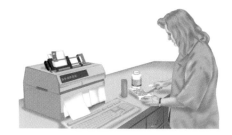

filling prescriptions

The Pharmacy Technician

The activities on these pages may be part of a pharmacy technician's job responsibilities. However, **specific responsibilities and tasks for pharmacy technicians differ by setting and are described in writing by each employer** through job descriptions, policy and procedure manuals, and other documents. What individuals may and may not do in their jobs is often referred to as their "scope of practice." The pharmacist's scope of practice is of course much greater than the technician's. As part of their job requirement, all technicians are required to know specifically what tasks they may and may not perform, as well as which tasks must be performed by the pharmacist.

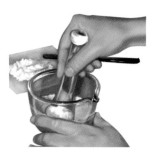

compounding

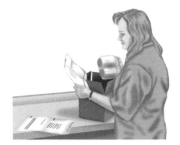

ordering

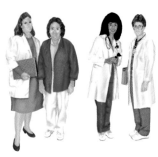

working with a team of health care professionals

PERSONAL STANDARDS

There are personal standards for pharmacy technicians.

Employers may specify these standards as part of the job requirement. Many, though not all, are outlined on these pages. There are standards for behavior, skill, health, hygiene and appearance. Anyone seeking to become a pharmacy technician should consider how they compare in each of these areas and what they must do to excel in them.

The pharmacy technician is a member of a team, the patient's health care team.

For this team to succeed, all its members, including the technician, must work together for the welfare of the patient. If a member of the team fails to perform as required, including the technician, there can be serious consequences for the patient. Anyone wishing to become a pharmacy technician must be able to work cooperatively with others, communicate effectively, perform as expected, and act responsibly. The patient's welfare depends upon it.

Technicians should have these personal qualities:

✔ **Dependable**

The patient, the pharmacist, and the patient's health care team will depend upon you performing your job as required, including showing up on time for scheduled work hours. You must do what you are required to do, whether anyone is observing you or not.

✔ **Detail Oriented**

Patients must receive medications exactly as they have been prescribed. Drugs, whether prescription or over the counter, can be dangerous if misused, and mistakes by pharmacy technicians can be life-threatening.

✔ **Trustworthy**

You will be entrusted with confidential patient information, dangerous substances, and perishable products. In addition, many drugs are very expensive and you will be trusted to handle them appropriately.

Respect for the Patient

The patient's welfare is the most important consideration in health care. To ensure this, there are various government laws and professional standards which guarantee basic **patient rights** and require health care providers to explain these rights to each patient.

The 1996 **Health Insurance Portability and Accountability Act** makes health care providers responsible for the privacy and security of all identifiable patient health information (also called Protected Health Information or PHI), in any form, whether it is electronic, on paper or orally communicated. Among other things, this means that computer files must be protected; any electronic transmission of health information, including claims and billing, must be done via HIPAA-compliant electronic data interchange (EDI); there can be no discussion of patient information within earshot of others; no casual discussion with anyone, including a patient's family members or friends, of a patient or patient information; directing patients to a private area when discussing medications or other personal health issues; making sure files and documents are securely stored where no unauthorized person can access them.

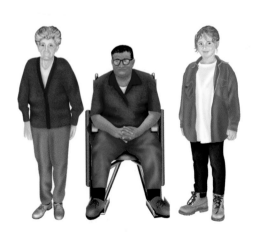

inventory to make an accounting of items on hand; also, with people, to assess characteristics, skills, qualities, etc.

confidentiality the requirement of health care providers to keep all patient information private among the patient, the patient's insurer, and the providers directly involved in the patient's care.

THE TECHNICIAN: A PERSONAL INVENTORY

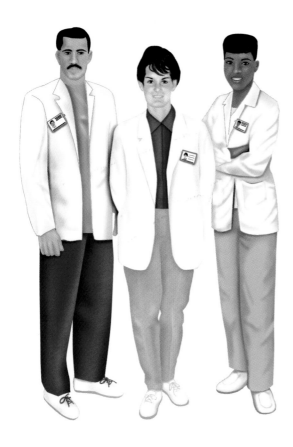

Technicians must follow these personal guidelines:

✔ Health
You must maintain good physical and mental health. If you become physically or mentally run-down, you increase the chance of making serious mistakes.

✔ Hygiene
Practice good hygiene. You will interact closely with others. Poor hygiene may hurt your ability to be effective. You will also be expected to perform in infection free conditions and poor hygiene can violate this requirement.

✔ Appearance
Your uniform and personal clothing should be neat, clean, and functional. Shoes should be comfortable. Clothes should allow the freedom of movement necessary to perform your duties. Hair should be well-groomed and pulled back if long. Fingernails should be neat and trim.

Technicians must be capable and competent in the following skill areas:

✔ Mathematics And Problem Solving
You will routinely perform mathematical calculations in filling prescriptions and other activities.

✔ Language and Terminology
You must learn the specific pharmaceutical terminology and medical abbreviations (e.g., QID, QS) that will be used on your job.

✔ Computer Skills
You will regularly use computers for entering patient information, maintaining inventory, filling prescriptions, and so on.

✔ Interpersonal Skills
You will interact with patients/customers, your supervisor, co-workers, physicians, and others. You must be able to communicate, cooperate, and work effectively.

 There are legal aspects to many of these standards. Failing to follow them can hurt your job performance and result in legal violations.

TRAINING & COMPETENCY

Training and competency requirements for pharmacy technicians differ from setting to setting.

Technician training is generally based on job requirements for the specific workplace, particular skills involved, any applicable professional standards, and state regulations. Regulations vary considerably but the number of states requiring some form of technician training has grown from 19 to 26 (or 34%) between 1996 and 2001 and six states now require certification for registration or licensure.

An example of a model curriculum for technician training is that of The American Society of Health-System Pharmacists (ASHP).

The ASHP is the leading association for pharmacists practicing in hospitals, and other health care systems. Their curriculum provides a national standard for developing technician competency. It can be adapted to different pharmacy settings and the specific needs of an individual training program. Training programs that meet ASHP standards can receive accreditation from it in recognition of having done so. The ASHP curriculum is also endorsed by the Pharmacy Technician Educator's Council (PTEC).

Your training program will prepare you to do your job.

Approximately 247 schools and training institutions offer a range of programs and credentials. Approximately 36% of these programs are accredited by the ASHP, and most are found in community, technical, and career colleges. Training programs are also offered in on-the-job settings such as community pharmacies, hospitals and other institutional settings.

Your employer will monitor and document your competency.

Your employer is legally responsible for your performance and therefore your competency. In addition to monitoring this on a daily basis, you will receive regularly scheduled performance reviews. The frequency of performance reviews will vary by employer and be indicated in your job description or other employee information. Through these reviews and other means, your employer will document your competency to perform your job.

TRAINING

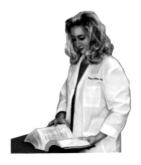 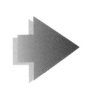

Training Program

Depending upon your setting, you will receive training in some or all of the following areas:

- drug laws
- terminology
- prescriptions
- calculations
- drug routes and forms
- drug dosage and activity
- infection control
- compounding
- preparing IV admixtures
- biopharmaceutics
- drug classifications
- inventory management
- pharmacy literature

An important part of training is exposure to actual workplace settings. Many technicians receive this in the form of **on-the-job** training from their employer or as internships through community colleges or other training programs.

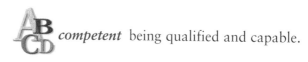

ABCD *competent* being qualified and capable.

COMPETENCY

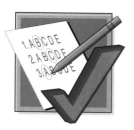 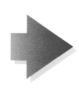 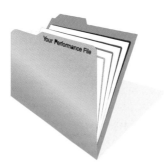

Testing

Demonstration of competency during training will generally be through written tests and practical demonstrations. In on-the-job training or internships, your performance will be directly judged by the supervising pharmacist.

Continuing Education

Pharmacy is a dynamic field that changes constantly. There are always new drugs, treatments, methods and other developments. As a result, continuing education is a critical element in maintaining competency for pharmacy technicians. In order to perform your job as required, you must continually learn new information. Ultimately, this will make your job more interesting and you more effective.

Performance

After you have qualified as competent, your employer will continue to monitor and document your performance and competency throughout your employment. These files may include:

➡ performance reviews
➡ complaints
➡ comments by your supervisor and and other appropriate personnel.

Most jobs also have a probation period during which time the pharmacy technician is expected to learn certain skill sets. If competency is not met, the technician may receive an extended probation period or be dismissed from the job.

 For information regarding ASHP accredited programs, contact:
The American Society of Health-System Pharmacists
7272 Wisconsin Ave.
Bethesda, MD 20814
301-657-3000
http://www.ashp.org

CERTIFICATION

Since there is no federal standard for training or competency, a valuable career step for pharmacy technicians is getting national *certification*.

In the United States, pharmacy technician certification is performed by the **Pharmacy Technician Certification Board (PTCB)**. To receive certification, technicians must pass a standardized national examination called the **Pharmacy Technician Certification Exam (PTCE)** which tests their knowledge and competency in basic pharmacy function and activity areas. As of November, 2003, there were 163,793 Certified Pharmacy Technicians. Although certification is mainly voluntary, some state boards of pharmacy are now requiring that pharmacy technicians earn certification.

Certification is a mark of achievement that employers, colleagues, and others will recognize.

If you pass the examination, you will be able to use the **CPhT** designation after your name. This designation stands for Certified Pharmacy Technician. Beyond verifying your competence as a technician, this indicates that you have a high level of knowledge and skill and can be given greater responsibilities. This in turn means that you may earn more, and will probably cost your employer less time and money for training. Studies have also shown that certified technicians have lower turnover, higher morale, greater productivity, and make fewer errors. Some employers may pay for the cost of the PTCE (if successfully completed) and/or provide training assistance for the PTCE.

Certification must be renewed every two years.

Because pharmacy is a constantly changing field, maintaining skills and competence requires continuing education. In order to renew their certification every two years, CPhTs must meet requirements of 20 contact hours of pharmacy-related continuing education, including at least one hour in pharmacy law. Up to ten contact hours of continuing education can occur at the CPhT's practice site under the supervision of a registered pharmacist, and these hours can be customized to fit the specific needs of the CPhT.

THE EXAMINATION

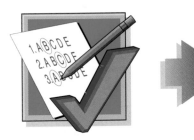

The certification exam tests these areas:

- ➡ assisting the pharmacist in serving patients (64% of the exam);
- ➡ maintaining medication and inventory control systems (25% of the exam);
- ➡ participating in the administration and management of pharmacy practice (11% of the exam).

Other facts about the exam:

- ➡ It contains 125 multiple choice questions for which the best answer must be chosen.
- ➡ Exams last three hours and are conducted by the Professional Examination Service, a non-profit company which performs national certification and licensure examinations.
- ➡ To take the exam, candidates must have a high school diploma or GED by the application deadline and have never been convicted of a felony.
- ➡ To pass the exam, candidates must score at least 650 out of a possible 900.

certification a legal proof or document that an individual meets certain objective standards, usually provided by a neutral professional organization.

Sample Exam Questions

The sample questions below reflect the "choose the best answer" format of the exam. This type of question requires careful reading and judgment. In some cases, there may be more than one answer that is at least partially correct. However, there will only be one correct answer that is the best and most complete answer.

1. Pharmacies located in hospitals are required to follow regulations of this organization:

1. ASHP

2. USP

3. ASCP

4. JCAHO

2. Of the following schedules of drugs, which is for drugs with no accepted medical use in the United States?

1. Schedule I

2. Schedule II

3. Schedule III

4. Schedule IV

3. Of the following needles, which size is the most likely to cause coring?

1. 13 G

2. 16 G

3. 20 G

4. 23 G

4. A solution of Halperidol (Haldol®) contains 2 mg/ml of active ingredient. How many grams would be in 473 ml of this solution?

1. 9.46 gm

2. 0.946 gm

3. 0.0946 gm

4. 0.00946 gm

5. You have a 70% solution of Dextrose 1000 ml. How many Kg of Dextrose is in 400 ml of this solution?

1. 280 Kg

2. 28 Kg

3. 2.8 Kg

4. 0.28 Kg

6. Which is the largest capsule size?

1. size 5

2. size 3

3. size 1

4. size 0

More sample exam questions and practice exams can be found in the workbook accompanying this text, the *Pharmacy Technician Workbook and Certification Review, second edition.*

 For information regarding technician certification contact:
The Pharmacy Technician Certification Board
2215 Constitution Avenue, N.W.
Washington, DC 20037
202-429-7576
http://www.ptcb.org

answers:
1. 4
2. 1
3. 1
4. 2
5. 4
6. 4

REVIEW

KEY CONCEPTS

PHARMACY TECHNICIAN

✔ Pharmacy technicians perform essential tasks that do not require the pharmacist's skill or expertise.

✔ Pharmacy technicians work under the direct supervision of a licensed pharmacist who is legally responsible for their performance.

✔ The specific responsibilities and tasks for pharmacy technicians differ by setting and are described in writing by each employer through job descriptions, policy and procedure manuals, and other documents.

✔ Having technicians perform these tasks gives the pharmacist more time for activities which require a greater level of expertise, such as consulting with patients.

✔ What individuals may and may not do in their jobs is often referred to as their "scope of practice."

✔ Like pharmacists, most pharmacy technicians are employed in community pharmacies and hospitals.

✔ However, they are also employed in clinics, home care, long term care, mail order prescription pharmacies, and various other settings.

✔ In various hospital and other environments, there are specialized technician jobs which require more advanced skills developed from additional education, training and experience.

PERSONAL STANDARDS

✔ Pharmacy technicians are entrusted with confidential patient information, dangerous substances, and perishable products.

✔ Drugs, whether prescription or over the counter, can be dangerous if misused, and mistakes by pharmacy technicians can be life-threatening.

✔ Pharmacy technicians routinely perform mathematical calculations in filling prescriptions and other activities.

✔ Pharmacy technicians must learn the specific pharmaceutical terminology that will be used on the job.

✔ Pharmacy technicians must be able to communicate, cooperate, and work effectively with others.

TRAINING AND COMPETENCY

✔ There is no federal standard for pharmacy technician training or competency.

CERTIFICATION

✔ In the United States, a valuable career step for pharmacy technicians is getting national certification by the Pharmacy Technician Certification Board (PTCB).

✔ The CPhT designation, Certified Pharmacy Technician, is good for two years. It verifies an individual's competence as a technician, and indicates a high level of knowledge and skill.

SELF TEST

MATCH THE TERMS.   *answers can be checked in the glossary*

certification

competent

confidentiality

personal inventory

professionals

scope of practice

technicians

- what individuals may and may not do in their jobs.

- to make an accounting of items on hand; also, with people, to assess characteristics, skills, qualities, etc.

- the requirement of health care providers to keep all patient information private among the patient, the patient's insurer, and the providers directly involved in the patient's care.

- being qualified and capable to perform a task or job.

- a legal proof or document that an individual meets certain objective standards, usually provided by a neutral professional organization.

- individuals who are given a basic level of training designed to help them perform specific tasks.

- individuals who receive extensive and advanced levels of education before being allowed to prac tice, such as physicians and pharmacists.

CHOOSE THE BEST ANSWER.   *the answer key begins on page 347*

1. In health care, _____ are individuals who are given a basic level of training designed to help them perform specific tasks.
   a. LPNs
   b. DOs
   c. professionals
   d. technicians

2. In pharmacy, technicians perform essential tasks that do not require _____ skill or expertise.
   a. the clerk's
   b. the pharmacist's
   c. scientific
   d. mathematical

3. Specialized technician jobs in hospitals have _____ compensation that entry level positions.
   a. less
   b. about the same
   c. greater

4. Specific responsibilities and tasks for pharmacy technicians differ by setting and are described in writing by each
   a. technician.
   b. local police department.
   c. employer.
   d. state board of pharmacy.

REVIEW

5. The pharmacy technician can do the following functions except:
   a. take patient information
   b. fill prescription orders
   c. compound prescription orders
   d. advise patients on medications

6. In the pharmacy setting, any procedure involving professional discretion or judgement is the responsibility of the
   a. pharmacy technician
   b. lead pharmacy technician
   c. store manager
   d. pharmacist

7. The term that describes making an accounting of items on hand is
   a. policy.
   b. inventory.
   c. ordering.
   d. re-ordering.

8. The requirement of health care workers to keep all patient information private among the patient, the insurer, and the providers directly involved in the patients care is called
   a. compliance.
   b. confidentiality.
   c. secrecy.
   d. portability.

9. Pharmacy technicians should be detail oriented. This means
   a. patients must receive medications exactly as they have been prescribed.
   b. an incorrect strength will always be detected by the pharmacist.
   c. technicians do not need to be careful because the pharmacist is supposed to find and correct all technician errors.

10. Pharmacy technicians should be trustworthy. This means
    a. pharmacy technicians cannot count controlled substances.
    b. pharmacy technicians should never obtain confidential information.
    c. that pharmacy technicians are entrusted with confidential information, dangerous substances, and perishable products.
    d. pharmacy technicians should not handle perishable products.

11. Good hygiene is important for pharmacy technicians because of the interactions with other persons and the expectation of performing in _____ conditions
    a. warm
    b. cold
    c. infection free
    d. sunny

12. Pharmacy technicians must be capable and competent in mathematics and problem solving because
    a. all medications that are available on prescription cannot lead to overdose death.
    b. pharmacists always check their work.
    c. all medications come pre-mixed and pre-packaged.
    d. mathematical calculations are routinely used.

13. Pharmacy technicians must be capable and competent with computer skills because
    a. pharmacists will check their data entry.
    b. pharmacists do all of the computer work.
    c. pharmacists should operate the computer.
    d. technicians regularly use computers.

14. Pharmacy technicians must be capable and competent in the area of interpersonal skills. This means
   a. they must be able to communicate, cooperate, and work effectively.
   b. they must socialize with their co-workers.
   c. the pharmacist should obtain all confidential information from the patient.
   d. they must make friends with every patient.

15. _____ typically monitor and document competency of pharmacy technicians.
   a. Employers
   b. Technicians
   c. Pharmacists
   d. PTCB

16. Any complaints received regarding an employee's employment
   a. are discarded after two weeks.
   b. are discarded after one year.
   c. are discarded within one week after the complaint was received.
   d. may be kept in the employee's performance/personnel file.

17. Training that occurs in actual workplace settings is called
   a. performance-based training.
   b. on-the-job training.
   c. community college training.
   d. certified training.

18. _____ is another term for being qualified and capable.
   a. Realistic
   b. Competent
   c. Professional
   d. Technical

19. In the United States, pharmacy technician certification is performed by the
   a. APhA.
   b. PTCB.
   c. ASHP.
   d. PTEC.

20. PTCB Certification must be renewed every
   a. three years.
   b. year.
   c. two years.
   d. four years.

21. After passing the Pharmacy Technician National Certification exam, pharmacy technicians may use the following designation after their name:
   a. PT
   b. RPhT
   c. CPhT
   d. none of the above

22. CPhTs need _____ of continuing education every _____ years to renew certification.
   a. 30 hours, 2
   b. 10 hours, 1
   c. 30 hours, 3
   d. 20 hours, 2

23. Continuing education for CPhTs must contain _____ in pharmacy law every _____ years.
   a. one hour, one
   b. two hours, one
   c. one hour, two
   d. two hours, two

DRUG REGULATION

— A Timeline —

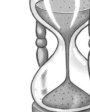

There are many laws in the United States concerning the safety and effectiveness of food, drugs, medical devices and cosmetics. Regardless of whether a product is produced in the United States or is imported, it must meet the requirements of these laws. The leading enforcement agency at the federal level for these regulations is the Food and Drug Administration. On these pages are brief descriptions of U.S. federal laws and their significance.

Food and Drug Act of 1906

Prohibited interstate commerce in adulterated or misbranded food, drinks, and drugs. Government pre-approval of drugs is required.

1927 Food, Drug and Insecticide Administration

The law enforcement agency is formed that would be renamed in 1930 as the Food and Drug Administration.

1950 Alberty Food Products v. U.S.

The United States Court of Appeals rules that the purpose for which a drug is to be used must be included on the label.

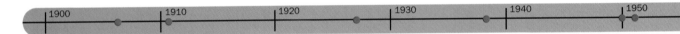

1911 Sherley Amendment

This law was enacted in response to the Supreme Court's interpretation that the 1906 Food and Drugs Act only applied to misleading information about the ingredients of a drug, as opposed to its effects. It prohibits false and misleading claims about the **therapeutic** effects of a drug.

1938 Food, Drug and Cosmetic (FDC) Act

In response to the fatal poisoning of 107 people, primarily children, by an untested sulfanilamide concoction, this comprehensive law requires new drugs be shown to be safe before marketing.

1951 Durham-Humphrey Amendment

This law defines what drugs require a prescription by a licensed practitioner and requires them to include this **legend** on the label: "Caution: Federal Law prohibits dispensing without a prescription.

The Thalidomide Lesson

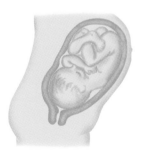

In 1962, a new sleeping pill containing the drug, thalidomide, was found to cause severe birth defects when used by pregnant women. This included lost limbs and other major deformities that affected thousands of children in Europe, where the drug had been widely used. In the United States, the drug was not yet approved for marketing and was only being used in tests, so it affected a small number of children. However, the nature of the defects and the number of children affected created a public demand in the U.S. for tighter drug regulation that resulted in the Kefauver-Harris Amendment. From then on, drugs would have to be shown to be both safe and effective before they could be marketed in the United States.

Later studies found Thalidomide to be safe and effective in treating multiple myeloma and it is now approved for that use.

therapeutic serving to cure or heal.

legend drug any drug which requires a prescription and either of these "legends" on the label: "Caution: Federal law prohibits dispensing without a prescription," or "Rx only."

1962 Kefauver-Harris Amendment

Requires drug manufacturers to provide proof of both safety and effectiveness before marketing the drug.

1966 Fair Packaging and Labeling Act

This requires all consumer products in interstate commerce to be honestly and informatively labeled.

1970 Controlled Substances Act (CSA)

The CSA classifies drugs that may be easily abused and restricts their distribution. It is enforced by the Drug Enforcement Administration (DEA) within the Justice Department.

1987 Prescription Drug Marketing Act

Restricts distribution of prescription drugs to legitimate commercial channels and requires drug wholesalers to be licensed by the states.

1990 Omnibus Budget Reconciliation Act (OBRA)

Among other things, this act requires pharmacists to offer counseling to Medicaid patients regarding medications.

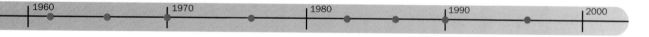

1960 1970 1980 1990 2000

1970 Poison Prevention Packaging Act

Requires child-proof packaging on all controlled and most prescription drugs dispensed by pharmacies. Non-child-proof containers may only be used if the prescriber or patient requests one.

1976 Medical Device Amendment

Requires pre-market approval for safety and effectiveness of life-sustaining and life-supporting medical devices.

1983 Orphan Drug Act

Provides incentives to promote research, approval and marketing of drugs needed for the treatment of rare diseases.

1996 Health Insurance Portability and Accountability Act

Among other things this act defined the scope of health information that may and may not be not be shared among health care providers without patient consent and provided for broad and stringent regulations to protect patients' right to privacy. All "covered entities", meaning any health care provider using electronic claims transmissions, billing or other electronic transfer of patient information, were required to be compliant with HIPAA privacy and security regulations by April 14, 2003. These regulations govern the transfer of patient health information whether it is communicated electronically, on paper or orally.

NEW DRUG APPROVAL

All new drugs, whether made domestically or imported, require FDA approval before they can be marketed in the United States.

A new drug is any drug proposed for marketing after 1938 that was not already recognized as safe and effective. This represents the vast majority of drugs on the market.

Before it will be approved, a new drug must be shown to be both safe and effective and that its benefits substantially outweigh its risks.

It is the responsibility of the drug manufacturer (not the FDA) to provide proof of this to the FDA's **Center for Drug Evaluation and Research (CDER)**. The proof is based on extensive testing which begins in the laboratory, where chemical analysis is performed, and moves on to animal testing and then clinical trials with people. The FDA estimates that the testing process currently takes 8.5 years.

"Clinical trials" involve testing the drug on people.

Clinical tests begin with small numbers of participants over a short period of time and eventually expand into large groups of participants over long periods. Trial participants must give their informed consent. Among other things, it means the person must be told of the risks of the treatment along with other treatment options in language they can understand. Participants are also free to leave the trial at any time they wish.

placebo an inactive substance given in place of a medication.

pediatric having to do with the treatment of children.

Testing Children

Children are not included in trials until a drug has been fully tested on adults. Drugs which have not been tested on children generally state on the label that their safety and effectiveness has not been established for children. Some drugs, however, may carry label information for pediatric use that is based on studies of adults and other pediatric treatment information. The Pediatric Labeling Rule in 1994 mandated that all drugs have pediatric dosing and safety information on their labels if the drug has potential use for pediatric patients.

TESTING

Animal Testing

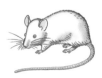

Once laboratory testing of a proposed new drug is finished, the drug is tested on animals before it will be tested on humans. Drug companies try to use as few animals and to treat them as humanely as possible. Since different species often react differently, more than one species is usually tested. Drug absorption into the bloodstream is monitored carefully. Only a fraction of a percent of drugs tested on animals are ever tested on humans.

Placebos

Placebos are inactive substances, not real medications, that are administered to give the patient the impression he or she is receiving a potentially effective medication. This provides a valuable comparison against patients who receive a test drug. Patients in trials must freely agree to the possibility that they may be given a placebo. They must also be informed of an effective treatment if one is available.

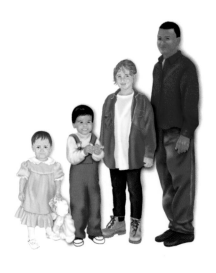

Testing Phases in Humans

There are **three phases** of testing a new drug in humans. Testing begins with a small number of participants for a short time and this gradually increases to a large number of participants over long periods of time. The goals of each phase also change from indicating a minimal level of safety to ultimately verifying the safety, effectiveness and dosage for widespread use. Only about 25% of drugs tested in phase 1 successfully complete phase 3.

phase 1

➡ **20-100 patients**
➡ **time: several months**
➡ **purpose: mainly safety**

phase 2

➡ **up to several hundred patients**
➡ **time: several months to two years**
➡ **purpose: short-term safety but mainly effectiveness**

phase 3

➡ **several hundred to several thousand patients**
➡ **time: one to four years**
➡ **purpose: safety, dosage, and effectiveness**

source: Food and Drug Administration

D uring the trial phase, a proposed new drug is called an investigational new drug (IND).

It is available for use only within the trial groups unless granted a special "treatment" status which is sometimes given to provide relief to critically ill patients outside of clinical trials. An example of this is AZT, which was used on thousands of AIDS patients who were not part of a clinical trial prior to the drug receiving FDA approval. It is worth noting, however, that such drugs are extremely expensive and are excluded from coverage by most insurers and HMOs.

Tests are "controlled" by comparing the effect of a proposed drug on one group of patients with the effect of a different treatment on other patients.

Patients have the same condition and similar characteristics and are placed in either treatment groups or control groups at random to make sure the groups have essentially the same characteristics. The control group may receive no drug at all, a placebo, a drug known to be effective, or a different dose of the same drug.

The patients in a trial are always "blind" to the treatment.

They are not told which group (controlled or treatment) they are in. In a "double-blind" test, neither the patients nor the physicians know whether the patient is receiving the active drug or a placebo. This prevents patients and/or their physicians from imagining effects one way or the other. Medical results alone determine the drug's effectiveness and its safety.

Medical Products Other Than Drugs

Medical devices and biological products such as insulin and vaccines must also meet FDA testing and approval requirements. The **Center for Devices and Radiological Health (CDRH)** is responsible for devices. The **Center for Biologics Evaluation and Research (CBER)** is responsible for biological products made from living organisms.

MARKETED DRUGS

A patent for a new drug gives its manufacturer an exclusive right to market the drug for a specific period of time under a brand name. During this time, the manufacturer attempts to recover the costs of the drug's research and development. A drug patent is in effect for 17 years from the date of the drug's discovery. Since the testing and approval process takes years to complete, for many years drugs reached the market with only half their patent time left. To compensate for this, the Hatch-Waxman Act of 1984 provided for up to five year extensions of patent protection to the patent holders to make up for time lost while products went through the FDA approval process.

Once a patent for a brand drug expires, other manufacturers may copy the drug and release it under its pharmaceutical or "generic" name.

Manufacturers of generic drugs do not need to perform the safety and effectiveness testing required of new drugs. However, they need to demonstrate that the drug is **pharmaceutically equivalent** to the proprietary (patented brand) drug—that it has same active ingredients, same dosage form, same route of administration, and same strength, and that it is **therapeutically equivalent**—that the body's use of the drug is the same. This is measured by the rate and extent to which the active ingredients are absorbed into the bloodstream.

Over-The-Counter (OTC) drugs are drugs which do not require a prescription.

They can be used upon the judgment of the consumer. There are over 100,000 OTC drugs in 80 therapeutic categories marketed. The FDA publishes acceptable ingredients for OTC drugs in "Drug Monographs." The manufacturer of an OTC drug must follow monograph requirements to be able to market their drug without undergoing the FDA new drug approval process. Though some OTC drugs were available before FDA approval was required, the FDA has been reviewing them under the "OTC Drug Review Program," and all new OTC drugs require FDA approval.

LABELS AND LABELING

While all drugs are required to have clear and accurate information for all labels, inserts, packaging, and so on, there are different information requirements for various categories of drugs. Information requirements for OTC drugs are designed to enable consumers to use them without medical advice. Manufacturers of prescription drugs do not have to include directions for use on their labels since such directions must be supplied by the prescriber and dispenser. In many cases, important associated information may not fit on the label itself, and it will be provided in the form of an insert, brochure, or other document that is referred to as **labeling.** We'll look at labels and label information requirements on these next few pages.

Look Alike, Sound Alike

Federal laws require that a drug and/or its container not be imitative of another drug so that the consumer will be misled. Nevertheless, there are many drugs with similar sounding names in similar looking packages. It is therefore essential for pharmacy technicians to pay close attention to the details of drug names and packaging. Using the wrong drug can have very serious consequences. A list of some Look-Alike and Sound-Alike drugs is in the Classifications Appendix.

 labeling important associated information that is not on the label of a drug product itself, but is provided with the product in the form of an insert, brochure, or other document.

OTC LABELS

Active Ingredient (In Each Tablet)　　　Purpose

Chlorpheniramine Maleate 4 mg...Antihistamine

Uses: for the temporary relief of these symptoms of hay fever
▶ sneezing　　　▶ runny nose　　　▶ itchy, watery eyes

Warnings

**Ask a Doctor Before Use
If You Have:**

▶ glaucoma
▶ a breathing problem such as emphysema or chronic bronchitis
▶ difficulty in urination due to enlargement of the prostate gland

If You Are:

▶ taking sedatives or tranquilizers

When Using This Product:

▶ marked drowsiness may occur
▶ alcohol, sedatives, and tranquilizers may increase the drowsiness effect
▶ avoid alcoholic beverages
▶ use caution when driving a motor vehicle or operating machinery
▶ excitability may occur, especially in children

If pregnant or breast-feeding, ask a health professional before use.
Keep out of reach of children. In case of overdose, get medical help right away.

Directions:

Adults and children over 12 years:	Take 1 tablet every 4 to 6 hours as needed. Do not take more than 6 tablets in 24 hours.
Children 6 to under 12 years:	Take 1/2 tablet every 4 to 6 hours as needed. Do not take more than 3 tablets in 24 hours.
Children under 6 years:	Ask a doctor.

FDA label format for OTC medications

Many over-the-counter products have labels that are difficult to read, understand, or both. To the left is a label format adopted by the FDA to make it easier to read and understand the information currently contained on over-the-counter medication labels. Note that it may take until 2005 before all OTC products have the new label format.

Over-the-counter medications do not require a prescription but sometimes prescriptions are written for them for insurance or other reasons. In addition, patients often seek counseling regarding the use of over-the-counter medications. As a result, the pharmacy technician will deal with OTC medications regularly and should be familiar both with their label information and how to handle inquiries about them.

Since OTC medications are not without risks, all patients requesting information on them should be referred to the pharmacist. OTC medications may have significant drug interactions with prescription drugs the patient may be taking which could lead to serious adverse effects, including death.

The following information should be contained on the labels of over-the counter-medications.

➡ product name
➡ name and address of manufacturer or distributor
➡ list of all active and other ingredients
➡ amount of contents
➡ adequate warnings
➡ adequate directions for use

SAMPLE LABELS

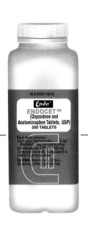

MANUFACTURER STOCK LABEL

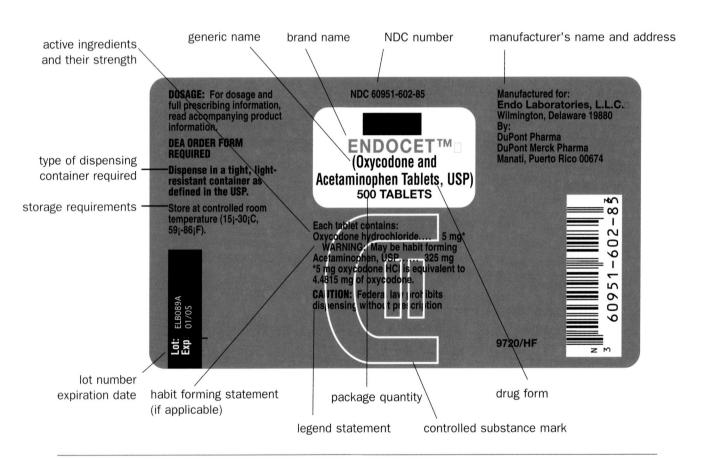

active ingredients and their strength

generic name

brand name

NDC number

manufacturer's name and address

type of dispensing container required

storage requirements

lot number
expiration date

habit forming statement (if applicable)

package quantity

drug form

legend statement

controlled substance mark

DOSAGE: For dosage and full prescribing information, read accompanying product information.

DEA ORDER FORM REQUIRED

Dispense in a tight, light-resistant container as defined in the USP.

Store at controlled room temperature (15¡-30¡C, 59¡-86¡F).

NDC 60951-602-85

ENDOCET™
(Oxycodone and Acetaminophen Tablets, USP)
500 TABLETS

Each tablet contains:
Oxycodone hydrochloride.... 5 mg*
 WARNING: May be habit forming
Acetaminophen, USP..... 325 mg
*5 mg oxycodone HCl is equivalent to 4.4815 mg of oxycodone.

CAUTION: Federal law prohibits dispensing without prescription

Manufactured for:
Endo Laboratories, L.L.C.
Wilmington, Delaware 19880
By:
DuPont Pharma
DuPont Merck Pharma
Manati, Puerto Rico 00674

Lot: ELB089A
Exp: 01/05

9720/HF

3 N 60951-602-85

Labeling

In addition to a container label, manufacturer prescription drugs must also be accompanied by labeling which includes information on the following: clinical pharmacology, indications and usage, contraindications, warnings, precautions, adverse reactions, drug abuse and dependence, dosage, and packaging. This information is designed to inform both the prescriber and the dispenser regarding the drug.

NDC (National Drug Code) Numbers

An NDC number is an identification number assigned by the manufacturer to a drug product. Each NDC number has 3 sets of numbers: the first set indicates the manufacturer; the second set indicates the medication, its strength, and dosage form; and the third set indicates the package size. Note that depending on whether it is an older or newer drug product, the first set of numbers could have four or five digits and the second set of numbers could have three or four digits. The last set of numbers always has two digits.

controlled substance mark the mark (CII-CV) which indicates the control category of a drug with a potential for abuse.

DISPENSED PRESCRIPTION DRUG LABEL

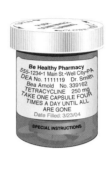

Minimum requirements on prescription labels for most drugs generally are as follows:

✔ name and address of dispenser

✔ prescription serial number.

✔ date of prescription or filling

✔ expiration date

✔ name of prescriber

And any of the following that are stated in the prescription:

✔ name of patient

✔ directions for use

✔ cautionary statements

Certain drugs have greater requirements, and many states impose greater requirements.

Typical elements on a prescription label:

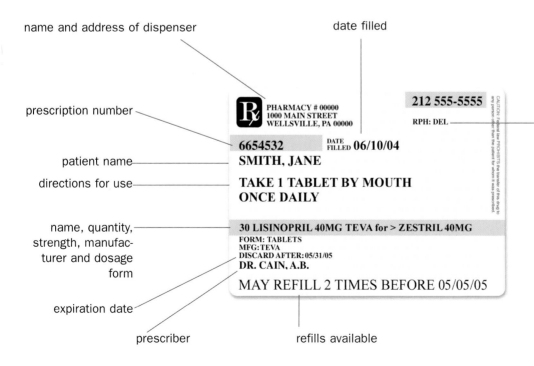

name and address of dispenser

date filled

prescription number

patient name

directions for use

name, quantity, strength, manufacturer and dosage form

expiration date

prescriber

refills available

initials of the person who keyed the information into the computer

PHARMACY # 00000
1000 MAIN STREET
WELLSVILLE, PA 00000

212 555-5555

RPH: DEL

6654532   DATE FILLED **06/10/04**

SMITH, JANE

TAKE 1 TABLET BY MOUTH ONCE DAILY

30 LISINOPRIL 40MG TEVA for > ZESTRIL 40MG

FORM: TABLETS
MFG: TEVA
DISCARD AFTER: 05/31/05
DR. CAIN, A.B.

MAY REFILL 2 TIMES BEFORE 05/05/05

CONTROLLED SUBSTANCES

The government tightly controls the use of drugs that can be easily abused.

The 1970 Controlled Substances Act (CSA) identified five groups or schedules of such drugs as **controlled substances** and put strict guidelines on their distribution. It required manufacturers, distributors, or dispensers of controlled substances to register with the Drug Enforcement Administration (DEA) of the Justice Department. This created a "closed system" in which only registered parties can distribute these drugs.

The five control schedules are as follows*:

Schedule I:
➡ Each drug has a high potential for abuse and no accepted medical use in the United States. It may not be prescribed. Heroin, various opium derivatives, and hallucinogenic substances are included on this schedule.

Schedule II:
➡ Each drug has a high potential for abuse and may lead to physical or psychological dependence, but also has a currently accepted medical use in the United States. Amphetamines, opium, cocaine, methadone, and various opiates are included on this schedule.

Schedule III:
➡ Each drug's potential for abuse is less than those in Schedules I and II and there is a currently accepted medical use in the U.S., but abuse may lead to moderate or low physical dependence or high psychological dependence. Anabolic steroids and various compounds containing limited quantities of narcotic substances such as codeine are included on this schedule.

Schedule IV:
➡ Each drug has a low potential for abuse relative to Schedule III drugs and there is a current accepted medical use in the U.S., but abuse may lead to limited physical dependence or psychological dependence. Phenobarbital, the sedative chloral hydrate, and the anesthetic methohexital are included in this group.

Schedule V:
➡ Each drug has a low potential for abuse relative to Schedule IV drugs and there is a current accepted medical use in the U.S., but abuse may lead to limited physical dependence or psychological dependence. Compounds containing limited amounts of a narcotic such as codeine are included in this group.

*21 USC Sec. 812 as of 1/96. Note: these schedules are revised periodically. It is important to refer to the most current schedule.

REGULATIONS

Labels

Manufacturers must clearly label controlled drugs with their control classification.

Record keeping

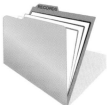

Distributors are required to maintain accurate records of all controlled substance activity. This includes accurate records of inventory as well as drugs dispensed. Schedule-II prescription records must be kept separate from non-controlled drug records, though in some cases they may be kept with other controlled drug records.

Security for Controlled Drugs

Schedule II drugs must be stored in a locked tamper-proof narcotics cabinet that is usually secured to the floor or wall. Schedule III, IV, and V drugs may be kept openly on storage shelves in retail and hospital settings.

Joint responsibility

By law, both the prescriber and the dispenser of the prescription have joint responsibility for the legitimate medical purpose of the prescription. This is primarily intended to ensure that controlled substances not be prescribed for inappropriate reasons.

DEA Number

All prescribers of controlled substances must be authorized by the DEA. They are assigned a DEA number which must be used on all controlled drug prescriptions.

SAMPLE LABELS AND ORDER FORM

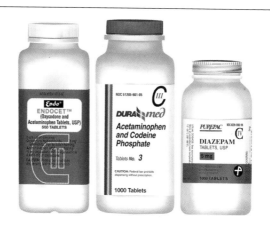

Manufacturer containers and labels for C-II, C-III, and C-IV controlled drug products . Note that the control substance marks are prominent.

At right is a sample DEA Form 222 which is used to order C-I and C-II substances. It must be signed by a registered person, in triplicate. Note that C-III-C-V don't require federal order forms. Because of the lower potential for abuse they are controlled by the record keeping requirements for all controlled substances.

This form can be requested on-line from http://www.deadiversion.usdoj.gov/drugreg/index.html. Each form has its own unique serial number issued when the form is requested. The form must be completed in writing.

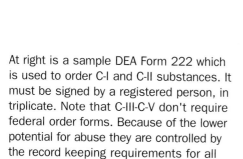

CONTROLLED SUBSTANCE PRESCRIPTIONS

Controlled-Substance Prescriptions

Controlled-substance prescriptions have greater requirements at both federal and state levels than other prescriptions, particularly Schedule II drugs. On controlled substance prescriptions, the DEA number must appear on the form and the patient's full street address must be entered.

On Schedule II prescriptions, the form must be signed by the prescriber. In many states, there are specific time limits that require Schedule II prescriptions be promptly filled. Quantities are limited and no refills are allowed. When the prescription is filled, the pharmacist draws a line across it indicating it has been filled.

Federal requirements for Schedules III-V are less stringent than for Schedule II. For example, faxed

prescriptions are allowed and they may be refilled up to five times within a six month period. However, state and other regulations may be stricter than federal requirements, so it is necessary to know the requirements for your specific job setting.

DEA Formula

DEA numbers are required by federal law. They have two letters followed by seven single-digit numbers, e.g., AB1234563. **Following is a formula for validating a DEA number on a prescription form:** If the sum of the first, third and fifth digits is added to twice the sum of the second, fourth, and sixth digits, the total should be a number whose *last digit* is the same as the last digit of the DEA number.

PUBLIC SAFETY

Though the FDA approval process is quite thorough, it is impossible to fully prove that a drug is safe for use.

No matter how many people participate in the clinical trials, the number is always just a fraction of how many will use a drug once it is approved. So there is always the risk that the drug may produce adverse side effects when used on a larger population. To monitor this, the FDA maintains a reporting program called **MedWatch** which encourages health care professionals to report adverse effects that occur from the use of an approved drug or other medical product. MedWatch does not monitor vaccines. That is performed by the Vaccine Adverse Event Reporting System (VAERS).

The FDA has several options if it determines that a marketed drug presents a risk of illness, injury, or gross consumer deception.

It may seek an *injunction* that prevents the manufacturer from distributing the drug; it may seize the drug; or it may issue a *recall* of the drug or certain lots of the drug. Of these, recalls are considered the most effective, largely because they involve the cooperation of the manufacturer, which after all is the only party that knows where the drugs have been distributed. As a result, recalls are the FDA's preferred means of removing dangerous drugs from the market.

---

 adverse effect an unintended side effect of a medication that is negative or in some way injurious to a patient's health.

injunction a court order preventing a specific action, such as the distribution of a potentially dangerous drug.

recall the action taken to remove a drug from the market and have it returned to the manufacturer.

A Manufacturer Recall

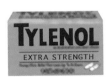 When someone tampered with a small number of Tylenol capsule packages and fatally poisoned seven people, Johnson & Johnson immediately recalled the capsules from the market. This swift and responsible action resulted in a highly favorable public response and increased popularity for Tylenol—and Johnson & Johnson.

RECALLS

Recalls are, with a few exceptions, voluntary on the part of the manufacturer. However, once the FDA requests a manufacturer recall a product, the pressure to do so is substantial. The negative publicity from not recalling would significantly damage a company's reputation, and the FDA would probably take the manufacturer to court, where criminal penalties could be imposed. The FDA can also require recalls in certain instances with infant formulas, biological products, and devices that pose a serious health hazard. Manufacturers may of course recall drugs on their own and do so from time to time for any number of reasons.

Recall Classifications

There are three classes of recalls:

Class I

Where there is a strong likelihood that the product will cause serious adverse effects or death.

Class II

Where a product may cause temporary but reversible adverse effects, or in which there is little likelihood of serious adverse effects.

Class III

Where a product is not likely to cause adverse effects.

How an FDA requested recall works:

Reports of adverse effects

The FDA receives enough reports of adverse effects or misbranding that it decides the product is a threat to the public health. It contacts the manufacturer and recommends a recall.

Manufacturer agrees to recall

If the manufacturer agrees to a recall, they must establish a recall strategy with the FDA that addresses the depth of the recall, the extent of public warnings, and a means for checking the effectiveness of the recall. The depth of the recall is identified by wholesale, retail, or consumer levels. The effectiveness may require anything from no follow-up to a complete follow-up check of everyone who should have been notified of the recall. Checks can be made by personal visit, phone calls, or letters.

Customers contacted

Once the strategy is finalized, the manufacturer contacts its customers by telegram, mailgram, or first-class letters with the following information:

✔ the product name, size, lot number, code or serial number, and any other important identifying information.

✔ reason for the recall and the hazard involved.

✔ instructions on what to do with the product, beginning with ceasing distribution.

Recalls listed publicly

Recalls are listed in the weekly FDA Enforcement Report.

LAW AND THE TECHNICIAN

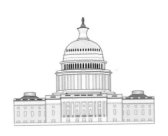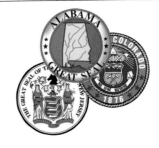

FEDERAL LAW

Federal laws provide a foundation for the state laws which govern pharmacy practice. In addition to the specific drug laws enforced by the FDA and DEA, there are federal laws regulating the treatment of patients (especially in nursing homes) that apply to various aspects of pharmacy practice. These laws guarantee certain patient rights including privacy and confidentiality, right to file complaints, information necessary for informed consent, and the right to refuse treatment.

A major piece of legislation affecting patients' privacy rights and how health care providers may or may not use patient health information is the **Health Insurance Portability and Accountability Act** of 1996. In an effort to streamline health care costs, this act encourages providers to use electronic transactions and allows a minimum amount of patient health information to be transferred among providers, without patient consent, for purposes of treatment, payment or administrative operations. At the same time, to protect patients' rights, HIPAA makes the health care provider responsible for maintaining the privacy and security of patient information, informing the patient of their privacy policies and procedures, and allowing the patient to both review and correct any records.

STATE LAW

In each state, the State Department of Professional Regulation is responsible for licensing all prescribers and dispensers. There are also state boards of pharmacy that administer state regulations for the practice of pharmacy in the state. In many cases, state regulations are stricter than federal, and the stricter state regulation must be followed. By definition, this means that the lesser Federal requirements are also being met. Following both state and federal regulations is mandatory.

Each state has specific regulations which may or may not be different from other states. For example, a few states allow pharmacists to prescribe under limited conditions. Many allow nurse practitioners and physician assistants to prescribe. When states allow non-physicians to prescribe, they limit their **scope of authority.** That is, a non-physician prescriber may only prescribe for certain conditions and must follow a strict set of rules (called a **protocol**) that determines the prescription. Non-physician prescribers include dentists, veterinarians, pharmacists, nurse practitioners, and physician assistants. Since states differ on many aspects of pharmacy practice, including who may and may not prescribe, it is necessary to know your own state's regulations, a copy of which can be obtained from your state's Board of Pharmacy.

States regulate the work of pharmacy technicians largely by holding the pharmacist supervising a technician responsible for the technician's performance. If a technician fails to observe any relevant law, the supervising pharmacist is subject to a penalty by the state board. As a result, the supervising pharmacist must explain all the regulations (federal, state, and local) that apply to the technician as part of the job description, and must work with the technician to assure **compliance** with those regulations.

compliance doing what is required.

negligence failing to do something that should or must be done.

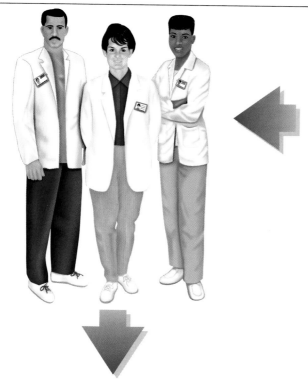

LIABILITY

Legal liability means you can be prosecuted for misconduct. This is true even if you are directed to do it by a supervisor, physician, patient, or customer. Misconduct doesn't necessarily mean you intended to do something, or even that you actively did it. You can be guilty of misconduct by simply failing to do something you should have done. This is called **negligence**, and is the most common form of misconduct. Here are some ways the pharmacy technician can be negligent:

➡incorrectly labeling the prescription;
➡failing to maintain patient confidentiality;
➡failing to recognize expired drugs;
➡calculation errors;
➡dispensing the wrong medication;
➡incorrect handling of controlled substance;
➡inaccurate record keeping.

For information about a pharmacy technician liability insurance policy, see page 261 in Chapter 12.

OTHER STANDARDS

Besides the FDA, DEA, and the State Board of Pharmacy, there are various professional bodies and associations which set and maintain pharmacy standards. These include:

➡**American Society of Health-System Pharmacists:** The ASHP is a 30,000 member association for pharmacists practicing in hospitals, HMOs, long-term care facilities, home care agencies, and other health care systems. It is an accrediting organization for pharmacy residency and pharmacy technician training programs.

➡**United States Pharmacopeia:** The USP is a voluntary not-for-profit organization that sets standards for the manufacture and distribution of drugs and related products in the United States. These standards are directly referred to by federal and state laws and are published in the "United States Pharmacopeia and the National Formulary."

➡**Joint Commission on Accreditation of Health Care Organizations:** JCAHO is an independent non-profit organization that establishes standards and monitors compliance for nearly twenty thousand health care programs in the United States. JCAHO-accredited programs include hospitals, health care networks, hmos, and nursing homes, among others.

➡**The American Society for Consultant Pharmacists:** The ASCP sets standards for practice for pharmacists who provide medication distribution and consultant services to nursing homes.

Basic criminal and civil laws also apply to pharmacy technicians, which means that crimes like theft, discrimination, sexual harassment, fraud, etc. are punishable just as they would be outside of your job.

REVIEW

KEY CONCEPTS

DRUG REGULATION

✔ In the United States, the leading enforcement agency at the federal level for regulations concerning drug products is the Food and Drug Administration.

✔ The distribution of drugs that may be easily abused is controlled by the Drug Enforcement Administration (DEA) within the Justice Department.

✔ Before it is approved for marketing, a new drug must be shown to be both safe and effective and that its benefits substantially outweigh its risks.

✔ Federal law defines what drugs require a prescription by a licensed practitioner.

✔ Manufacturers' containers for prescription drugs must have this legend on the label: "Caution: Federal Law prohibits dispensing without a prescription." By 2003, this was changed to "Rx only."

✔ Pharmacists must offer counseling to patients regarding medications.

✔ Federal law requires child-proof packaging on all controlled and most prescription drugs dispensed by pharmacies.

NEW DRUG APPROVAL

✔ Placebos are inactive substances, not real medications, that are used to test the effectiveness of drugs.

MARKETED DRUGS

✔ Once a patent for a brand drug expires, other manufacturers may copy the drug and release it under its pharmaceutical or "generic" name.

SAMPLE LABELS

✔ The minimum requirements on prescription labels for most drugs are as follows: name and address of dispenser, prescription serial number, date of prescription or filling, name of prescriber, name of patient, directions for use, and cautionary statements.

CONTROLLED SUBSTANCES

✔ Controlled drugs have greater requirements for labeling.

✔ Manufacturers must clearly label controlled drugs with their control classification.

✔ All prescribers of controlled substances are assigned a DEA number which must be used on all controlled drug prescriptions.

PUBLIC SAFETY

✔ There is always the risk that an approved drug may produce adverse side effects when used on a larger population.

✔ Recalls are, with a few exceptions, voluntary on the part of the manufacturer.

LAW AND THE TECHNICIAN

✔ Federal laws provide a foundation for the state laws which govern pharmacy practice in every state.

✔ State boards of pharmacy are responsible for licensing all prescribers and dispensers and administering regulations for the practice of pharmacy in the state.

✔ Legal liability means you can be prosecuted for misconduct.

SELF TEST

MATCH THE TERMS.

answers can be checked in the glossary

adverse effect

controlled substance mark

injunction

labeling

legend drug

liability

NDC (National Drug Code)

negligence

pediatric

placebo

recall

therapeutic

- a court order preventing a specific action, such as the distribution of a potentially dangerous drug.
- an inactive substance given in place of a medication.
- an unintended side affect of a medication that is negative or in some way injurious to a patient's health.
- any drug which requires a prescription and this "legend" on the label: Rx only.
- failing to do something you should have done.
- having to do with the treatment of children.
- important associated information that is not on the label of a drug product itself.
- legal responsibilty for costs or damages arising from misconduct or negligence.
- serving to cure or heal.
- the action taken to remove a drug from the market and have it returned to the manufacturer.
- the mark (CII-CV) which indicates the control category of a drug with a potential for abuse.
- the number on a manufacturer's label indicating the manufacturer and product information.

CHOOSE THE BEST ANSWER.

the answer key begins on page 347

1. Both domestic and imported drugs require approval by (a/the) _____ before they can be marketed in the United States.
   a. FDA
   b. US Marshal
   c. DEA
   d. US Customs

2. The _____ prohibited interstate commerce in adulterated or misbranded food, drinks, and drugs.
   a. 1938 Food, Drug and Cosmetic (FDC) Act
   b. Food and Drug Act of 1906
   c. Sherley Amendment
   d. 1990 Omnibus Budget Reconciliation Act (OBRA)

3. Because of fatal poisoning from liquid sulfanilamide, the _____ required new drugs be shown to be safe before marketing.
   a. Food and Drug Act of 1906
   b. 1938 Food, Drug and Cosmetic Act
   c. 1951 Durham Humphrey Amendment
   d. 1990 Omnibus Budget Reconciliation Act (OBRA)

4. The _____ required drug manufacturers to provide proof of safety and efficacy.
   a. 1938 Food Drug and Cosmetic Act
   b. Omnibus Budget Reconciliation Act (OBRA)
   c. Durham-Humphrey Amendment
   d. Kefauver-Harris Amendment

REVIEW

5. The _____ required child-proof packaging for most prescription drugs.
   a. Food, Drug and Cosmetic Act
   b. Poison Prevention Packaging Act
   c. Durham-Humphrey Amendment
   d. Kefauver-Harris Amendment

6. The Drug Enforcement Agency (DEA) is associated with the
   a. Kefauver-Harris Amendment.
   b. Durham-Humphrey Amendment.
   c. 1970 CSA.
   d. 1990 Omnibus Budget Reconciliation Act (OBRA).

7. Pharmacists were required to offer counseling to Medicaid patients by the
   a. Durham-Humphrey Amendment.
   b. 1990 Omnibus Budget Reconciliation Act (OBRA).
   c. Kefauver-Harris Amendment.
   d. Sherley Amendment.

8. Drugs that require prescriptions are _____ drugs.
   a. durham
   b. humphrey
   c. legend
   d. kefauver

9. An inactive substance given in place of a medication during clinical trials is a
   a. pediatric.
   b. phase 2.
   c. phase 3.
   d. placebo.

10. The FDA requires _____ phases of testing in humans.
    a. two
    b. three
    c. four
    d. five

11. The main purpose of phase 2 clinical trials is
    a. dosage.
    b. economics.
    c. animals.
    d. effectiveness.

12. Phase 3 clinical trials generally have _____ participants.
    a. several hundred to several thousand
    b. 20-100 patients
    c. less than 10
    d. up to several hundred patients

13. After a patent has expired for a medication, other manufacturers may copy the drug and release it under the _____ name.
    a. generic
    b. trade
    c. brand
    d. patent

14. Drugs that do not require a prescription are _____ drugs.
    a. FDA
    b. OTC
    c. Durham-Humphrey
    d. legend

15. The Drug Enforcement Administration (DEA) is within the _____ of the US government.
    a. Treasury Department
    b. Labor Department
    c. FDA
    d. Justice Department

16. Of the following Schedule of drugs, which one deals with drugs that have no accepted medical use in the United States?
    a. Schedule I
    b. Schedule II
    c. Schedule III
    d. Schedule IV

17. Amphetamines, opium, cocaine, and methadone are in DEA Schedule _____ because they have accepted medical use, but have a high potential for abuse and may lead to physical or psychological dependence.
    a. II
    b. III
    c. IV
    d. V

18. The FDA reporting system for adverse effects that occur from use of approved drugs is called
    a. Class I.
    b. MedWatch.
    c. VAERS.
    d. Class II.

19. _____ drug recalls are issued by manufacturers when there is a strong likelihood that the product will cause serious adverse effects or death.
    a. Class I
    b. Class II
    c. Class III
    d. Class IV

20. A technician could be prosecuted for misconduct called _____ if s/he incorrectly labeled a prescription.
    a. liability
    b. insubordination
    c. negligence
    d. compliance

21. Basic criminal and civil laws, like theft, discrimination, sexual harassment, and fraud, apply to pharmacy technicians.
    a. True
    b. False

22. Pharmacies located in the health care institutions (hospitals, etc.) are required to follow regulations of this organization:
    a. ASHP
    b. USP
    c. ASCP
    d. JCAHO

TERMINOLOGY

Root	Prefix
Suffix	C.V.

Medical dictionaries contain thousands of words that are used in medicine and pharmacy.

Many of the words don't look like words commonly used in literature or speech, and at first glance they can be quite intimidating. But the secret to learning medical science terminology is to learn that there is a system, or order, to it. The purpose of this chapter is to explain this system.

Medical science terminology is made up of a small number of *root words*.

Most of these root words originate from either Greek or Latin words. Words developed from the Greek language are most often used to refer to diagnosis and surgery. Words from the Latin language generally refer to the anatomy of the body.

Numerous *suffixes* and *prefixes* are attached to the root word.

The suffixes and prefixes give specifics to the meaning of the root word. The suffix is a modifier attached to the end of the root word, and the prefix is attached to the front of the root word. So each medical science term will have at least one root word and then a suffix or prefix to complete the meaning. It is not required that every root word have both a suffix and a prefix. Each root could have just one. In general, prefixes are used less frequently than suffixes.

Combining vowels are used to connect the prefix, root word, or suffix parts of the term.

In some cases the combining vowel can be used to combine two root words. And there are some cases where the combining vowels are not used at all. Sometimes a combining vowel is added to make the word easier to pronounce. The most common combining vowel is the letter "o".

root word the base component of a term which gives it a meaning that may be modified by other components.

prefix a modifying component of a term located before the other components of the term.

suffix a modifying component of a term located after the other components of the term.

ROOT WORDS

The root word is the foundation of medical science terminology. Root words can immediately identify what part of the body a term relates to. For example, consider this list of common root words and the parts of the body to which they refer:

Root	Part of Body
card	heart
cyst	bladder
gastr	stomach
hemat	blood
hepat	liver
my	muscle
pector	chest
neur	nerve
pneum	lung
ocul	eye
derma	skin
ven	vein
mast	breast
oste	bone
nephr	kidney
ot	ear

If a phrase contains the word "cardiac," it is referring to the heart, since "card" is the root word of the word cardiac. The word "ocular" would refer to the eye since "ocul" is the root word of the word ocular.

Learning the most popular roots, suffixes, and prefixes will help you to understand a large amount of pharmaceutical terminology.

Medical Term

Medical and pharmaceutical nomenclature is a system made up of these four elements:

- ➡ **root words**
- ➡ **prefixes**
- ➡ **suffixes**
- ➡ **combining vowels**

PREFIXES

A prefix is added to the beginning of a root word to clarify its meaning. For example, *"derma"* is the root word for skin, or things related to the skin, and *"xero"* is a prefix used to describe things that are dry. So:

xero + derma = xeroderma

➡ *meaning:* a "dry skin" condition

Consider another example. The root word for vision is *"opia,"* and the prefix for double is *"dipl."* So:

dipl + opia = diplopia

➡ *meaning:* double vision

For a final example, consider the prefix *"sub"* and the root *"lingu."* "Sub" means under or beneath, and "lingu" is the root word for tongue. So:

sub + lingu = sublingu

➡ *meaning:* under the tongue

However, there are few English words ending in "u," and so this combination is further modified with the typical suffix *"al"* which means "pertaining to," as in:

sub + lingu + al = sublingual

➡ *meaning:* pertaining to under the tongue

SUFFIXES

The suffix is added to the end of a root word to clarify the meaning. Sometimes the connection is made without the aid of a connecting vowel.

Root	Suffix
gastr (stomach)	**itis** (inflammation)

➡ **gastritis**: inflammation of the stomach

Root	Suffix
neur (nerve)	**algia** (pain)

➡ **neuralgia**: a pain in the nerve

Sometimes a **combining vowel** (CV) is used to complete the connection of the different word parts.

1st Root	2nd Root	Suffix	CV
pneum (lung)	**thorax** (chest)		**o**

➡ **pneumothorax**: area of the chest containing the lungs

1st Root	2nd Root	Suffix	CV
card (heart)	**my** (muscle)	**pathy** (disease)	**i, o**

➡ **cardiomyopathy**: disease in the heart muscle tissue

COMBINING THE ELEMENTS

The last combination possibility is to have a prefix and a suffix attached to a root word.

Prefix	Root	Suffix
hypo (low)	**glyc** (sugar)	**emia** (blood)

➡ **hypoglycemia**: low blood sugar

Prefix	Root	Suffix
hyper (high)	**thyroid** (thyroid)	**ism** (state of)

➡ **hyperthyroidism**: too much thyroid activity

And then there is always the possibility that a combining vowel (CV) will be used within a word.

Prefix	Root	Suffix	CV
peri (around)	**dont** (teeth)	**ic** (pertaining to)	**o**

➡ **periodontic**: around the teeth

ORGAN SYSTEM TERMINOLOGY

Agood way to learn medical science terminology is to learn it based on the different organ systems in the body.

There are names for structures and parts of organ systems that form the root words used in medical science terminology. These names have to be learned. Then they can be applied to understand or to construct words.

The cardiovascular system distributes blood throughout the body using blood vessels called arteries, capillaries, and veins. Blood transports nutrients to the body's cells and carries waste products away from them. Blood is made up of red blood cells, white blood cells, platelets, and plasma. **Erythrocytes** (red blood cells) transport oxygen from the lungs to the body and carbon dioxide from the cells to the lungs. **Leukocytes** (white blood cells) fight bacterial infections by producing antibodies.

Blood is pumped through the cardiovascular system by the heart. Valves within the heart maintain the flow of blood in only one direction. Conductive tissue which is unique to the heart muscle is responsible for the heartbeat.

When blood is forced out of the heart, the increased pressure on the system is called the **systolic** phase. When blood pressure is monitored, this pressure is reported (in mm Hg) as the first number of a two number sequence. The **diastolic** phase, or relaxation phase, is the second number reported in blood pressure monitoring. Blood pressures are reported as systole/diastole, i.e., 120/80. A sphygmomanometer is used to measure blood pressure.

CARDIOVASCULAR SYSTEM

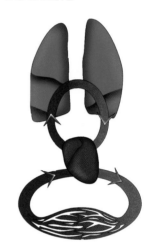

Root Words

angi	vessel
aort	aorta
card	heart
oxy	oxygen
pector	chest
phleb	vein
stenosis	narrowing
thromb	clot
vas(cu)	blood vessel
ven	vein

Prefix	Root Word	Suffix	CV	Term	Meaning
hyper (high)	tension (pressure)			**hypertension**	high blood pressure
	thromb (clot)	sis (abnormal condition)	o	**thrombosis**	condition of having blood clots in the vascular system
	phleb (vein)	itis (inflammation)		**phlebitis**	inflammation of a vein
	arter (artery)	sclerosis (hardening)	i, o	**arteriosclerosis**	hardening of the arteries
	card (heart) my (muscle)	pathy (disease)	i, o	**cardiomyopathy**	disease of the heart muscle
	my (muscle) card (heart)	ial (condition of)	o	**myocardial**	concerning heart muscle
tachy (fast)	card (heart)	ia (condition of)		**tachycardia**	abnormally rapid heart action

ENDOCRINE SYSTEM

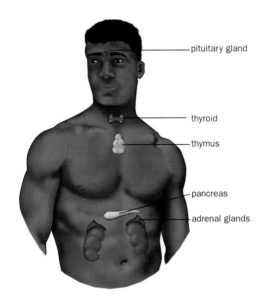

pituitary gland

thyroid

thymus

pancreas

adrenal glands

Root Words

lipid	fat
nephr	kidney
thym	thymus
adrena	adrenal
gluc	sugar
pancreat	pancreas
somat	body

The endocrine system consists of the glands that secrete **hormones**, chemicals that assist in regulating body functions.

Several organs act as endocrine glands as well as members of other organ systems. For example, the liver, stomach, pancreas, and kidneys are members of endocrine system as well as other organ systems. Organs that belong primarily to the endocrine system include the pituitary gland, the adrenal glands, the thyroid gland, and the gonads (ovaries and testes).

The pituitary gland produces multiple hormones and is located at the base of the brain. It controls the body's growth and releases hormones into the bloodstream that control much of the activity of the other glands. The thyroid gland is located just below the larynx and releases hormones important for regulating body metabolism. There are four smaller parathyroid glands located on the thyroid gland. The thymus gland is located beneath the sternum. The pancreas is best known for its production of insulin and glucagon. The small adrenal glands are located on top of the kidneys. They produce such hormones as aldosterone, cortisol (hydrocortisone), androgens, and estrogens. The medulla region of the adrenal glands produce the catecholamines adrenaline (epinephrine) and noradrenaline (norepinephrine).

Prefix	Root Word	Suffix	CV	Term	Meaning
end (within)	crine (secrete)		o	**endocrine**	pertaining to the glands that secrete hormones into the bloodstream
hyper (high)	lipid (fat)	emia (blood)		**hyperlipidemia**	increase of lipids in the blood
hypo (low)	thyroid (thyroid gland)	ism (condition)		**hypothyroidism**	a deficiency of thyroid secretion
	somat (body)	ic (pertaining to)		**somatic**	pertaining to the body

 The majority of the terms used in body system terminology are for disorders or conditions.

ORGAN SYSTEM TERMINOLOGY (cont'd)

GASTROINTESTINAL TRACT

The gastrointestinal (GI) tract is located in the abdomen, and is surrounded by the peritoneal lining. The GI tract contains the organs that are involved in the digestion of foods and the absorption of nutrients. These organs include the stomach, small and large intestine, gallbladder, liver, and pancreas.

The GI tract is sometimes inappropriately referred to as the **alimentary tract.** The alimentary tract refers to the system that goes from the mouth to the anus. The alimentary tract contains organs such as lips, tongue, teeth, salivary glands, pharynx, esophagus, rectum, and anus, in addition to the GI tract.

Several organs contribute to the digestion of foods by secreting enzymes into the small intestine when food is present. Ducts carry bile from the liver (hepatic duct) and the gallbladder (cystic duct) to the duodenum. The pancreas is located behind the stomach and also contributes enzymes to the digestive process.

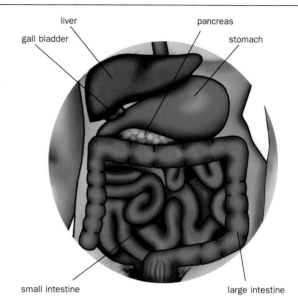

Root Words

chol	bile
col	colon
duoden	duodenum
enter	intestine
esophag	esophagus
gastr	stomach
hepat	liver
lapar	abdomen
pancreat	pancreas

Prefix	Root Word	Suffix	CV	Term	Meaning
an (no)	orexia (appetite)			**anorexia**	loss of appetite
a (no)	phagia (swallow)			**aphagia**	inability to swallow
	appendic (appendix)	itis (inflammation)		**appendicitis**	inflammation of the appendix
	col (colon)	itis (inflammation)		**colitis**	inflamed or irritable colon
dia (across, through)	rrhea (discharge)			**diarrhea**	liquid or unformed bowel movements
	duoden (duodenum)	al (pertaining to)		**duodenal**	pertaining to the duodenum
	hemat (blood)	emesis (vomit)		**hematemesis**	vomiting of blood
	hepat (liver)	itis (inflammation)		**hepatitis**	inflammation of the liver from various causes
	hepat (liver)	oma (tumor)		**hepatoma**	liver tumor
	gastr (stomach)	itis (inflammation)		**gastritis**	inflammation of the stomach
	gastr (stomach) } enter (abdomen)	itis (inflammation)	o	**gastroenteritis**	inflammation of the stomach and the intestinal tract

alimentary tract the organs from the mouth to the anus. The GI tract is a portion of the alimentary tract.

integumentary system the body covering, i.e., skin, hair, and nails.

INTEGUMENTARY SYSTEM

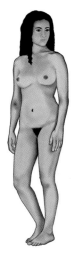

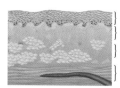

} epidermis
} dermis
} subcutaneous
} muscle

The covering of the body is referred to as the **integumentary system**. It is the body's first line of defense, acting as a barrier against disease and physical hazards. It also helps control body temperature by releasing heat through sweat or by constricting blood vessels to act as insulation. It includes the skin, hair, and nails.

Hair is made of keratinized cells. Finger nails and toenails are also composed of keratin. The mammary glands, or breasts, are also considered part of the integumentary system.

The skin is composed of the **epidermis** and **dermis.** The epidermis has no blood or nerves and is constantly discarding dead cells. The dermis, which is made of living cells, contains capillaries, nerves, and lymphatics. The dermis also contains the subaceous glands, sweat glands, and hair.

The subcutaneous layer of tissue is beneath the dermis but is closely interconnected to it. It separates the skin from the other organs (for example, the muscular system, as in the illustration).

Root Words

necr	death (of cells, body)
derma	skin
cutane	skin
mast	breast
onych	nail

Prefix	Root Word	Suffix	CV	Term	Meaning
	derma (skin)	itis (inflammation)		**dermatitis**	skin inflammation
erythro (red)	derma (skin)			**erythroderma**	abnormal redness of skin
	lact (milk)	tation (act of secreting)		**lactation**	secretion of milk
	mast (breast)	ectomy (removal)		**mastectomy**	surgical removal of breast
	onych (nail)	mycosis (fungal infection)	o	**onychomycosis**	fungal infection of nails
pach (thick)	derma (skin)		y	**pachyderma**	abnormal thickness of skin
sub (under)	cutane (skin)	ous (pertaining to)		**subcutaneous**	beneath the skin
trans (through)	derma (skin)	al (pertaining to)		**transdermal**	through the skin

ORGAN SYSTEM TERMINOLOGY (cont'd)

LYMPHATIC SYSTEM

The lymphatic system is responsible for collecting plasma water that leaves the blood vessels, filtering it for impurities through its lymph nodes, and returning the lymph fluid back to the general circulation. The lymphatic system is the center of the body's immune system.

The largest organ in the system is the spleen. It is responsible for removing old red blood cells from the circulation. It is also a storage organ for **lymphocytes,** a type of white blood cell that attacks bacteria and disease cells. Lymphocytes release antibodies that destroy disease cells and provide immunity against them.

The thymus, tonsils, spleen, and adenoids are lymphoid organs outside the network of the lymphatic system.

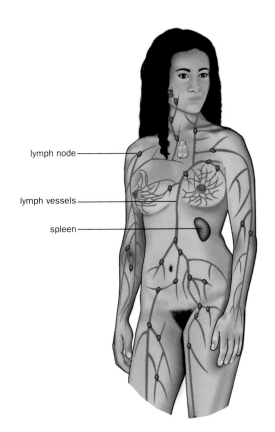

lymph node ——
lymph vessels ——
spleen ——

Root Words

aden	gland
cyt	cell
hemo, hemat	blood
lymph	lymph
splen	spleen

Prefix	Root Word	Suffix	CV	Term	Meaning
	aden (gland)	pathy (disease)	o	**adenopathy**	lymph node disease
	hemat (blood)	oma (tumor)		**hematoma**	a collection of blood, often clotted
	hemo (blood)	philia (attraction)		**hemophilia**	a disease in which the blood does not clot normally
	lymph (lymph tissue)	oma (tumor)		**lymphoma**	lymphatic system tumor
	leuk (white)	emia (blood condition)		**leukemia**	increase in white blood cells
	thym (thymus)	oma (tumor)		**thymoma**	tumor of the thymus

lymphocytes a type of white blood cells that helps the body defend itself against bacteria and diseased cells.

MUSCULAR SYSTEM

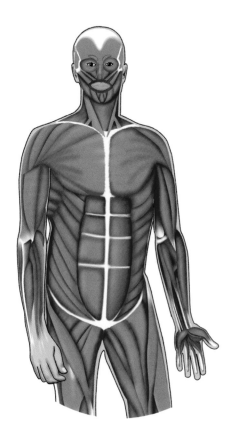

The word muscle comes from the Latin *mus* (mouse) and *cle* (little) because muscle movements resemble a mouse moving under a cover.

The body contains more than 600 muscles which give shape and movement to it. The skeletal muscles are attached to the bones by tendons. The muscles themselves are striated, i.e., made up of fibers.

The action of most muscles is called voluntary, because it is controlled consciously. Involuntary muscles operate automatically and are found in the heart, the stomach, or in walls of blood vessels.

Some muscles produce an outward or **flexor movement** and these are called agonist muscles. Antagonist muscles are the ones that contract or bring the limb back to the original position.

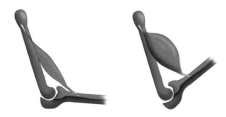

expansion and contraction of muscles

Root Words

my	muscle
fibr	fiber
tendin	tendon

Prefix	Root Word	Suffix	CV	Term	Meaning
	fibr (fiber) my (muscle) }	algia (pain)	o	**fibromyalgia**	chronic pain in the muscles
	my (muscle)	plasty (repair)	o	**myoplasty**	plastic surgery of muscle tissue
	tendin (tendon)	itis (inflammation)		**tendinitis**	inflammation of a tendon

flexor movement an expansion or outward movement by muscles.

ORGAN SYSTEM TERMINOLOGY (cont'd)

NERVOUS SYSTEM

The most complex of the body organ systems is the nervous system, the body's system of communication. The **neuron** (nerve cell) is the basic functional unit in this system. There are over 100 billion neurons in the brain alone. Neurons also transmit information from the brain to the entire body.

The primary parts of this system are the brain and the spinal cord, called the central nervous system (CNS). The peripheral nervous system is composed of nerves that branch out from the spinal cord.

There are subdivisions of the peripheral nervous system called the autonomic nervous system and the somatic nervous system. The autonomic nervous system controls the automatic functions of the body, e.g., breathing, digestion, etc. The somatic nervous system controls the voluntary actions of the body, e.g., muscle movements.

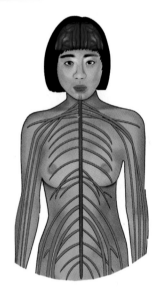

central and peripheral nervous systems

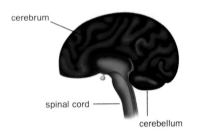

brain and spinal cord

Root Words

cerebr	cerebrum
encephal	brain
mening	meninges
myel	spinal cord
neur	nerve

Prefix	Root Word	Suffix	CV	Term	Meaning
	encephal (brain)	itis (inflammation)		**encephalitis**	inflammation of the brain
	neur (nerve)	algia (pain)		**neuralgia**	severe pain in a nerve
	neur (nerve)	oma (tumor)		**neuroma**	tumor of nerve cells

SKELETAL SYSTEM

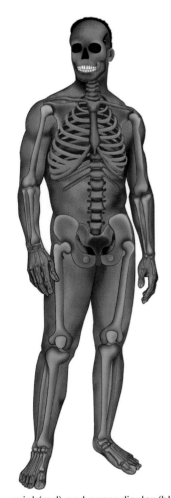

axial (red) and appendicular (blue) skeleton

The skeletal system protects soft organs and provides structure and support for the body's organ systems. Made up largely of hard **osseus** tissue, it is a living system that undergoes dynamic changes throughout life.

The system's 206 bones are called **axial** (skull and spinal column) or **appendicular** (arms, legs, and connecting bones). They are held together at joints by connective tissue called ligaments and cartilage. Joints range from rigid to those allowing full motion (e.g., the ball and socket joints of the hips and shoulders).

Root Words

arthr	joint
calcane	heel bone
carp	wrist
crani	cranium
dactyl	finger or toe
femor	thigh bone
fibul	small, outer lower leg bone
humer	humerus
myel	bone marrow, spinal cord
oste	bone
patell	kneecap
ped, pod	foot
pelv	pelvis
phalang	bones of fingers and toes
rachi	spinal cord, vertebrae
spondy	backbone, vertebrae
stern	sternum, breastbone
tibi	large lower leg bone
vertebr	backbone, vertebrae

Prefix	Root Word	Suffix	CV	Term	Meaning
	arthr (joint)	algia (pain)		**arthralgia**	joint pain
	arthr (joint)	itis (inflammation)		**arthritis**	inflammation of a joint
	carp (wrist)	al (pertaining to)		**carpal**	pertaining to the carpus in the wrist
	crani (cranium)	malacia (softening)	o	**craniomalacia**	softening of the skull
	oste (bone) arthr (joint)	itis (inflammation)	o	**osteoarthritis**	chronic disease of bones and joints
	oste (bone) carcin (cancer)	oma (tumor)	o	**osteocarcinoma**	cancerous bone tumor
	rachi (vertebrae)	itis (inflammation)		**rachitis**	inflammation of the spine

ORGAN SYSTEM TERMINOLOGY (cont'd)

FEMALE REPRODUCTIVE SYSTEM

The female reproductive system produces hormones (e.g., estrogen, progesterone), controls menstruation, and provides for childbearing. The system contains the vagina, uterus, fallopian tubes, ovaries, and the external genitalia.

The mammmary glands (located in breast tissue) are also associated with the female reproductive system, The mammary glands produce and secrete milk at child-birth.

The vagina is a muscular tube that leads from an external opening to the cervix and uterus. The uterus is a hollow, pear-shaped organ. The fallopian tubes transport eggs from the ovary to the uterus. The ovaries are located on each side of the uterus. In sexually mature females, the uterus is prepared for the possibility of fertilization and pregnancy each month during the menstrual cycle.

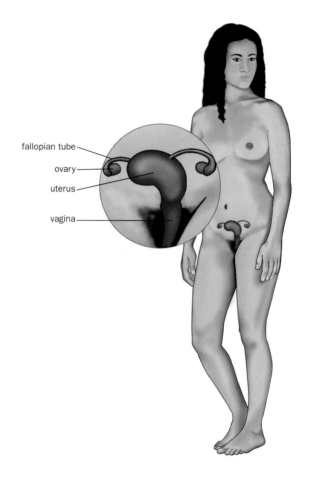

fallopian tube

ovary

uterus

vagina

Root Words

gynec	woman
hyster	uterus
lact	milk
mamm	breast
mast	breast
metr	uterus
ovari	ovary
salping	fallopian tube
toc	birth
uter	uterine

Prefix	Root Word	Suffix	CV	Term	Meaning
a (no)	men (menstrual)	orrhea (discharge)		**amenorrhea**	absence of menstruation
dys (difficult)	men (menstrual)	orrhea (discharge)		**dysmenorrhea**	menstrual pain
dys (difficult)	toc (birth)	ia (condition of)		**dystocia**	difficult labor
end (within)	metri (uterus)	sis (abnormal)	o	**endometriosis**	abnormal growth of uteral tissue within the pelvis
	gynec (woman)	logy (study of)	o	**gynecology**	the study of the female reproductive organs
	mast (breast)	itis (inflammation)		**mastitis**	inflammation of the breast
	salping (fallopian)	cyesis (pregnancy)	o	**salpingocyesis**	fetal development in the fallopian tube
	vagin (vagina)	itis (inflammation)		**vaginitis**	inflammation of the vagina

MALE REPRODUCTIVE SYSTEM

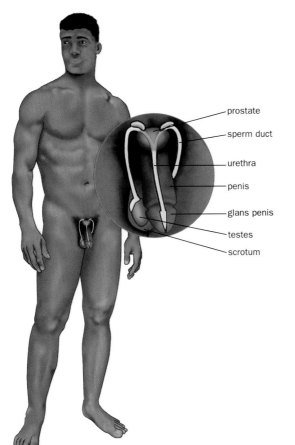

prostate
sperm duct
urethra
penis
glans penis
testes
scrotum

The male reproductive system produces sperm and secretes the hormone testosterone. The primary male sex organs are the testicles. They are the oval shaped organs enclosed in the scrotum.

The seminal glands, located at the base of the bladder, produce part of the seminal fluid. They have ducts that lead into sperm ducts called the vas deferens which carry the sperm from the testes. The prostate gland is located at the upper end of the urethra. The penis (glans penis) is the external organ for urination and sexual intercourse. The tip of the penis is covered by the prepuce (foreskin). The urethra, by which urine and semen leave the body, is inside the penis.

Root Words

andr	male
balan	glans penis
orchid, test	testis, testicle
prostat	prostate gland
sperm	sperm
vas	vessel, duct
vesicul	seminal vescles

Prefix	Root Word	Suffix	CV	Term	Meaning
a (no)	sperm (sperm)	ia (condition of)		**aspermia**	inability to produce semen
	balan (glans penis)	itis (inflammation)		**balanitis**	inflammation of the glans penis
crypt (hidden)	orchid (testis)	ism (state of)		**cryptorchidism**	failure of testes to drop into the scrotum
	prostat (prostate)	itis		**prostatitis**	inflammation of prostate
	prostat (prostate)	lith (stone)	o	**prostatolith**	a prostate stone
	semin (testis)	oma (tumor)		**seminoma**	tumor of the testes

ORGAN SYSTEM TERMINOLOGY (cont'd)

RESPIRATORY SYSTEM

The respiratory system brings oxygen into the body through inhalation and expels carbon dioxide gas through exhalation. It produces sound for speaking and helps cool the body.

The lungs have specialized tissues called **alveoli** that exchange the gases between the blood and the air. Respiratory muscles (especially the diaphragm) expand the lungs automatically, causing air to be inhaled into the upper respiratory tract. As air enters through the nose, it is warmed, moistened, and filtered. The pharynx directs food into the esophagus and air into the trachea. The larynx contains the vocal cords. The trachea, or windpipe, connects to the two bronchi (bronchial tubes) that enter the lungs.

Inside the lungs, the bronchial tubes branch out and lead to the alveolar sacs that are the site of gas exchange within the lungs. The pleural cavity surrounds the lungs and provides lubrication for respiration.

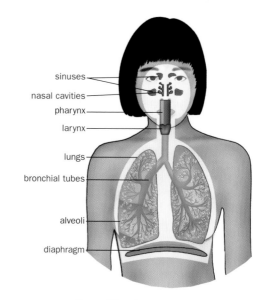

Root Words

aer	air
aero	gas
pneum	lung, air
pulmon	lung
pector	chest
nasal	nose
sinus	sinus
laryng	larynx
bronch	bronchus
ox	oxygen
capnia	carbon dioxide

Prefix	Root Word	Suffix	CV	Term	Meaning
a (no)	pnea (to breathe)			**apnea**	temporary failure to breathe
	bronch (bronchus)	itis (inflammation)		**bronchitis**	inflammation of bronchial membranes
cyan (blue)		sis (condition of)	o	**cyanosis**	blue discoloration of skin
dys (difficult)	pnea (to breathe)			**dyspnea**	labored breathing
hyper (high)	capnia (CO_2)			**hypercapnia**	excessive carbon dioxide in the blood
hypo (low)	ox (oxygen)	ia (condition of)		**hypoxia**	abnormally low blood oxygen level
	laryng (larynx)	itis (inflammation)		**laryngitis**	inflammation of the larynx
para (around)	nasal (nose)			**paranasal**	near or along the nasal cavities
	pector (chest)	algia (pain)		**pectoralgia**	chest pain
	pneum (lung)	nia (condition of)	o	**pneumonia**	inflammation of the lungs
	pulmon (lung)	ary (pertaining to)		**pulmonary**	pertaining to the lungs
	sinus (sinus)	itis (inflammation)		**sinusitis**	inflammation of the sinuses

URINARY TRACT

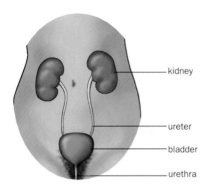

kidney

ureter

bladder

urethra

The urinary tract is responsible for removing wastes from the blood. The urinary tract includes the kidneys, ureters, urinary bladder, and urethra.

The primary organ of the urinary tract is the kidney, which removes waste materials from the blood. The **nephron** is the functional unit of the kidney. There are several million nephrons in the kidneys. As the blood passes through the nephrons, plasma water is filtered through the glomerulus. Waste materials may be contained in the filtrate or may be secreted into the filtrate at other sites in the nephron. Urine is formed as some filtered plasma water is reabsorbed, and waste materials continue to be filtered or secreted into the nephron.

Urine leaves the kidney through the ureters and collects in the bladder. It is excreted from the bladder through the urethra.

Root Words

cyst	bladder
vesic	bladder
ren	kidney
nephr	kidney
uria	urine, urination

Prefix	Root Word	Suffix	CV	Term	Meaning
an (no)	uria (urine)			**anuria**	inability to produce urine
	cyst (bladder)	itis (inflammation)		**cystitis**	inflammation of the bladder
	cyst (bladder)	lith (stone)	o	**cystolith**	a bladder stone
	nephr (kidney)	itis (inflammation)		**nephritis**	inflammation of the kidney
poly (much)	uria (urine)			**polyuria**	excessive urination
	ure (urine)	emia (blood condition)		**uremia**	toxic blood condition caused by kidney insufficiency or failure

alveoli a part of the lungs where gases are exchanged between blood and the air.

nephron the functional unit of the kidney responsible for removing wastes from the blood and producing urine.

ORGAN SYSTEM TERMINOLOGY (cont'd)

SENSES: HEARING

The sense of hearing, as well as the maintenance of body equilibrium, is performed by the ear. The external ear consists of a funnel shaped structure which captures sound waves and channels them through an opening to the **tympanic membrane** (eardrum). The opening also contains glands that make earwax that protects the external ear.

The **middle ear** consists of three bony structures (malleus, incus, and stapes) that transmit sound from a vibrating tympanic membrane to the cochlea. The eustachian tube connects the middle ear to the nose and throat, serving to equalize the air pressure on both sides of the tympanic membrane.

The inner ear is called the **labyrinth** for obvious reasons. It consists of three areas: vestibule, cochlea, and semicircular canals. The cochlea contains the organ of hearing. When sound waves are transmitted to it, it converts them into nerve impulses that are sent to the brain for interpretation. The semicircular canals are responsible for body equilibrium.

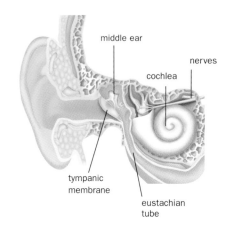

middle ear

nerves

cochlea

tympanic membrane

eustachian tube

Root Words

ot	ear
cusis	hearing condition
acous	hearing
audi	hearing
salping	eustachian tube
tympan	eardrum
myring	eardrum
cerumin	wax-like, waxy

Prefix	Root Word	Suffix	CV	Term	Meaning
	labyrinth (inner ear)	itis (inflammation)		**labyrinthitis**	inflammation of the inner ear
	ot (ear)	algia (pain, ache)		**otalgia**	pain in the ear
	ot (ear)	mycosis (fungal infection)	o	**otomycosis**	fungal ear infection
	ot (ear)	orrhea (drainage)		**otorrhea**	ear infection with discharge
para (partial)	cusis (hearing condition)			**paracusis**	hearing disorder
	tympan (eardrum)	itis (inflammation)		**tympanitis**	inflammation of the middle ear

SENSES: SIGHT

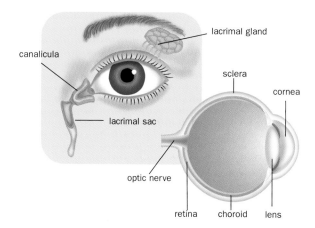

The eyes are the organs that provide sight. The eyelids protect the eye and assist in its lubrication. The conjunctiva is the blood-rich membrane between the eye and the eyelid. There are several glands that secrete fluids to protect and lubricate the eye: the **lacrimal glands** above each eye secrete tears and the meibomian glands produce sebum. Excess fluid drains into the canalicula (tear ducts).

The eye has three layers. The outer layer is composed of the **sclera** and the **cornea.** The sclera is the white part of the eye. The cornea is transparent so the iris (the color of the eye) and the pupil (the opening of the eye) are visible. The middle layer is called the **choroid** and contains blood vessels that nourish the entire eye. In the third layer, the lens focuses light rays on the **retina.** The vitreous humor (one of two fluids in the eye) lies between the retina and the lens. Rods and cones within the retina are responsible for visual reception. The optic nerve within the retina transmits the nerve impulses to the brain.

Root Words

blephar	eyelid
cor	pupil
dacry, lacrim	tear, tear duct
corne, kerat	cornea
retin	retina
irid, iri	iris
bi, bin	two
opia	vision

Prefix	Root Word	Suffix	CV	Term	Meaning
ambly (dull)	opia (vision)			**amblyopia**	reduction in vision
	blephar (eyelid)	itis (inflammation)		**blepharitis**	inflammation of eyelids
	blephar (eyelid)	optosis (drooping)		**blepharoptosis**	drooping of upper eyelid
	conjunctiv (conjunctiva)	itis (inflammation)		**conjunctivitis**	inflammation of the conjunctiva
end (within)	ophthalm (eye)	itis (inflammation)		**endophthalmitis**	inflammation of the inside of the eye
	irid (iris)	plegia (paralysis)	o	**iridoplegia**	paralysis of the iris
	ocul (eye)	mycosis (fungus infection)	o	**oculomycosis**	fungal disease of the eye
	retin (retina)	itis (inflammation)		**retinitis**	inflammation of the retina

PREFIXES

Root	Prefix
Suffix	C.V.

Below are common prefixes used in medical and pharmaceutical science terminology.

a	without
ambi	both
an	without
ante	before
anti	against
bi	two or both
brady	slow
chlor	green
circum	around
cirrh	yellow
con	with
contra	against
cyan	blue
dia	across or through
dis	separate from or apart
dys	painful, difficult
ec	away or out
ecto	outside
end	within
epi	upon
erythr	red
eu	good or normal
exo	outside
heter	different
hom	same
hyper	above or excessive
hypo	below or deficient
im	not
immun	safe, protected
in	not
infra	below or under
inter	between
intra	within
is	equal
leuk	white
macro	large

medi	middle
melan	black
meso	middle
meta	beyond, after, changing
micro	small
mid	middle
mono	one
multi	many
neo	new
pan	all
para	alongside or abnormal
peri	around
polio	gray
poly	many
post	after
pre	before
pro	before
pseudo	false
purpur	purple
quadri	four
re	again or back
retro	after
rube	red
semi	half
sub	below or under
super	above or excessive
supra	above or excessive
sym	with
syn	with
tachy	fast
trans	across, through
tri	three
ultra	beyond or excessive
uni	one
xanth	yellow
xer	dry

SUFFIXES

Root	Prefix
Suffix	C.V.

Below are common suffixes used in medical and pharmaceutical science terminology.

ac	pertaining to		oi	resembling
al	pertaining to		ole	small
algia	pain		oma	tumor
ar	pertaining to		opia	vision
ary	pertaining to		opsia	vision
asthenia	without strength		osis	abnormal condition
cele	pouching or hernia		osmia	smell
cyesis	pregnancy		ous	pertaining to
cynia	pain		paresis	partial paralysis
eal	pertaining to		pathy	disease
ectasis	expansion or dilation		penia	decrease
ectomy	removal		phagia	swallowing
emia	blood condition		phasia	speech
gram	record		philia	attraction for
graph	recording instrument		phobia	fear
graphy	recording process		plasia	formation
ia	condition of		plegia	paralysis, stroke
iasis	condition, formation of		rrhea	discharge
iatry	treatment		sclerosis	narrowing, constriction
ic	pertaining to		scope	examination instrument
icle	small		scopy	examination
ism	condition of		spasm	involuntary contraction
itis	inflammation		stasis	stop or stand
ium	tissue		tic	pertaining to
lith	stone, calculus		tocia	childbirth, labor
logy	study of		tomy	incision
malacia	softening		toxic	poison
megaly	enlargement		tropic	stimulate
meter	measuring instrument		ula	small
metry	measuring process		y	condition, process

MEDICAL ABBREVIATIONS

Many medical and pharmaceutical terms are abbreviated for ease of communication and record notation.

It has been estimated that about 10,000 abbreviations are used in the medical sciences. Many abbreviations are specific for one institution or one area of the country. It is also possible that one abbreviation may have more than one meaning. When in doubt, the pharmacy technician should verify the meaning of an abbreviation.

Common Medical Abbreviations

AAA	Abdominal aortic aneurysm		KVO	Keep vein open
ABG	Arterial blood gases		LBW	Low birth weight
ADD	Attention deficit disorder		LDL	Low density lipoprotein
AIDS	Acquired immunodeficiency syndrome		LKS	Liver, kidney, spleen
ALL	Acute lymphocytic leukemia		LOC	Loss of consciousness
AV	Atrial-ventricular		MG	Myasthenia gravis
AMI	Acute myocardial infarction		MI	Myocardial infarction
ANS	Autonomic nervous system		MICU	Medical intensive care unit
BM	Bowel movement		MRI	Magnetic resonance imaging
BP	Blood pressure		NKO	No known allergies
BPH	Benign prostatic hyperplasia		NPO	Nothing by mouth
BSA	Body surface area		NVD	Nausea, vomiting, diarrhea
CA	Cancer		OTC	Over the counter pharmaceuticals
CAD	Coronary artery disease		PAP	Pulmonary artery pressure
CF	Cardiac failure		PUD	Peptic ulcer disease
CHF	Congestive heart failure		PVD	Peripheral vascular disease
CMV	Cytomegalovirus		RA	Rheumatoid arthritis
CNS	Central nervous system		RBC	Red blood count or red blood cell
COPD	Chronic obstructive pulmonary disease		ROM	Range of motion
CV	Cardiovascular		s	Without
CVA	Cerebrovascular accident (stroke)		SaO2	Systemic arterial oxygen saturation
DI	Diabetes insipidus		SOB	Short of breath
DM	Diabetes melitus		STD	Sexually transmitted diseases
DOB	Date of birth		T	Temperature
DX	Diagnosis		T&C	Type and cross-match
ECG, EKG	Electrocardiogram		TAH	Total abdominal hysterectomy
ENT	Ears, nose, throat		TB	Tuberculosis
GERD	Gastroesophageal reflux disease		TPN	Total parenteral nutrition
GI	Gastrointestinal		Tx	Treatment
H	Hypodermic		U	Units
HA	Headache		U/A	Urinalysis
HBP	High blood pressure		UCHD	Usual childhood diseases
HDL	High density lipoprotein		URD	Upper respiratory diseases
HIV	Human immunodeficiency virus		UTI	Urinary tract infection
HR	Heart rate		VD	Venereal disease
ID	Infectious diseases		WBC	White blood count or white blood cell
IH	Infectious hepatitis		WT	Weight
IO, I/O	Fluid intake and output		XX	Female sex chromosome
IOP	Intraocular pressure		XY	Male sex chromosome

DRUG CLASSIFICATIONS

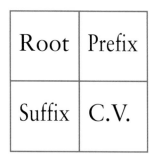

Root	Prefix
Suffix	C.V.

Drug classification names can be understood by identifying their components.

The same system used to interpret medical science terminology can be used to interpret drug classification names.

A classification is a grouping of drugs that have some properties in common.

For example, penicillin, cefoxitine, and ciprofloxacin are used to treat bacterial infections, so they are grouped in a class called anti-infectives.

Each of the drugs mentioned above has unique properties, but they all share the property of being effective against bacterial infections. So the classification name "anti-infective" is created by combining "anti" and "infective" into anti-infective, meaning "against infection." Since much of drug therapy is based on opposing some physiological process in the body, many drugs classes begin with the prefix "anti" or "ant."

THE "AGAINST" CLASSES

Some examples of the "anti" classes of drugs

antacids	relieves gastritis, ulcer pain, indigestion and heartburn
antianginals	relieves heart pain
anticoagulant	dissolves or prevents blood clots
anticonvulsants	prevents seizures
antidepressants	prevents depression
antidiarrheals	stops diarrhea
antiemetics	prevents nausea and vomiting
antihistamine	blocks the effects of histamine
antihyperlipidemics	lowers high cholesterol levels
antihypertensive	reduces blood pressure
anti-inflammatory	reduces inflammation
antipruritics	prevents or relieves itching
antispasmodics	relieves intestinal cramping
antitussive	relieves coughing by inhibiting cough reflex

OTHER CLASSES

Here are examples of other classification names which can be understood by breaking down the term into its medical terminology components.

de + conges + tant	**decongestant:**	reduces nasal congestion
an + alges + ics	**analgesics:**	without pain, kills pain
hypo + glyc + emics	**hypoglycemics:**	reduces blood sugar levels
hypo + lipid + emics	**hypolipidemics:**	reduces blood lipid (cholesterol) levels
kerat + o + lytics	**keratolytics:**	destroys skin layers such as warts
contra + cep + tives	**contraceptives:**	prevents pregnancy
psych + o + tropic	**pyschotropic:**	changes mental states
sperm + i + cide	**spermicide:**	destroys sperm

REVIEW

KEY CONCEPTS

TERMINOLOGY

✔ Much of medical science terminology is made up of a combination of root words, suffixes, and prefixes that originated from either Greek or Latin words.

✔ A prefix is added to the beginning of a root word and a suffix is added to the end of a root word to clarify the meaning.

✔ Combining vowels are used to connect the prefix, root word, or suffix parts of the term.

✔ It is not necessary that a root word have a prefix, suffix, and combining vowel.

ORGAN SYSTEM TERMINOLOGY

✔ The cardiovascular system circulates blood throughout the body in blood vessels called arteries, capillaries, and veins.

✔ The endocrine system consists of the glands that secrete hormones (chemicals that assist in regulating body functions).

✔ The GI tract contains the organs that are involved in the digestion of foods and the absorption of nutrients.

✔ The integumentary system (i.e., the body's covering) is the first line of defense against disease and physical hazards.

✔ The lymphatic system is the center of the body's immune system.

✔ The body contains more than 600 muscles which give it shape and allow movement.

✔ The nervous system is the body's system of communication. The neuron (nerve cell) is its basic functional unit.

✔ The skeletal system protects soft organs and provides structure and support for the body's organ systems.

✔ The female reproductive system produces hormones (estrogens, progesterone), controls menstruation, and provides for childbearing.

✔ The male reproductive system produces sperm and secretes the hormone testosterone.

✔ The respiratory system brings oxygen into the body through inhalation and expels carbon dioxide gas through exhalation.

✔ The primary organ of the urinary tract is the kidney; each kidney has millions of nephrons that collect waste materials.

✔ The sense of hearing, as well as maintenance of the body's equilibrium, is the function of the ear.

✔ The eye is the sensitive organ involved in sight. Several body mechanisms are involved in protecting this organ.

MEDICAL ABBREVIATIONS/DRUG CLASSIFICATIONS

✔ There are an estimated 10,000 medical abbreviations used in medical science. Many abbreviations are specific to an institution or area of the country.

✔ The same system used in medical science terminology can be applied to the names given to various drug classes.

SELF TEST

MATCH THE TERMS.   *the answer key begins on page 347*

1. through the skin   a) athersclerosis
2. blood tumor   b) kidney
3. ven   c) chest
4. ot   d) transdermal
5. gastr   e) eye
6. hardening of
    artery   f) heart
7. muscle repair   g) hematoma
8. black cell tumor   h) myoplasty
9. liver tumor   i) encephalitis
10. card   j) bladder
11. cyst   k) blood
12. derma   l) bone
13. fallopian pregnancy   m) breast

14. hemat   n) ear
15. hepat   o) melanocytoma
16. mast   p) vein
17. high fat content
    in blood   q) liver
18. nephr   r) salpingocyesis
19. neur   s) lung
20. ocul   t) muscle
21. oste   u) nerve
22. brain inflammation   v) skin
23. pector   w) stomach
24. pneum   x) hyperlipidemia
25. my   y) hepatoma

MULTIPLE CHOICE.   *the answer key begins on page 347*

1. Medical science terminology requires that
    a _____ be present in every
    word.
    a. root word
    b. suffix
    c. combining vowel
    d. all of the above

2. Words from the _____ lan-
    guage are most often used to refer to diag-
    nosis and surgery; words from the
    _____ language generally
    refer to the anatomy of the body.
    a. Latin, Greek
    b. Greek, Latin
    c. Latin, Latin
    d. Greek, Greek

3. The _____ is a modifier
    attached to the end of the root word and
    the _____ is a modifier
    attached to the front of the root word.
    a. prefix, suffix
    b. suffix, prefix
    c. suffix, root
    d. prefix, root

4. Red blood cells are called
    _____ and white blood
    cells are called _____.
    a. leukocytes, lymphocytes
    b. erythrocytes, leukocytes
    c. leukocytes, erythrocytes
    d. erythrocytes, lymphocytes

REVIEW

5. A _____ is used to measure blood pressure.
   a. tachometer
   b. otoscope
   c. barometer
   d. sphygmomanometer

6. Which is not part of the endocrine system?
   a. adrenal glands
   b. lacrimal glands
   c. thymus gland
   d. pituitary gland

7. The root word "somat" refers to the
   a. body.
   b. skin.
   c. abdomen.
   d. neurons.

8. The alimentary tract contains which organs?
   a. gastrointestinal tract
   b. esophagus
   c. rectum
   d. all of the above

9. Which class of drugs would be used to treat high blood pressure?
   a. hypolipidemics
   b. antihypertensives
   c. antianginals
   d. hypoglycemics

10. Flexor movement is
   a. expansion or outward movement by muscles.
   b. contraction or inward movement by muscles.
   c. tightening of muscles in any direction.
   d. clockwise rotation of muscles.

11. The bones in the foot are _____ bones.
   a. carpal
   b. flexor
   c. axial
   d. appendicular

12. Hepatitis is inflammation of the
   a. heart.
   b. spleen.
   c. kidneys.
   d. liver.

13. Hemophilia is
   a. a condition where the blood does not clot normally.
   b. a special type of anemia.
   c. the fear of donating blood.
   d. a tumor in the blood system.

14. The neuron is the basic functional unit in the _____ system.
   a. olfactory
   b. skeletal
   c. urinary tract
   d. nervous

15. The skeletal system root word dactyl means
   a. finger or toe.
   b. bone.
   c. large lower leg bone.
   d. wrist.

16. Dysmenorrhea means
   a. absence of menstruation.
   b. inflammation of the breast.
   c. menstrual pain.
   d. fetal development in the fallopian tube.

17. Alveoli are located in the
    a. liver.
    b. kidney.
    c. lungs.
    d. bladder.

18. Bronchitis means
    a. temporary failure to breathe.
    b. inflammation of bronchial membranes.
    c. labored breathing.
    d. chest pain.

19. Cystitis is inflammation of the
    a. kidney.
    b. bowel.
    c. liver.
    d. bladder.

20. Otomycosis means a/an
    a. viral ear infection.
    b. bacterial ear infection.
    c. ear infection with discharge.
    d. fungal ear infection.

21. The prefix "immun" means
    a. safe, protected.
    b. red.
    c. good or normal.
    d. gray.

22. The prefix "pseudo" means
    a. true.
    b. with.
    c. false.
    d. across or through.

23. The suffix "sclerosis" means
    a. pain.
    b. narrowing, constriction.
    c. involuntary contraction.
    d. across or through.

24. The suffix "itis" means
    a. small.
    b. treatment.
    c. tumor.
    d. inflammation.

25. Which layer in the integumentary system is next to muscle tissue?
    a. epidermis
    b. dermis
    c. subcutaneous
    d. subdermis

26. How many muscles are in the human body?
    a. more than 600
    b. more than 10,000
    c. 206
    d. 316

27. Which part of the nervous system controls the automatic function of the body?
    a. somatic nervous system
    b. autonomic nervous system
    c. cerebrum
    d. brain and spinal cord

28. Lacrimal glands can be found in the
    a. female reproductive system.
    b. eye.
    c. ear.
    d. endocrine system.

PRESCRIPTIONS

A prescription is a written order from a practitioner for the preparation and administration of a medicine or a device.

Medical doctors (MD), doctors of osteopathy (DO), dentists (DDS), and veterinarians (DVM) are the primary practitioners allowed to write prescriptions. Opticians and podiatrists are also allowed to write prescriptions for drugs relative to their field of practice. In some states, however, nurse practitioners, physicians assistants and/or pharmacists are also allowed limited rights to prescribe medications based on predetermined protocols (specific guidelines for practice) and in collaboration with one of the primary practitioners mentioned above.

Prescriptions are subject to many federal and state rules and regulations.

These regulations have been developed to protect the patient and to provide for certain minimum standards of practice. The rules and regulations that govern both community and hospital pharmacy practice are continually evaluated and updated as new technologies, new medications, and new protocols are developed and adopted.

Community pharmacists dispense directly to the patient and the patient is expected to administer the medication according to the pharmacist's directions.

This requires clear communication between the pharmacist and the patient. The patient receives information from the pharmacist on the prescription label, and from an information sheet supplied with the medication. In addition, the pharmacist counsels the patient or the patient's representative when the prescription is purchased.

In institutional settings, nursing staff generally administer medications to patients.

As a result, the rules and regulations that govern prescription dispensing in institutional settings are quite different from those rules that apply to community practice. Labeling is quite different and many medications are packaged in individual doses.

Prescription Products

Prescriptions sometimes require the pharmaceutical preparation of a medication from ingredients (an activity called **extemporaneous compounding**). However, they are usually written for commercially available products that are specified by brand or generic name, strength, and route of administration. The pharmacist fills the prescription with that exact product or, if allowed (by the prescriber, insurer, etc.), a product that is determined to be equivalent.

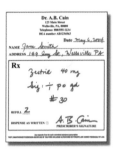

1. **A prescription is written by a prescriber.**

A physician/practitioner determines that a medication is necessary and communicates the details in the written form known as a prescription.

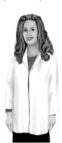

10. **Pharmacist provides counseling.**

The pharmacist is called to the counter to counsel the patient or the patient representative regarding the medications as required by OBRA '90 and by other state or provincial statutes.

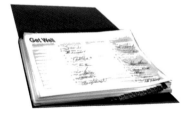

9. **Patient receives the prescription.**

The patient or the patient representative accepts the prescription, the sale is rung through the cash register, and the insurance log is signed. If the patient has not signed the pharmacy's notice of HIPAA compliance, they do so at this time.

The process illustrated here occurs in the community pharmacy. It is somewhat different in institutional settings where medications are administered by nursing staff, instead of the patients themselves.

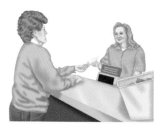

2. The written prescription is presented at the pharmacy.

The patient or a representative presents the written prescription at the pharmacy counter.

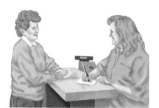

3. Prescription information is checked.

The prescription is assessed for completeness, e.g. prescriber information, drug name, strength, dosage form, directions.

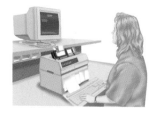

4. Patient and prescription data is entered into system.

Patient data is collected (correct spelling of name, address, insurance information, etc.) and entered into the computerized prescription system.

THE PRESCRIPTION PROCESS

5. Prescription is processed.

The prescription is interpreted and confirmed by the system. If third party billing is involved, this is done online simultaneously.

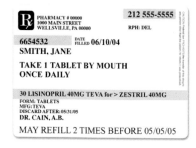

PHARMACY # 00000
1000 MAIN STREET
WELLSVILLE, PA 00000   212 555-5555
RPH: DEL

6654532   DATE FILLED 06/10/04
SMITH, JANE

TAKE 1 TABLET BY MOUTH
ONCE DAILY

30 LISINOPRIL 40MG TEVA for > ZESTRIL 40MG
FORM: TABLETS
MFG: TEVA
DISCARD AFTER: 05/31/05
DR. CAIN, A.B.

MAY REFILL 2 TIMES BEFORE 05/05/05

6. Label is generated.

Once the prescription and third-party billing is confirmed, the label and receipt are printed.

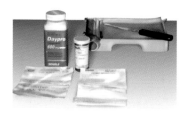

8. Prescription is checked.

If the prescription has been prepared by a technician, there is a final check by the pharmacist to make sure that it is as prescribed.

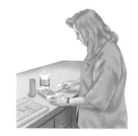

7. Prescription is prepared.

The correct product is selected and the prescribed amount of it is measured and placed into a suitable container and labeled appropriately.

PHARMACY ABBREVIATIONS

Abbreviations for many medical terms are regularly used in the pharmacy.

Many of these abbreviations are from Latin words, though a number are from English. They are commonly used on prescriptions to communicate essential information on formulations, preparation, dosage regimens, and administration of the medication. The technician must know these abbreviations and their meanings.

MOST COMMON ABBREVIATIONS

Note that while it is not necessary to know the latin term from which an abbreviation comes, it has been included for reference.

	Abbreviation	Meaning	Latin term
ROUTE	a.d.	right ear	auris dexter
	a.s., a.l.	left ear	auris sinister
	a.u.	each ear	auris utro
	i.m., IM	intramuscular	
	i.v., IV	intravenous	
	i.v.p., IVP	intravenous push	
	IVPB	intravenous piggyback	
	o.d.	right eye	oculus dexter
	o.s., o.l.	left eye	oculus sinister
	o.u.	each eye	oculus utro
	per neb	by nebulizer	
	p.o.	by mouth	per os
	p.r.	rectally, into the rectum	
	p.v.	vaginally, into the vagina	
	SC, subc, subq	subcutaneously	
	S.L.	sublingually, under the tongue	
	top.	topically, locally	
FORM	aq, aqua	water	aqua
	caps	capsules	capsula
	cm.	cream	
	elix.	elixir	
	liq.	liquid	liquor
	supp.	suppository	suppositorum
	SR,XR, XL	slow/extended release	
	syr.	syrup	syrupus
	tab.	tablet	tabella
	ung., oint	ointment	ungentum
TIME	a.c.	before food, before meals	ante cibum
	a.m.	morning	ante meridien
	b.i.d.,bid	twice a day	bis in die
	h	hour, at the hour of	hora
	h.s.	at bedtime	hora somni
	p.c.	after food, after meals	post cibum
	p.m.	afternoon or evening	
	p.r.n., prn	as needed	pro re nata
	q.i.d., qid	four times a day	quater in die
	q	each, every	quaque
	q.d.	every day	quaque die
	q__h	every__ hour(s)	
	qod	every other day	
	stat.	immediately	statim
	t.i.d., tid	three times a day	ter in die

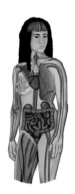

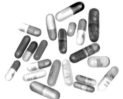

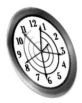

Note that some prescribers will leave out periods in written abbreviations, and that some may use capital letters, while others may not.

MEASUREMENT

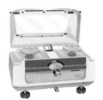

Abbreviation	Meaning	Latin term
ī , ǐī	one, two, etc.	
a.a. or aa	of each	ana
ad	to, up to	ad
aq. ad	add water up to	
dil.	dilute	dilutus
f, fl.	fluid	
fl. oz.	fluid ounce	
g., G., gm.	gram	
gtt.	drop	guttae
l, L	liter/Litre	
mcg.	microgram	
mEq.	milliequivalent	
mg.	milligram	
ml., mL	milliliter/millilitre	
q.s.	a sufficient quantity	quantum sufficiat
q.s. ad	add sufficient quantity to make	quantum sufficiat ad
ss̈	one-half	
tbsp.	tablespoon	
tsp.	teaspoon	

OTHER

c	with	cum
disp.	dispense	
f, ft.	make, let it be made	fac, fiat, fiant
gtt	drop	
NR	no refill	
s̄	without	sine
ut dict., u.d.	as directed	ut dictum

LESS COMMON ABBREVIATIONS

The following abbreviations are also used in pharmacy, though less frequently than the others on these pages.

ad lib.	at pleasure		gr.	grain (1 gr ≃ 65 mg)
a.	before		lot.	lotion
amp.	ampule		N.F.	National Formulary
aur.; a	ear		NS	normal saline
b.	twice		per g. button	per gastric button
brach.	the arm		per n.g.t.	per naso-gastric tube
BSA	body surface area		Sig.	write, label
c.c.	cubic centimeter (1 cc ≃ 1 ml)		SOB	shortness of breath
c.	food		sol.	solution
comp.	compound		tinc.; tr.	tincture
c.c.	with food; with meals		troche	lozenge
D5W	Dextrose 5% in water		tuss.	cough
emuls.	emulsion		USP	United States Pharmacopea

PRESCRIPTION INFORMATION

The modern prescription has stringent requirements designed to inform the pharmacist and protect the patient.

Today's prescription regulations vary from state to state and province to province, but generally a prescription for a community pharmacy will contain the information illustrated below.

ELEMENTS OF THE PRESCRIPTION

Prescriber information:
Name, title, office address, and telephone number

Drug Enforcement Agency (DEA) registration number of prescriber (required for all controlled substances)

Name and address of patient.

Other patient information such as age or weight is optional, but may be important in verifying the correct dosing of the medication. Also, the date of birth is often added to ensure that the prescription is filled for the correct patient.

Note: If a compound is prescribed, a list of ingredients and directions for mixing is included.

Refill instructions

DAW: Dispense As Written and/or Generic Substitution Allowed instructions (optional).

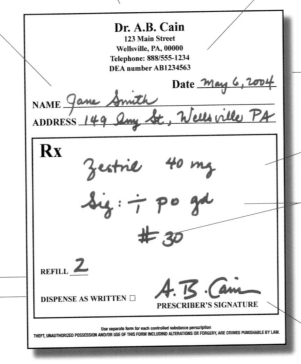

Dr. A.B. Cain
123 Main Street
Wellsville, PA, 00000
Telephone: 888/555-1234
DEA number AB1234563

Date _May 6, 2004_

NAME _Jane Smith_
ADDRESS _149 Any St., Wellsville PA_

Rx

Zestril   40 mg

Sig: ī po qd

30

REFILL _2_

DISPENSE AS WRITTEN ☐   _A. B. Cain_
PRESCRIBER'S SIGNATURE

Use separate form for each controlled substance prescription
THEFT, UNAUTHORIZED POSSESSION AND/OR USE OF THIS FORM INCLUDING ALTERATIONS OR FORGERY, ARE CRIMES PUNISHABLE BY LAW.

Date the prescription is written.

Inscription: Name (brand or generic), strength of medication and quantity.

Signa: This comes from the latin word signa, meaning "to write." It is abbreviated to **Sig** or **S** and indicates the directions for use and the administration route (e.g., p.o., p.r., sc).

Signature of prescriber (not required on a verbal prescription).

Note: Prescriptions are written in ink, never pencil. They may be hand written or electronically produced.

Additional Information

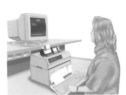

In addition to the above, the information at right must be added to the prescription in the pharmacy. This information is a product of the computerized prescription filling process. Some data are automatically assigned by the computer (e.g., prescription number), while other information is added by the pharmacist or pharmacy technician as they input the data necessary for the proper filling of the prescription (e.g., the product selected).

- ➡ Date the product is dispensed.
- ➡ Identity of the product by manufacturer and NDC (National Drug Code)—DIN (Drug Identification Number) in Canada.
- ➡ Prescription and/or transaction number.
- ➡ Insurance information for the patient.
- ➡ Price charged.
- ➡ Initials of the technician and pharmacist involved in the filling of the prescription.
- ➡ Signature of the pharmacist receiving the prescription if it is a verbal order.

*The prescription information on these pages applies to the community pharmacy setting. In institutions, **medication orders** are used instead of a prescription form. See chapter 16 for more information on institutional practices.*

PRESCRIPTION INFORMATION CHECKLIST

Consider these factors

➡ Is the patient's full name clear on the prescription? Has a nickname or initial been used?

➡ Is the patient's date of birth, street address, telephone number, insurance information, preference for brand or generic drugs, and allergy information already on file in the pharmacy?

➡ Is the medication for an over-the-counter product that the patient can receive without a prescription? Is the prescription for a Schedule II drug that has very special prescription requirements?

➡ When was the prescription written? How many days or weeks has it been since it was written?

➡ Is the drug available in the pharmacy in the quantity written? Does it require compounding?

➡ Is the prescription suspicious in any way? Is it written on a legitimate prescription blank and all in the same hand writing and with the same ink? Are there any signs of alteration of quantities, strength, or the name of the drug? Is this a possible drug of abuse and if so do the quantities and directions seem appropriate?

Take this action

✔ **Determine the exact name** so that multiple files are not created for one patient.

✔ **Always confirm the information on file as current.** Record the date of birth of the patient on the prescription as a double check when filling the prescription.

✔ **Check with the pharmacist on all OTC and Schedule II prescriptions.** Only the pharmacist should recommend an OTC medicine or determine which OTC medicine is requested on the prescription.

✔ **Check with the pharmacist to determine if the prescription can be filled if it is more than a few days old.** Some prescriptions may be valid for months, but others must be verified if they are more than a few days old.

✔ **Inform the patient if there might be a delay in filling the prescription.**

✔ **Alert the pharmacist to any potential forgeries.** Let the pharmacist follow through with the patient and the prescriber..

Note that although the prescription shown here is hand written, more prescribers are using computers and hand-held devices to document and produce prescriptions. In some states prescriptions are transmitted electronically from the prescriber to the pharmacy.

 signa the directions for use to be printed on the prescription label.

 R$_x$ is an abbreviation of the Latin word "recipe", which means "take." As we use it today, "recipe" has a broader meaning in that it is a description of the amounts and steps involved in preparing a mixture of different elements.

THE FILL PROCESS

Once prescription information is finalized in the computerized prescription system, a label and receipt are printed out.

At this point, the correct medication must be selected from pharmacy stock and the prescribed amount measured or counted and packaged. If the prescription calls for a compounded product, the technician must follow pharmacy policy of its preparation.

The pharmacy technician completes the fill process by placing the correct amount of medication into an appropriate container and labeling it correctly.

This includes placing the computer-generated label on the container so it sticks firmly, is straight, and is easy to read. It also includes placing the appropriate **auxiliary labels** on the container. These are the additional warning labels that are placed on filled prescription containers.

A pharmacist must check the final product and label.

When finished with preparation, the technician initials the pharmacy copy of the label and organizes the finished product, prescription order, and the stock bottle that the medication was taken from for the pharmacist to check and verify. If the prescription is correctly filled, the pharmacist initials the pharmacy copy of the label information to indicate that the prescription was correctly filled. The prescription may then be released to the patient.

Avoiding Errors

If the technician is unsure about any aspect of a prescription, he or she must ask the pharmacist for direction. Never dispense guesswork! The careful screening of prescription orders by the technician can prevent medication errors and other errors. Medication errors can be very serious. They include, but are not limited to the dispensing of:

➡ the wrong medication
➡ the wrong strength, dosage form, or quantity
➡ the wrong directions
➡ the medication to the wrong patient,
➡ the dispensing of medications on the order of a forged or altered prescription.

An awareness that medication errors exist and that they are very serious is the first step in preventing medication errors from happening.

CONSIDERATIONS

The technician should consider these factors when filling prescriptions:

Are the fill instructions clear and reasonable?

Do the directions, quantity, and strength fit with what is usual for this medication? Are there any opportunities for confusion (e.g. is the dosing schedule q.i.d. or q.d.)? Does the Sig. read: 2 hs or q hs?

Are the administration directions clear?

Are the directions clearly translated in an unambiguous fashion in order to avoid any misinterpretation by the patient (e.g. does take two tablets daily mean that the patient is to take one tablet twice daily or two tablets once daily)?

Are there look-alike names?

Are there any look-alike drug names that could be confused with the intended medication? For example, did the prescriber write HCTZ 50mg (hydrochlorothiazide) or HCT 250mg (hydrocortisone)?

Don't add information!

Never add information that is not indicated based on what you assume the prescriber meant when writing the prescription. The prescriber has knowledge of the patient's condition that you don't. Adding directions that you assume to be correct may not be appropriate.

Pay attention to warnings!

When warning screens appear regarding potential insurance claim errors, dosing irregularities, or drug interactions, **call the pharmacist to evaluate each warning.** An ignored warning might result in the patient being over-billed, undermedicated, or hospitalized due to a severe drug-drug interaction. Only the pharmacist determines which warnings require intervention and which are for informational purposes.

Check against the original!

During the fill process, always refer to the original prescription first and then refer to the label.

THE PHARMACIST'S ROLE

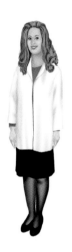

The pharmacist's role is multifaceted and includes:

✔ using his/her knowledge and expertise in order to assure that the physicians' orders are carried out accurately and safely,

✔ ensuring that the correct medication, strength and dosage form is dispensed,

✔ ensuring that the directions for the patient are clear, accurate, and unambiguous,

✔ ensuring that there are no potential problems with drug allergies, drug-drug or drug-disease interactions,

✔ ensuring that there are no misunderstandings by the patient with respect to how to take the medication,

✔ ensuring that the patient understands the beneficial effects that can be expected from the medication and the potential side effects that he/she should be cautious about while taking the medication,

✔ ensuring that the prescriber has been contacted regarding the prescription if appropriate,

✔ ensuring that the prescription has been accurately and fairly billed to the patient or the appropriate third party,

✔ counseling the patient on the use of OTC medications.

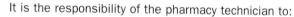

THE PHARMACY TECHNICIAN'S ROLE

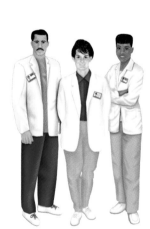

It is the responsibility of the pharmacy technician to:

✔ assist the pharmacist in the technical (non-judgment requiring) aspects of prescription filling;

✔ treat each patient, their personal information, and their medication with respect;

✔ gather all appropriate information needed in a timely, efficient, and professional manner;

✔ quickly and accurately locate the appropriate medication for dispensing, calculate quantities, and re-package medication for the prescription;

✔ quickly, accurately, and efficiently key patient data and prescription information into the computer;

✔ request the advice of the pharmacist whenever a warning screen appears during the filling of a prescription;

✔ request the advice of the pharmacist whenever judgment is required, e.g., for counseling on the use of a medications, questions regarding therapy, and so on;

✔ answering the telephone and "in-house" patient queries, and passing the patient on to the pharmacist when appropriate.

Prescriptions for OTC Medications

Prescriptions may be written for over-the-counter (OTC) medications. When this happens, consult the pharmacist. The prescription is generally not filled. The pharmacist instead helps the patient locate the product on the shelf and then counsels the patient with respect to the prescriber's orders. The patient then purchases the medication as an over-the-counter product.

LABELS

The general purpose of the prescription label is to provide information to the patient regarding the dispensed medication and how to take it. Additionally, the label includes information about the pharmacy, the patient, the prescriber, and the prescription or transaction number assigned to the prescription.

As with prescriptions, requirements for prescription labels vary from state to state (and in Canada from province to province). Generally, however, a prescription label contains the information indicated below.

the name, address, and telephone number of the pharmacy

a prescription and/or transaction number

the name of the patient for whom the medication is dispensed

directions for use that are clear, accurate and unambiguous

the name, quantity, strength, manufacturer, and dosage form of the medication dispensed

expiration date of the medication

the name of the prescriber

the date dispensed

the initials of the person who keyed the information into the computer and often the handwritten initials of the pharmacist who checked the prescription.

refill information.

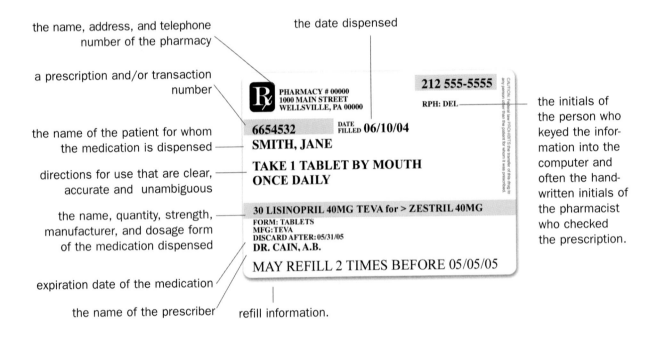

PHARMACY # 00000
1000 MAIN STREET
WELLSVILLE, PA 00000

212 555-5555

RPH: DEL

6654532   DATE FILLED 06/10/04

SMITH, JANE

TAKE 1 TABLET BY MOUTH
ONCE DAILY

30 LISINOPRIL 40MG TEVA for > ZESTRIL 40MG
FORM: TABLETS
MFG: TEVA
DISCARD AFTER: 05/31/05
DR. CAIN, A.B.

MAY REFILL 2 TIMES BEFORE 05/05/05

DIRECTIONS FOR USE

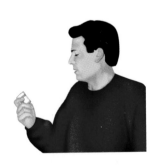

✔ **Directions should start with a verb** (take, instill, inhale, insert, apply) **and completely, clearly, and accurately describe the administration of the medication.**

✔ **Indicate the route of administration.** For example, "take one capsule by mouth", "apply to affected area", "insert rectally", etc.

✔ **Use whole words, not abbreviations.** For example, use "tablets" not "tabs."

✔ **Use familiar words, especially in measurements.** For example, use "two teaspoonfuls" or "10 ml" as most measuring droppers and spoons are calibrated in teaspoons and ml.

 In community pharmacy, a label that is easily understood by the patient is absolutely essential.

AUXILIARY LABELS

Colored auxiliary labels may also be applied to the prescription container in order to provide additional information to the patient (e.g. Shake Well, Keep Refrigerated, Take With Food or Milk). Many computerized prescription systems will automatically print out the appropriate labels to use.

Prescriptions for controlled substances from schedules II, III and IV must carry the following warning:

Caution: Federal law prohibits the transfer of this drug to any person other than the patient for whom it was prescribed. This warning is pre-printed on many labels.

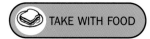 TAKE WITH FOOD

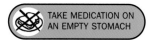 TAKE MEDICATION ON AN EMPTY STOMACH

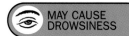 MAY CAUSE DROWSINESS

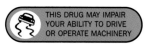 THIS DRUG MAY IMPAIR YOUR ABILITY TO DRIVE OR OPERATE MACHINERY

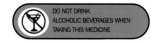 DO NOT DRINK ALCOHOLIC BEVERAGES WHEN TAKING THIS MEDICINE

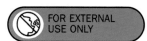 FOR EXTERNAL USE ONLY

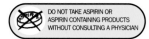 DO NOT TAKE ASPIRIN OR ASPIRIN CONTAINING PRODUCTS WITHOUT CONSULTING A PHYSICIAN

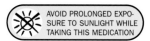 AVOID PROLONGED EXPOSURE TO SUNLIGHT WHILE TAKING THIS MEDICATION

PLACING THE LABEL

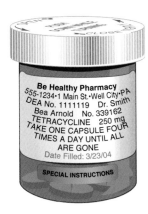

Be Healthy Pharmacy
555-1234•1 Main St.•Well City•PA
DEA No. 1111119   Dr. Smith
Bea Arnold   No. 339162
TETRACYCLINE   250 mg
TAKE ONE CAPSULE FOUR
TIMES A DAY UNTIL ALL
ARE GONE
Date Filled: 3/23/04

SPECIAL INSTRUCTIONS

Labeling the container correctly includes:

✔ placing the computer-generated label on the container so it is parallel to the edges of the container, easy to locate, and easy to read;

✔ making sure the label sticks adequately to the container and is without creases. (Some pharmacies place transparent tape over the label to protect the label from spills and prevent accidental smudging or obliteration of information.);

✔ placing the appropriate auxiliary labels on the container;

✔ placing labels on prescription vials into which eye drops, ear drops and eye ointments have been placed;

✔ in some states, placing the label on the actual container rather than the box in which it is packaged.

INSTITUTIONAL LABELS

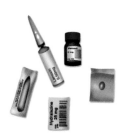

Rules for institutional pharmacy prescription labels vary by institution but often do not contain much more than the name, strength, manufacturer, lot number, expiration date, and dosage form of the medication. Since the condition of a patient in the hospital can change relatively quickly, their medication orders may be regularly updated. As a result, the nursing staff refers to the most recent physician's instructions in the patient's chart to verify prescribing information. It is also worth noting that unit dose packaging is widely used in institutional settings, and such packaging often has space for only essential identifying information about the medication.

EXAMPLES

PRESCRIPTION TO LABEL

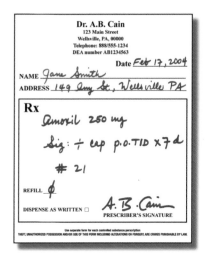

➡ Amoxil is a brand name for Amoxicillin.
➡ 250 mg is the strength.
➡ ᵢ̄ cap means "take one capsule."
➡ P.O. means "by mouth."
➡ TID means "three times a day."
➡ x7d means "for seven days."
➡ #21 means a "quantity of 21."
➡ there are no refills; generic substitution may be used.

Therefore, the prescription is for a week's supply of Amoxicillin 250mg capsules: 21 capsules, one capsule to be taken three times daily for seven days.

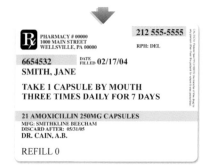

The label for the above prescription.

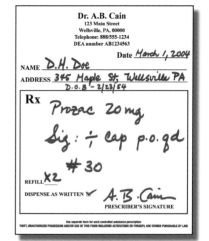

➡ The drug is Prozac.
➡ 20mg is the strength.
➡ ᵢ̄ cap means "take one capsule."
➡ P.O. means "by mouth."
➡ qd means "each day" or "once daily"
➡ #30 means a "quantity of 30."
➡ there are 2 refills; dispense as written; generic substitution not allowed.

Therefore, the prescription is for a 30 day supply of Prozac 20mg capsules: 30 capsules, one capsule to be taken each day, with two refills.

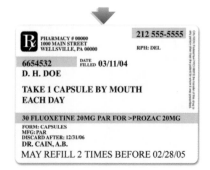

℞ Note that "D.O.B." on this prescription means the date of birth. While this is optional, it is important, and sometimes necessary, as with online adjudication of a claim.

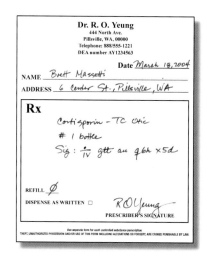

Dr. R. O. Yeung
444 North Ave.
Pillsville, WA, 00000
Telephone: 888/555-1221
DEA number AY1234563

Date *March 18, 2004*

NAME *Brett Massetti*
ADDRESS *6 Center St., Pillsville, WA*

Rx

Cortisporin - TC Otic
1 bottle
Sig : i̅v̅ gtt au q6h x5d

REFILL Ø
DISPENSE AS WRITTEN ☐

R O Yeung
PRESCRIBER'S SIGNATURE

Use separate form for each controlled substance prescription
THEFT, UNAUTHORIZED POSSESSION AND/OR USE OF THIS FORM INCLUDING ALTERATIONS OR FORGERY, ARE CRIMES PUNISHABLE BY LAW.

➡ The drug is Cortisporin - TC Otic drops.

➡ No strength is needed as it is a combination of several drugs and it comes only in one formulation.

➡ #1 bottle means "dispense one bottle."

➡ Sig means "The directions are..."

➡ i̅v̅ gtt au q6h x5d means "Instill 4 drops into each ear every six hours for 5 days."

➡ Note that Cortisporin - TC comes in only one size (10 ml). When several sizes are available, ask the pharmacist to get his/her selection. Most often an appropriate package size can be selected by examining the directions.

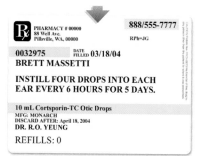

℞ PHARMACY # 00000
88 Well Ave.
Pillsville, WA, 00000
RPh=JG

888/555-7777

0032975 DATE FILLED **03/18/04**
BRETT MASSETTI

**INSTILL FOUR DROPS INTO EACH
EAR EVERY 6 HOURS FOR 5 DAYS.**

10 mL Cortsporin-TC Otic Drops
MFG: MONARCH
DISCARD AFTER: April 18, 2004
DR. R.O. YEUNG

REFILLS: 0

Dr. J. P. Hoyt
321 Center Street
Healthtown, NV, 00000
Telephone: 775/555-1221
DEA number BH1111119

Date *02/04/04*

NAME *Teresa Sanchez*
ADDRESS *10 West 2nd Ave, Healthtown, NV*

Rx

Metro gel Vag.
i̅ pv hs
x7

REFILL *1*
DISPENSE AS WRITTEN ☐

J P Hoyt
PRESCRIBER'S SIGNATURE

Use separate form for each controlled substance prescription
THEFT, UNAUTHORIZED POSSESSION AND/OR USE OF THIS FORM INCLUDING ALTERATIONS OR FORGERY, ARE CRIMES PUNISHABLE BY LAW.

➡ The drug is MetroGel Vaginal Gel.

➡ No strength is needed as it only comes in one strength.

➡ i̅ pv hs means "insert one applicatorful vaginally at bedtime."

➡ x7 means "for seven doses" or "for seven nights.

➡ There is one refill; note, however, that many states place a time limit on refills such as one year for legend drugs and six months for controlled drugs (Sch III & IV).

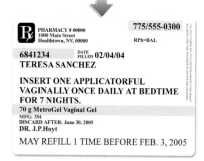

℞ PHARMACY # 00000
1000 Main Street
Healthtown, NV, 00000
RPh=BAL

775/555-0300

6841234 DATE FILLED **02/04/04**
TERESA SANCHEZ

**INSERT ONE APPLICATORFUL
VAGINALLY ONCE DAILY AT BEDTIME
FOR 7 NIGHTS.**
70 g MetroGel Vaginal Gel
MFG: 3M
DISCARD AFTER: June 30, 2005
DR. J.P.Hoyt

MAY REFILL 1 TIME BEFORE FEB. 3, 2005

EXAMPLES (cont'd)

MEDICATION ORDERS

There are various formats for the medication orders used in institutional settings. Here are two samples. Note the following factors that are indicated by one or both of the examples:

➡ multiple medications are often used.

➡ abbreviations are used.

➡ orders are indicated by time of order.

➡ orders are revised to include changes in therapy.

➡ administration times are noted and signed by nursing staff.

➡ allergies are indicated.

These and other aspects of medication orders reflect the special characteristics of the institutional environment.

DOCTOR'S ORDERS

PATIENT IDENTIFICATION

099999999   675-01
SMITH, JOHN
12/06/1950

DR P JOHNSON

DATE	TIME	DOCTOR'S ORDERS 1	DATE/TIME INITIALS	DATE/TIME INITIALS
1/31/04	2200	Admit patient to 6th floor		
		Pneumonia, Dehydration		
		All: PCN-Rash		
		Order CBC, chem-7, blood cultures stat		
		NS @ 125ml/hr IV		
		Dr Johnson X2222		

DATE	TIME	DOCTOR'S ORDERS 2	DATE/TIME INITIALS	DATE/TIME INITIALS
2/01/04	330	Tylenol 650mg po q4-6 hrs PRN for Temp>38°C		
		Verbal Order Dr Johnson/Jane Doe, RN		

DATE	TIME	DOCTOR'S ORDERS 3	DATE/TIME INITIALS	DATE/TIME INITIALS
2/01/04	600	Start Clarithromycin 500mg po q 12°		
		Multivitamin po qd		
		Order CXR for this am		
		Dr Johnson X2222		

COMMUNITY HOSPITAL
Medication Administration Record

Room/Bed: 675-01
Patient: SMITH, JOHN
Account #: 099999999
Sex: M
Age: 48Y
Doctor: JOHNSON, P.

From 0730 on 02/01/04 to 0700 on 02/02/04

Diagnosis: PNEUMONIA; DEHYDRATION
Height: 5'11"   weight: 75KG

Verified By: _Susie Smith, RN_

Allergies: PENICILLIN-->RASH

	0730–1530	1600–2300	2330–0700
0.9% SODIUM CHLORIDE 1 LITER BAG DOSE 125 ML/HR IV ORDER #2	800 JD	1600 SS	2400
MULTIVITAMIN TABLET DOSE: 1 TABLET P.O. QD ORDER #4	1000 ® Given @ 9AM JD		
CLARITHROMYCIN 500 MG TABLET DOSE: 500MG P.O. Q 12 HRS ORDER #5	1000 JD	2200 SS	
ACETAMINOPHEN 325 MG TABLET DOSE: 650 MG P.O. Q 4-6 H P.R.N. FOR TEMP>38°C ORDER # 17	1200 JD		

Init / Signature	Init / Signature
SS / Susie Smith, RN	___ / _____
JD / Jane Doe, RN	___ / _____
___ / _____	___ / _____

℞ There are rules for written information on institutional documents which generally include the requirement to use black ink; red ink is also required for some information such as patient allergies.

HIPAA

HIPAA: The Health Insurance Portability and Accountability Act

The Health Insurance Portability and Accountability Act (HIPAA) of 1996 came into effect on April 14, 2003 with wide reaching consequences for health care professionals. HIPAA is a large statute that primarily concerns the continuation of health insurance coverage for workers who leave their jobs. However, there are a number of regulations relating to privacy and protected health information ("PHI") that all health care providers ("covered entities"), including pharmacies, must follow.

Rules have been established to regulate how and when pharmacies and other covered entities may use and disclose a patient's protected health information. Other rules require administrative, physical and technical safeguards to prevent illicit access to patient information while it is stored or transmitted electronically. Examples of PHI are name and address, date of birth, social security number, payment history, account number, name and address of health care provider and/or health plan, and medical/prescription drug histories.

Under HIPAA, pharmacies and other covered entities are required to provide a written notice of their privacy practices to their patients. This notice must describe the pharmacy's privacy procedures and patients' privacy rights, and must describe how the pharmacy intends to use and disclose patients' PHI. Each pharmacy must make a good faith effort to have every patient sign an "acknowledgement" that the patient has received the pharmacy's notice of privacy practices. This acknowledgement may be signed when the patient picks up his or her medication. The acknowledgement must be maintained separately from the consultation log that all patients sign when picking up their medication. Acknowledgement signatures must remain on file for six years from the last date of service to the patient.

HIPAA also states that a pharmacy may disclose PHI, without patient approval, to business associates that perform services on behalf of the patient. Examples of such business associates would be physicians' offices and pharmacy benefits management (prescription insurance) companies. However, these disclosures must follow the "minimum necessary" requirement which means that covered entities may use, disclose and request only the minimum necessary amount of PHI to other covered entities.

All personnel who have access to PHI must be formally trained regarding HIPAA. This includes pharmacists, pharmacy technicians, pharmacy clerks, and any other employee who may come into contact with PHI. Even the computer specialists who come to the pharmacy to service computers must be HIPAA trained and HIPAA compliant. No one is exempt.

Penalties for violations of HIPAA rules range from fines ($100 to $250,000) to jail (up to ten years). As you can see, it is very important for all pharmacy personnel to familiarize themselves with HIPAA policies and procedures established and practiced at their workplace.

REVIEW

KEY CONCEPTS

PRESCRIPTIONS

✔ A prescription is a written or verbal order from a practitioner for the preparation and administration of a medicine or a device.

✔ Medical doctors (MD), doctors of osteopathy (DO), dentists (DDS), and veterinarians (DVM) are the primary practitioners allowed to write prescriptions. Podiatrists and optomotrists are also allowed to write prescriptions. All practitioners must write within the scope of their practice.

✔ In many states, nurse practitioners, physicians assistants and/or pharmacists are also allowed limited rights to prescribe medications.

✔ In community pharmacies, pharmacy technicians generally receive the prescription, collect patient data (correct spelling of name, address, allergy and insurance information, etc.) and enter them into a computerized prescription system.

PRESCRIPTION INFORMATION

✔ The pharmacist should be consulted on all OTC and Schedule II prescriptions.

✔ The prescription is entered into the computer and drug-drug, drug-disease, and drug-allergy information is automatically checked by the pharmacy software. If third party billing is involved, this is done online simultaneously.

THE FILL PROCESS

✔ Once the prescription and third-party billing is confirmed by the on-line computer system, the label and receipt are printed and the prescription is prepared.

✔ Since the patient is expected to self-administer the medication, the label's directions for use must be clear, unambiguous and concise.

✔ Pharmacists must provide counseling to patients on all new prescriptions and on any refilled prescriptions where clarification is required. A patient may refuse counseling.

✔ In institutional settings, nursing staff generally administer medications to patients.

✔ Technicians must request the advice of the pharmacist whenever judgment is required.

LABELS

✔ Many computerized prescription systems will automatically indicate which auxiliary labels to use with each drug.

HIPAA

✔ The Health Insurance Portability and Accountability Act (HIPAA) contains regulations related to privacy and protected health information (PHI).

✔ Examples of PHI are name and address, date of birth, social security number, payment history, account number, name and address of health care provider and/or health plan, and medical or prescription history.

✔ Under HIPAA, pharmacies and other covered entities are required to provide a written notice of their privacy practices to their patients.

✔ A pharmacy may disclose PHI to business associates that perform services on behalf of the patient.

✔ All personnel who have access to PHI must be formally trained regarding HIPAA.

SELF TEST

MATCH THE TERMS.   *answers can be checked in the glossary*

auxiliary labels

extemporaneous compounding

look-alikes

medication orders

DEA number

prescription

protocols

signa, sig

HIPAA

OBRA '90

- a written order from a practitioner for the preparation and administration of a medicine or a device.
- the pharmaceutical preparation of a medication from ingredients.
- a federal act that is generally credited with states mandating pharmacist counseling on all new prescriptions.
- required on all controlled drug prescriptions; identifies the prescriber.
- specific guidelines for practice.
- the directions for use on a prescription that should be printed on the label.
- the additional warning labels that are placed on filled prescription containers.
- a federal act that, among other things, protects the privacy of individuals and the sharing of protected health information.
- the form used to prescribe medications for patients in institutional settings.
- drug names that have similar appearance, particularly when written.

MATCH THE TERMS.   *the answer key begins on page 347*

1. ointment	a) prn	8. one-half	h) ung
2. drop	b) gtt	9. at bedtime	i) hs
3. twice a day	c) tid	10. by mouth	j) q
4. three times a day	d) bid	11. topically, locally	k) p.c.
5. four times a day	e) qid	12. every day	l) po
6. as needed	f) $\overline{ss}$	13. each, every	m) top.
7. each ear	g) au	14. after food, after meals	n) qd

REVIEW

CHOOSE THE BEST ANSWER.   *the answer key begins on page 347*

1. Primary practitioners allowed to write prescriptions without a requirement for collaboration and protocols include
   a. nurse practitioners and physician assistants.
   b. medical doctors, doctors of osteopathy, dentists, and veterinarians.
   c. pharmacists and physician assistants.
   d. nurse practitioners and pharmacists.

2. _____ are allowed to write some prescriptions in some states, as determined by protocols and collaboration with a primary prescriber.
   a. Medical doctors
   b. Doctors of osteopathy
   c. Pharmacists, nurse practitioners, and/or physician assistants
   d. Doctors of veterinary medicine

3. _____ dispense directly to the patient and the patient is expected to administer the medication according to the pharmacist's directions.
   a. Hospital pharmacists
   b. Nursing home pharmacists
   c. Community pharmacists
   d. Institutional pharmacists

4. In institutional settings, _____ generally administer(s) medications to patients.
   a. nursing staff
   b. pharmacists
   c. medical doctors
   d. doctors of osteopathy

5. Counseling, as required by OBRA '90, is provided by
   a. physicians
   b. pharmacy technicians
   c. pharmacists
   d. nurses

6. All of the following duties may be performed by the pharmacy technician except:
   a. requesting PHI from a patient such as date of birth, address, allergy and insurance information.
   b. selecting an OTC product for a patient.
   c. inputting and updating patient information in the computer.
   d. placing the medication in a vial and attaching the prescription label to the vial.

7. A medication error may involve
   a. the wrong dosage form.
   b. the wrong directions.
   c. the wrong patient
   d. all of the above.

8. The two drug names Accupril 40 mg and Accutane 40 mg exemplify
   a. Signa.
   b. extemporaneous compounding.
   c. look-alike names.
   d. OTC medications.

9. The directions for use (such as $\bar{\imath}$ cap t.i.d.) make-up the
   a. DAW indicator.
   b. insigna.
   c. inscription.
   d. Signa.

10. Directions for use should start with a/an
   a. adjective.
   b. verb.
   c. noun.
   d. adverb.

11. When the Sig. contains q.d., the medication should be taken (every)
    a. hour.
    b. four times daily.
    c. day.
    d. week.

Questions 12-14 are based on this information from a prescription:

    Amoxil   250 mg/5ml
    Sig: ī̄ tsp tid x10d
    M: qs

12. The medication should be taken:
    a. twice daily.
    b. every 10 hours.
    c. three times daily.
    d. none of the above.

13. The amount of medication to be dispensed is:
    a. 100 ml.
    b. 150 ml.
    c. 250 ml.
    d. the amount of medication is not indicated.

14. The following auxiliary labels should be placed near the medication label:
    a. shake well
    b. may cause drowsiness
    c. do not take with milk or other dairy products
    d. discard unused portion after 5 days

15. "Caution: Federal law prohibits the transfer of this drug to any person other than the patient for whom it was prescribed" must be on the label for
    a. only Schedule V controlled substances.
    b. Schedule II, III, and IV controlled substances.
    c. legend drugs.
    d. only Schedule II controlled substances.

16. If a prescription is written for Tenormin 50 mg D.A.W., this means that
    a. the insurance may require the patient to receive the generic.
    b. the patient may switch to generic for refills.
    c. the patient may choose the generic.
    d. the brand name must be dispensed.

17. Medication orders in institutional settings are ordered by
    a. pharmacy technicians.
    b. pharmacists.
    c. doctors.
    d. nurses.

18. For the prescription: Prozac 20 mg #30 ī̄ qd NR, how many refills are allowed?
    a. zero
    b. one
    c. 20
    d. 3

19. "Take with Food" is an example of a/an
    a. auxiliary label.
    b. extemporaneous compound.
    c. route of administration.
    d. drug-food interaction.

20. For the prescription: Clarithromycin 500 mg #20 ī̄ b.i.d. nr, what is the Sig?
    a. ī̄ b.i.d
    b. nr
    c. Clarithromycin 500 mg
    d. #20

NUMBERS

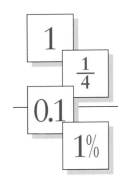

The amount of a drug in its manufactured or prescribed form is always stated numerically — that is, with numbers.

Knowing how to work with numbers is essential to the proper handling of drugs and preparation of prescriptions. This involves understanding the different number forms, measurement units, and mathematical operations that are regularly used. In pharmacy we use two different number systems: Arabic (such as 1, 1/2, 0.5, or 50%) and Roman (such as I, V, X, L, C, D or M). Most of the time we use Arabic numerals, although Roman numerals are often used to indicate quantities in prescription order writing.

ROMAN NUMERALS

Roman numerals are letters that represent numbers. They were originally developed and used by the Roman Empire. They can be capital or lower case letters, and are:

$$ss = \frac{1}{2}$$

L or l = 50

I or i = 1   C or c = 100

V or v = 5   D or d = 500

X or x = 10   M or m = 1000

When grouped together, these few letters can express a large range of numbers, using a simple *positional notation*. That means the position of the letters has a mathematical importance, as determined by these rules:

When the second of two letters has a value equal to or smaller than that of the first, their values are to be added.

EXAMPLE:

xx = 20	or	10 plus 10
dc = 600	or	500 plus 100
lxvi = 66	or	50 plus 10 plus 5 plus 1

When the second of two letters has a value greater than that of the first, the smaller is to be subtracted from the larger.

EXAMPLE:

iv = 4	or	1 subtracted from 5
xxxix = 39	or	30 plus (1 subtracted from 10)
xc = 90	or	10 subtracted from 100

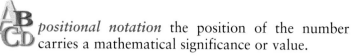 *positional notation* the position of the number carries a mathematical significance or value.

℞ *Answers for these problems can be found in the answer key beginning on page 347.*

PRACTICE PROBLEMS — ROMAN NUMERALS

Write the following in Roman numerals:

1. 18   _____
2. 64   _____
3. 72   _____
4. 126   _____
5. 100   _____
6. 7   _____
7. 28   _____

Write the following in Arabic numbers:

8. xxxiii _____
9. CX   _____
10. mc   _____
11. iss   _____
12. XIX   _____
13. xxiv   _____

Interpret the quantity in each of these phrases taken from prescriptions:

14. Caps. no. xiv.   _____
15. Gtts. ix.   _____
16. Tabs. no. XLVIII. _____
17. Tabs. no. xxi   _____

— I V X L C D M —

FRACTIONS

$$\dfrac{1}{4}$$

FRACTIONS

Fractions are commonly used in the Arabic system. A fraction is a numerical representation (as 3/4, 5/8, 3.234) indicating there is part of a whole. A fraction also represents the division of two numbers.

Numerators and Denominators

In a fraction, the denominator (number below the bar) tells us how many parts the whole is divided into, and the numerator (number above the bar) tells us how many of those parts exist.

In a fraction, the numerator can be zero, but the denominator cannot be zero. Division by zero is undefined, therefore no denominator can be zero.

One way to think of a fraction is as division that hasn't been completed.

Fractions can be used to indicate equal parts of a whole unit.

EXAMPLE

We can read $\dfrac{2}{5}$ as two-fifths, two over five or two divided by five.

Every fraction can be converted to a decimal by dividing. Using a calculator to divide 2 by 5

$$\dfrac{2}{5} \quad = \quad 0.4.$$

Here are some other fractions and their decimal equivalents. Remember, you can find the decimal equivalent of any fraction by dividing.

$$\dfrac{1}{2} \quad = \quad 0.5$$

$$\dfrac{2}{3} \quad = \quad 0.67$$

$$\dfrac{3}{4} \quad = \quad 0.75$$

℞ *Answers for the problems on the following page can be found in the answer key beginning on page 347.*

numerator the top or left number in a fraction that indicates a portion of the denominator to be used.

denominator the bottom or right number in a fraction which is divided into the numerator to give the fraction's value.

Reciprocals

Reciprocals are two different fractions that equal 1 when multiplied together. Every fraction has a reciprocal (except those fractions with zero in the numerator). The easiest way to find the reciprocal of a fraction is to switch the numerator and denominator, or just turn the fraction over.

To find the reciprocal of a whole number, just put 1 over the whole number.

EXAMPLE:

The reciprocal of 2 is $\frac{1}{2}$

EXAMPLE:

The reciprocal of 3 is $\frac{1}{3}$

EXAMPLE:

The reciprocal of 4 is $\frac{1}{4}$

EXAMPLE:

The reciprocal of 2/3 is $\frac{3}{2}$

PRACTICE PROBLEMS -- NUMERATORS, DENOMINATORS, AND RECIPROCALS

Use a calculator to convert the following fractions to decimals:

1. $\frac{1}{3}$ = _____

2. $\frac{1}{2}$ = _____

3. $\frac{1}{4}$ = _____

4. $\frac{3}{10}$ = _____

5. $\frac{1}{10}$ = _____

Determine the reciprocal of the following fractions:

6. $\frac{1}{5}$ = _____

7. $\frac{2}{3}$ = _____

8. $\frac{2}{5}$ = _____

9. $\frac{2}{9}$ = _____

10. $\frac{1}{15}$ = _____

FRACTIONS (cont'd)

$$\frac{1}{4}$$

ADDING AND SUBTRACTING FRACTIONS

In order to add or subtract fractions the fractions must have the same denominator or common denominators. Addition and subtraction of like fractions is easy. To add or subtract like fractions just add or subtract the numerators and write the sum or difference over the common denominator.

To add or subtract fractions with different denominators, you must first find equivalent fractions with common denominators: First find the smallest multiple for the denominator of both numbers. Then rewrite the fractions as equivalent fractions with the smallest multiple of both numbers as the denominator. (The smallest multiple of both numbers is called the **least common denominator**.)

EXAMPLE: $\frac{1}{3} + \frac{3}{5}$

The smallest multiple for the denominator of both numbers is 15

$$\frac{1}{3} = \frac{1 \times 5}{3 \times 5} = \frac{5}{15}$$

$$\frac{3}{5} = \frac{3 \times 3}{5 \times 3} = \frac{9}{15}$$

The problem can now be rewritten

$$\frac{5}{15} + \frac{9}{15}$$

Since the denominators are equal, we only have to add the numerators to get the answer:

$$\frac{5 + 9}{15} = \frac{14}{15}$$

PRACTICE PROBLEMS -- ADDING AND SUBTRACTING FRACTIONS

Add or subtract the following fractions.

1. $\frac{1}{4} + \frac{1}{4} = $ _____

2. $\frac{3}{8} + \frac{5}{8} = $ _____

3. $\frac{2}{5} - \frac{1}{5} = $ _____

4. $\frac{7}{8} - \frac{3}{8} = $ _____

5. $\frac{2}{5} + \frac{3}{5} = $ _____

6. $\frac{1}{8} + \frac{3}{8} = $ _____

7. $\frac{1}{4} + \frac{1}{5} = $ _____

8. $\frac{4}{15} + \frac{1}{5} = $ _____

9. $\frac{1}{4} + \frac{3}{16} = $ _____

10. $\frac{5}{8} - \frac{1}{4} = $ _____

Multiplying fractions is frequently stated by using the word "of." If you must determine 1/2 of 10, you would multiply 1/2 X 10. 1/2 X 10 = 5.

MULTIPLYING AND DIVIDING FRACTIONS

To multiply fractions, first multiply the numerators of the fractions to get the new numerator. Then multiply the denominators of the fractions to get the new denominator.

EXAMPLE: $\frac{2}{3}$ of 24

Multiply $\frac{2}{3}$ X $\frac{24}{1}$

$= \frac{48}{3}$

$\frac{48}{3}$ can be reduced to 16.

To divide a number by a fraction multiply the number by the reciprocal of the fraction.

EXAMPLE: 24 DIVIDED BY $\frac{1}{3}$

Find the reciprocal of the fraction:

The reciprocal of $\frac{1}{3}$ is 3

Multiply the number by the reciprocal of the fraction:

24 X 3 = 72

EXAMPLE: Divide $\frac{1}{3}$ by 8.

First, find the reciprocal of the fraction:

The reciprocal of 8 is $\frac{1}{8}$.

Second, multiply the number by the reciprocal of the fraction:

$\frac{1}{3}$ X $\frac{1}{8}$ = $\frac{1}{24}$

PRACTICE PROBLEMS -- MULTIPLYING AND DIVIDING FRACTIONS

Multiply the following fractions:

1. $\frac{1}{4}$ of $\frac{1}{4}$ = _____

2. $\frac{1}{3}$ of $\frac{3}{8}$ = _____

3. $\frac{2}{3}$ of $\frac{1}{3}$ = _____

4. $\frac{3}{8}$ of $\frac{5}{8}$ = _____

Divide the following fractions:

5. $\frac{1}{3}$ divided by $\frac{1}{2}$ = _____

6. $\frac{1}{4}$ divided by $\frac{3}{4}$ = _____

7. $\frac{2}{5}$ divided by $\frac{1}{5}$ = _____

8. $\frac{3}{8}$ divided by $\frac{3}{8}$ = _____

DECIMAL NUMBERS

ADDING AND SUBTRACTING DECIMALS

To add decimal numbers, first put the numbers in a vertical column, aligning the decimal points Then add each column of digits, starting on the right and working left. If the sum of a column is more than ten, "carry" digits to the next column on the left. Place the decimal point in the answer directly below the decimal points in the terms.

EXAMPLE: Add 324.5678 to 1.2345

Step 1:

```
  324.5678
    1.2345
         3  (carry the 1)
```

Step 2:

```
  324.5678
    1.2345
        23  (carry the 1)
```

Step 3:

```
  324.5678
    1.2345
       023  (carry the 1)
```

Step 4:

```
  324.5678
    1.2345
     .8023
```

Step 5:

```
  324.5678
    1.2345
    5.8023
```

Step 6:

```
  324.5678
    1.2345
   25.802
```

Step 7:

```
  324.5678
    1.2345
  325.8023
```

PRACTICE PROBLEMS -- ADDING DECIMALS

Add the following decimal fractions:

1. 0.6 + 0.4 + 0.3   = _____

2. 4 + 3.1 + 0.3   = _____

3. 0.39 + 3.92 + 0.03   = _____

4. 3.365 + 15.432 + 5.001   = _____

5. 37.02 + 25 + 6.4 + 3.89   = _____

6. 4.0086 + 0.034 + 0.6 + 0.05   = _____

7. 43.766 + 9.33 + 17 + 206   = _____

8.
```
  354.2312
  +5.1092
```

9.
```
  224.0021
  +6.4444
```

10.
```
  5223.2312
   +65.3217
```

To subtract decimal numbers, first put the numbers in a vertical column, aligning the decimal points. Then subtract each column, starting on the right and working left. If the digit being subtracted in a column is larger than the digit above it, "borrow" a digit from the next column to the left. Place the decimal point in the answer directly below the decimal points in the terms.

EXAMPLE: Subtract 1.203 from 32.55

Step 1:

$$
\begin{array}{r}
32.255 \\
\underline{1.203} \\
2
\end{array}
$$

Step 2:

$$
\begin{array}{r}
32.255 \\
\underline{1.203} \\
52
\end{array}
$$

Step 3:

$$
\begin{array}{r}
32.255 \\
\underline{1.203} \\
.052
\end{array}
$$

Step 4:

$$
\begin{array}{r}
32.255 \\
\underline{1.203} \\
1.052
\end{array}
$$

Step 5:

$$
\begin{array}{r}
32.255 \\
\underline{1.203} \\
31.052
\end{array}
$$

PRACTICE PROBLEMS -- SUBTRACTING DECIMALS

Subtract the following decimal fractions:

1. 3.2 - 3.36 = _____

2. 14.33 - 5.7 = _____

3. 25.5 - 11.21 = _____

4. 1.0026 - 0.03 = _____

5. 75.013 - 3.048 = _____

6. 30.313 - 15.721 = _____

7.
$$
\begin{array}{r}
254.2311 \\
\underline{-3.1082}
\end{array}
$$

8.
$$
\begin{array}{r}
24.0032 \\
\underline{-3.3333}
\end{array}
$$

9.
$$
\begin{array}{r}
523.2309 \\
\underline{-63.3467}
\end{array}
$$

10.
$$
\begin{array}{r}
372.21 \\
\underline{-3.89}
\end{array}
$$

DECIMAL NUMBERS
(cont'd)

MULTIPLYING DECIMALS

To multiply decimal numbers, first multiply the numbers just as if they were whole numbers. Then line up the numbers on the right (do not align the decimal points). Next, starting on the right, multiply each digit in the top number by each digit in the bottom number. Then add the products.

Finally, place the decimal point in the answer by starting at the right and moving the point the number of places equal to the sum of the decimal places in both numbers that were multiplied together.

EXAMPLE: Multiply 47.2 by 5.5

```
        47.2    (has 1 decimal place)
    x    5.5    (has 1 decimal place)
       2360
       2360
     259.60    (has 2 decimal places)
```

EXAMPLE: Find the product (9.683)(6.1)

```
       9.683    (has 3 decimal places)
    x    6.1    (has 1 decimal place)
       9683
      58098
     59.0663   (has 3 + 1 = 4 decimal places)
```

PRACTICE PROBLEMS -- MULTIPLYING DECIMALS

Multiply the following decimals:

1. (0.5)(0.7)   =   _____

2. (0.4)(0.8)   =   _____

3. (0.3)(0.3)   =   _____

4. (0.5)(0.3)   =   _____

5. 6(3.7)   =   _____

6. 5.3(0.03)   =   _____

7. 7.2(0.02)   =   _____

8. 0.22(0.12)   =   _____

9.   25.24
     x 23.02

10. 123.444
      x 3.1

SIGNIFICANT FIGURES

SIGNIFICANT FIGURES

In pharmacy, we usually use a calculator to perform our calculations. Calculators are useful because they help us to avoid mathematical errors. We use decimal fractions when we use calculators.

In pharmacy, we also often perform calculations using measured amounts (for example, we may need to measure 80 mL of water to prepare an oral suspension). The actual value that we can use in our calculations that contain measured amounts depends on the sensitivity of the measuring device. When we multiply and divide decimal fractions using calculators, we must be careful to *include only the significant figures in our calculations* and answers. That is to say, we must be careful to keep in mind the sensitivity of the measuring device that is used when we perform the calculations.

A significant figure (or significant digit) is one that is actually measured using the measuring device. For instance, in the example above, if the sensitivity of the graduate used to measure the water measures to the nearest mL, the measurement should be expressed as 80 mL and not 80.0 mL. Numbers that are not measured (for example 30 capsules) are not affected by the sensitivity of a measuring device, and therefore are not subject to the rules of significant figures. When a calculation (addition, subtraction, multiplication, etc.) involves several measurements, and each measurement has a different number of significant digits, the final answer should have the same number of significant figures as the measured term that has the least number of significant figures. Also, if a calculation contains both numbers that are measured and numbers that are not measured, only the numbers that are measured should be considered when determining the number of significant figures for the answer.

There are four rules for assigning significant figures:

1. Digits other than zero are always significant.

2. Final zeros after a decimal point are always significant.

3. Zeros between two other significant digits are always significant.

4. Zeros used only to space the decimal are never significant.

EXAMPLE

1.20 gm of hydrocortisone powder are needed to compound a prescription. How many significant figures are in this measured amount?

Since final zeros after a decimal point are always significant, the number of significant figures is 3.

MEASUREMENT

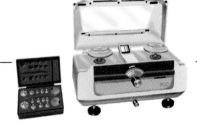

There are different systems of measurement used in pharmacy: metric, English, apothecary, and avoirdupois.

The metric system is the primary system used. Within these systems there are different measurements for weight, volume, and length, as well as for liquids and solids. It is necessary to know how to convert one type of measurement to another. There are also different measurement systems for temperature.

METRIC SYSTEM

The major system of weights and measures used in medicine is the metric system. It was developed in France in the late 18th century and is based on a decimal system. That is, **different measurement units are related by measures of ten.** Technicians need to know metric measures for both liquids and solids.

Liquids

Liquids (including lotions) are measured by **volume.** The most widely used metric volume measurements are liters or milliliters.

Unit	Symbol	Liquid Conversions		
liter	L	1 L	= 10 dl	= 1000 ml
deciliter	dl	1 dl	= 0.1 L	= 100 ml
milliliter	ml	1 ml	= 0.001 L	= 0.01 dl

Note: deciliters are rarely used in pharmacy, but are included here for reference and to illustrate the decimal relationship of these measures.

Solids

Solids (pills, granules, ointments, etc.) are measured by **weight.**

Unit	Symbol	Solid Conversions		
kilogram	kg	1 kg	= 1,000 g	
gram	g	1 g	= 0.001 kg	= 1000 mg
milligram	mg	1 mg	= 0.001 g	= 1000 mcg
microgram	mcg or μg	1 mcg	= 0.001 mg	= 0.000001 g

 Milliliters are sometimes referred to as *cubic centimeters (cc)*. They are not precisely the same but are quite close and are sometimes used interchangeably. Milliliter is the preferred usage for pharmacy.

℞ *To convert milligrams g to grams, move the decimal 3 places to the left (1 mg = 0.001 g).*

AVOIRDUPOIS SYSTEM

The Avoirdupois system is the system of weight (ounces and pounds) that we commonly use. However, one Avoirdupois unit used in pharmacy is rarely used elsewhere. It is the **grain.**

Unit	Symbol	Conversions		
pound	lb	1 lb	=	16 oz
ounce	oz	1 oz	=	437.5 gr
grain	gr	1 gr	=	64.8 mg

THE GRAIN

The grain is the same weight in several different measurement systems: Apothecary, Avoirdupois, and Troy. It is said to have been established as a unit of weight in 1266 by King Henry III of England when he required the English penny to weigh the equivalent of 32 dried grains of wheat. On the metric scale, one grain equals 64.8 milligrams. However, this is often rounded to 65 milligrams.

APOTHECARY SYSTEM

The Apothecary system is sometimes used in prescriptions, primarily with liquids. It includes the fluid ounce, pint, quart, and gallon. Although there are Apothecary weight units, they are generally not used, with the exception of the grain. The fluid ounce is a volume measure and is different than the weight ounce. It is always indicated by "fl oz."

Unit	Symbol	Conversions		
gallon	gal	1 gal	=	4 qt
quart	qt	1 qt	=	2 pt
pint	pt	1 pt	=	16 fl oz
ounce	fl oz	1 fl oz	=	8 fl dr
fluid dram	fl dr	1 fl dr	=	60 min
minim	min or M_x			

Note: drams and minims are rarely used in pharmacy today, but are included here for reference.

conversions the change of one unit of measure into another so that both amounts are equal.

MEASUREMENT (cont'd)

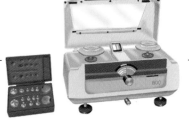

HOUSEHOLD UNITS

The teaspoon and tablespoon are common household measurement units that are regularly used in liquid prescriptions. Note that home teaspoons and tablespoons are not accurate for use in measuring medications.

Unit	Symbol	Conversions
teaspoon	tsp	1 tsp = 5 ml
tablespoon	tbsp	1 tbsp = 3 tsp = 15 ml
cup	cup	1 cup = 8 fl oz

TEMPERATURE

The **Centigrade** scale, which is also called **Celsius**, is used to measure temperature. The relationship of Centigrade (C) to Fahrenheit (F) is:

F temperature = **($1\frac{4}{5}$ times number of degrees C) + 32**

EXAMPLE   212°F = 100°C

because   a) $1\frac{4}{5}$ x 100 = 180

and   b) 180 + 32 = 212

C temperature = **$\frac{5}{9}$ x (number of degrees F - 32)**

EXAMPLE   100°C = 212°F

because $\frac{5}{9}$ x (212-32) = $\frac{5}{9}$ x 180 = 100

Note that the temperature of water freezing is 0°C and 32°F.

Some people find the following formula easier to remember and use:

9C = **5F - 160**

CONVERSIONS

Conversions are the change of one unit of measure into another so that both amounts are equal. Following are some commonly used unit conversions.

1 L	=	33.8 fl oz	1 lb	=	453.59 g
1 pt	=	473.167 ml	1 oz	=	28.35 g
1 fl oz	=	29.57 ml	1 g	=	15.43 gr
1 kg	=	2.2 lb	1 gr	=	64.8 mg

PRACTICE PROBLEMS — METRICS

Provide the abbreviation for these:

1. microgram _____
2. Liter _____
3. milliter _____
4. gram _____
5. milligram _____
6. kilogram _____

Convert these units to equivalents:

7. 1 kg = _____ g
8. 1 mg = _____ mcg
9. 2 gr = _____ mg
10. 1 L = _____ ml
11. 1 ml = _____ L
12. 1 mg = _____ g

PRACTICE PROBLEMS — CONVERSIONS

Convert these numbers using the conversions provided on the preceding pages as well as your knowledge of decimals:

1. 7 mg = _____ mcg
2. 3.2 g = _____ mg
3. 1 gr = _____ g
4. 2 tbsp = _____ ml
5. 0.3 L = _____ ml
6. 7 kg = _____ g

7. 1 oz = _____ gr
8. 0.5 kg = _____ lb
9. 10 ml = _____ tsp
10. 15 ml = _____ tbsp
11. 0°C = _____ °F
12. 250 ml = _____ L

CALCULATION SPACE

Answers for these problems can be found in the answer key beginning on page 347.

EQUATIONS & VARIABLES

EQUATIONS AND VARIABLES

In the calculations of Pharmacy related problems there is often an **unknown value** that needs to be determined. To solve the unknown value involves setting up a mathematical statement between the known amounts and the unknown. This statement is called an **equation**. The unknown fact in an equation is called a **variable**. The variable is often indicated by the letter, x.

> **An equation is a mathematical statement in which two terms are equal.**

Equations use the equal sign (=) to indicate equivalence. The following are equations:

$$1 = \tfrac{1}{2} + \tfrac{1}{2}$$
$$1 = \tfrac{1}{2} \times 2$$

EXAMPLE

You have a prescription for 120ml of Theophylline liquid and want to know how many fluid ounces is equal to 120ml. In this case, the number of ounces is the variable x that you want to determine. Since there are 29.57 ml in each fluid ounce, one way to state this problem mathematically is the following equation:

x fl oz = (total prescribed ml) ÷ (ml/fl oz conversion rate)

or

$$x \text{ fl oz} = \frac{\text{total prescribed ml}}{\text{ml/fl oz conversion rate}}$$

$$x \text{ fl oz} = \frac{120 \text{ ml}}{29.57 \text{ ml}}$$

x fl oz = 4 (approximately)

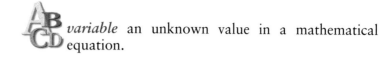 *variable* an unknown value in a mathematical equation.

EXAMPLE—FILLING A CAPSULE PRESCRIPTION

You have a prescription for amoxicillin 250mg, one capsule orally, three times a day for seven days. You want to know how many doses will be needed to fill this prescription. In this case doses needed is the unknown fact or variable that you are trying to solve for.

x (doses needed) = (capsules per dose) x (doses per day) x (days)

x = (1 capsule per dose) x (3 doses per day) x (7 days)

x = 21

You need 21 capsules of Amoxicillin 250 mg to fill the prescription.

EXAMPLE—INTRAVENOUS SOLUTION

You are preparing an Intravenous solution (IV) that requires the addition of Potassium Chloride (KCl). You have a vial of KCl containing a concentration of 20 mEq per 10ml. How many ml of this solution should you add to the IV if the IV should have a total of 45 mEq of KCl in it? This is made easier by first solving for the number of KCl per ml:

20 mEq divided by 10 ml = 2 mEq per ml

x (mls of KCl solution) = KCl needed ÷ KCl per ml

x = (45 mEq)÷ (2mEq)

x = 22.5

You need to add 22.5 ml of KCl solution to the IV.

RATIO & PROPORTION

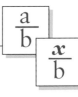

RATIO AND PROPORTION

Understanding ratios and proportions is important for pharmacy technicians. If you understand ratios and proportions, you will be able to perform most of the calculations necessary for your job.

Ratio

A ratio states **a relationship between two quantities**. The ratio of a to b can be stated as:

$$\frac{a}{b}$$

Proportion

Two equal ratios form a proportion: $\frac{a}{b} = \frac{c}{d}$

EXAMPLE

An example of this is the equation: $\frac{1}{2} = \frac{2}{4}$

$\frac{1}{2}$ and $\frac{2}{4}$ are equivalent ratios. 1 has the same relationship to 2 as 2 has to 4. Therefore, the equation is a proportion.

EXAMPLE

If one person has a bottle containing 5 tablets and another has 3 bottles each containing 5 tablets, one may have more tablets than the other but they both have the same proportion of tablets to bottles.

$$\frac{5 \text{ tablets}}{1 \text{ bottle}} = \frac{15 \text{ tablets}}{3 \text{ bottles}}$$

Each person has fives times as many tablets as bottles. The ratios are equivalent.

EXAMPLE

A solution of 5 g of a substance in 100 ml of water is equivalent to 50 g of the same substance in 1000 ml of water.

$$\frac{5 \text{ g}}{100 \text{ ml}} = \frac{50 \text{ g}}{1000 \text{ ml}}$$

Both numerators can be divided into their denominators twenty times. Therefore, the ratios are equivalent.

Solving Ratio and Proportion Problems

In a proportion equation, all four terms are related to each other and the relationship of each term to the others can be stated in different ways:

➤ $\dfrac{a}{b} = \dfrac{c}{d}$ *can be stated as* $\dfrac{b}{a} = \dfrac{d}{c}$

You can also state the equation for any one term by multiplying both sides of the equation by one of the other terms. For example:

➤ $b \times \dfrac{a}{b} = b \times \dfrac{c}{d}$ ➤ $\cancel{b} \times \dfrac{a}{\cancel{b}} = b \times \dfrac{c}{d}$

↳ *cancel out equal values*

➤ $a = \dfrac{bc}{d}$

These are also true: $b = \dfrac{ad}{c}$ $c = \dfrac{ad}{b}$ $d = \dfrac{bc}{a}$

Therefore, if three of the four terms in a proportion problem are known, an unknown fourth term (*x*) can also be calculated.

EXAMPLE

When you know the values of three of the four terms in a proportion equation, the unknown term is indicated by *x*, and the proportion equation can be written as:

$\dfrac{x}{b} = \dfrac{c}{d}$ ➡ *ratio you want = ratio you have*

Multiplying both sides of the equation by the value of b will then establish the relationship of the known terms to *x*.

$b \text{ times } \left(\dfrac{x}{b}\right) = b \text{ times } \left(\dfrac{c}{d}\right)$

$\cancel{b} \text{ times } \dfrac{x}{\cancel{b}} = b \text{ times } \dfrac{c}{d}$ ➡ $x = \dfrac{bc}{d}$

↳ *cancel out equal values*

You can then solve for the value of *x* by simple multiplication and division of the known values of b, c, and d.

$x = (b \text{ times } c) \text{ divided by } d$

RATIO & PROPORTION
(cont'd)

$$\frac{a}{b}$$

$$\frac{x}{b}$$

EXAMPLE

In one bottle there are four capsules. If every bottle contains the same number of capsules, how many capsules are in six bottles?

Steps

1. Define the variable and the correct ratios.

    a.   define the unknown variable ➡ x (total capsules)

    b.   establish the known ratio ➡ 4 capsules/1 bottle

    c.   establish the unknown ratio ➡ x capsules/6 bottles

2. Set up the proportion equation $\left(\frac{x}{b} = \frac{c}{d}\right)$.

$$\frac{x \text{ capsules}}{6 \text{ bottles}} = \frac{4 \text{ capsules}}{1 \text{ bottle}}$$

Note that the units must the same in both the numerator and denominator:

        numerator: capsules

        denominator: bottles

3. Establish the x equation.

$$6 \text{ bottles times } \frac{x \text{ capsules}}{6 \text{ bottles}} = 6 \text{ bottles times } \frac{4 \text{ capsules}}{1 \text{ bottle}}$$

$$6 \text{ bottles times } \frac{x \text{ capsules}}{6 \text{ bottles}} = 6 \text{ bottles times } \frac{4 \text{ capsules}}{1 \text{ bottle}}$$

➡ *cancel out equal values and units*

$$x \text{ capsules } = 6 \text{ times } 4 \text{ capsules}$$

4. Solve for x.

$$x \text{ capsules } = 24 \text{ capsules}$$

5. Express solution in correct units.

There are **24 capsules** in the six bottles.

1. Three of the four values must be known.

2. Numerators must have the same units.

3. Denominators must have the same units.

EXAMPLE—A PRESCRIPTION FOR TABLETS.

You receive a prescription for KTabs® one tablet BID x 30 days. How many tablets are needed to fill this prescription correctly?

Steps

1. Define the variable and correct ratios.

    a.   define the unknown variable ➡ x = total tablets needed

    b.   establish the known ratio ➡ 2 tablets / 1 day

    c.   establish the unknown ratio ➡ x tablets / 30 days

2. Set-up the proportion equation.

$$\frac{x \text{ tablets}}{30 \text{ days}} = \frac{2 \text{ tablets}}{1 \text{ day}}$$

3. Establish the x equation.

$$x \text{ tablets} = 30 \text{ days times } \frac{2 \text{ tablets}}{1 \text{ day}}$$

4. Solve for x.

$$x \text{ tablets} = 30 \cancel{\text{ days}} \text{ times } \frac{2 \text{ tablets}}{1 \cancel{\text{ day}}} = 60 \text{ tablets}$$

$$x \text{ tablets} = 60 \text{ tablets}$$

5. Express solution in correct units.

60 tablets of KTabs® are needed to fill the prescription.

RATIO & PROPORTION
(cont'd)

$$\frac{a}{b} \quad \frac{x}{b}$$

EXAMPLE—A LIQUID PRESCRIPTION

You receive a prescription for Amoxicillin 75 mg four times a day for ten days. You have available Amoxicillin 250 mg/5 ml 150 ml.

A. What is the correct individual dose?

1. Define the variable and correct ratios.

    a. define the unknown variable   ➡ x = ml per dose

    b. establish the known ratio   ➡   5 ml / 250 mg

    c. establish the unknown ratio   ➡ x ml / 75 mg

2. Set-up the proportion equation.

x ml / 75 mg = 5 ml / 250 mg

3. Establish the x equation

$$x \text{ ml} = 75 \text{ mg times } \frac{5 \text{ ml}}{250 \text{ mg}}$$

4. Solve.

$$x \text{ ml} = 75 \text{ \sout{mg} times } \frac{5 \text{ ml}}{250 \text{ \sout{mg}}} = \frac{375 \text{ ml}}{250} = 1.5 \text{ ml}$$

5. Express solution in correct units.

The dose is 1.5 ml of amoxicillin.

B. How many mls of amoxicillin do you need to last for ten days? A simple equation can determine this. Note that it is often useful to state the equation first in words, and then restate it in numbers. Using words to describe mathematical operations helps you to visualize and better understand the mathematics involved.

Word Equation:

amount needed = (dose amount) x (doses per day) x (number of days)

    Amoxicillin needed = 1.5 ml times 4 times 10 = 60 ml

C. Double check your answer.

$$1.5 \text{ ml of } \frac{250 \text{ mg}}{5 \text{ ml}} = 75 \text{ mg}$$

EXAMPLE—A MIXTURE DOSE

If a diarrhea mixture contains 3 ml of Paregoric in each 30 ml of mixture, how many ml of Paregoric would be contained in a teaspoonful dose of mixture?

conversion: 1 tsp = 5 ml

1. Define the variable and correct ratios.

    a. define the unknown variable   ➡ x ml of Paregoric

    b. establish the known ratio   ➡ 3 ml / 30 ml (mix)

    c. establish the unknown ratio   ➡ x ml/5 ml (mix)

2. Set-up the proportion equation

    x ml Paregoric/ 5 ml mix = 3 ml Paregoric/ 30 ml mix

3. Establish the x equation

$$x \text{ ml} = 5 \text{ ml mix times } \frac{3 \text{ ml Paregoric}}{30 \text{ ml mix}}$$

4. Solve.

$$x \text{ ml Paregoric} = 5 \text{ ml mix times } \frac{3 \text{ ml Paregoric}}{30 \text{ ml mix}} =$$

$$\frac{15 \text{ ml Paregoric}}{30 \text{ ml mix}} = 0.5 \text{ ml Paregoric}$$

5. Express solution in correct units.

There are 0.5 ml of paregoric in a teaspoon.

USING CALCULATORS

Though most of these examples can be solved without the use of a calculator, the use of calculators is essential in the correct computation of many dosage calculations. Their answers are precise and provided in decimals. Since it is relatively easy to make entry mistakes on a calculator, always recheck answers. Also, use judgment. If an answer doesn't appear to make sense, check it.

RATIO & PROPORTION
(cont'd)

$$\frac{a}{b} \quad \frac{x}{b}$$

EXAMPLE—IV FLOW RATE

In the pharmacy setting, you may be asked to provide information on **flow rate** or **rate of administration** for an IV solution. Flow rates are calculated using ratio and proportion equations. They are generally done in ml/hour, but for pumps used to dispense IV fluids to the patient, the calculation may need to be done in ml/min.

For example, if you have an order for KCl 10mEq and K Acetate 15 mEq in D5W 1000 ml to run at 80 ml/hour, you would determine the administration rate in ml/minute as follows:

1. Define the variable and correct ratios.

    a.   define the unknown variable ➡ x = ml

    b.   establish the known ratio ➡ 80 ml / 60 min

    c.   establish the unknown ratio ➡ x ml/ 1 min

2. Set-up the proportion equation

    x ml / 1 min = 80 ml / 60 min

3. Establish the x equation

    x ml   = 1 min times $\dfrac{80\ ml}{60\ min}$

4. Factor and solve.

    x ml   = 1 ~~min~~ times $\dfrac{80\ ml}{60\ \cancel{min}}$ = 1.33 ml

                         ➡ *80 divided by 60 = 1.33*

5. Express solution in correct units.

    The flow rate would be 1.33 ml/minute.

Note: IV Flow Rate calculations may involve *drops per ml* or *drops per minute* or involve calculating the amount of time before an IV bag will empty and require replacement. Using simple ratio and proportion equations will solve these problems.

PRACTICE PROBLEMS — RATIO AND PROPORTION

Use the space below the problem (and the rules you've learned from the preceding pages) to work out the answer.

1. A prescription calls for 100 mg of a drug that you have in a 250 mg/5 ml concentration. How many ml of the liquid do you need?

2. A prescription calls for 400 mg of a drug that you have in a 50 mg/ml concentration. How many ml of the liquid do you need?

3. A prescription calls for 10 mg of a drug that you have in a 2 mg/15 ml concentration. How many ml of the liquid do you need?

$$\frac{X\,mL}{1\,m} = \frac{1000}{480} \cdot \frac{1\,mol}{1} \qquad X\,mL/1\,min = \frac{1000\,mL}{480\,min}$$

4. KCl 10 mEq and K Acetate 15 mEq in D5W 1000 ml is ordered to be administered over 8 hours. What would the rate be in ml/min?

$$X/1\,mL = \frac{480\,min}{1}, \frac{1\,m}{1}$$

5. A prescription calls for 0.24 mg of a drug that you have in a 50 mcg/ml concentration. How many ml of the liquid do you need?

℞ *Answers for these problems can be found in the answer key beginning on page 347.*

PERCENTS & SOLUTIONS

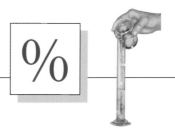

PERCENTS & SOLUTIONS

Percents are used to indicate the amount or **concentration** of something in a solution. Concentrations are indicated in terms of weight to volume or volume to volume.

Weight to Volume: grams per 100 milliliters   ➡   g/ml

Volume to Volume: milliliters per 100 milliliters ➡   ml/ml

EXAMPLE—IV SOLUTION

If there is 50% dextrose in a 1000 ml IV bag, how many grams of dextrose are there in the bag? You can solve this by developing a proportion equation. Since 50% dextrose means there are 50 grams of dextrose in 100 ml, the equation would be:

x g divided by 1000 ml   =   50 g divided by 100 ml

The x equation:

x g = 1000 ~~ml~~ times $\dfrac{50\ g}{100\ \cancel{ml}}$ = 10 times 50 g **= 500 g**

➡ *1000 divided by 100 = 10*

Answer: There are 500 grams of dextrose in the bag.

Another way to solve this is to **convert the percent to a decimal.** In a 50% solution, there are .5 g per ml:

50 g/100 ml = 0.5 g/ml

You can then multiply 0.5g by the total number of milliliters.

x = 0.5 g times 1000 = 500 g

Now how many ml will give you a 10 g of Dextrose?

The proportion equation:

x **ml/10 g = 100 ml /50 g**

The x equation:

x **ml = 10 ~~g~~ times $\dfrac{100\ ml}{50\ \cancel{g}}$ = $\dfrac{1000\ ml}{50}$ = 20 ml**

Answer: 20 ml of 50% solution contain 10 g of dextrose.

concentration the strength of a solution as measured by the weight-to-volume or volume-to-volume of the substance being measured.

Practice Problems — Percents

Convert the following fractions to percents:

   1. 60/100 = _____ %

   2. 80/100 = _____ %

   3. 12/100 = _____ %

Convert the following percents to decimals:

   4. 50% = _____

   5. 12.5% = _____

   6. 99% = _____

You have a 70% dextrose solution. How many grams in:

   7. 50 ml of solution

   8. 75 ml of solution

   9. 20 ml of solution

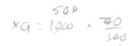

You have a 50% dextrose solution, how many ml will give you:

   10. 25 g of dextrose

   11. 35 g

   12. 10 g

13. You have a liquid that contains 12 mg /10 ml. What percent is this liquid? (Hint: To solve, you will need to convert mg to g per 100 ml using decimals.)

℞ *Answers for these problems can be found in the answer key beginning on page 347.*

PERCENTS & SOLUTIONS
(cont'd)

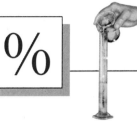

A PERCENT SOLUTION FORMULA

It is possible to set up a proportion equation specifically to convert concentrations for preparation of special intravenous solutions known as **hyperalimentation** or **total parenteral solutions TPNs.**

$$\frac{x \text{ volume needed}}{\text{want \%}} = \frac{\text{volume prescribed}}{\text{have \%}}$$

EXAMPLE—A DILUTION

The physician wants a 35% solution of dextrose 1000ml. You have a 50% solution of dextrose 1000ml. How will you make up what the physician wants ?

The terms for the formula are:

volume needed	➡ x ml
want %	➡ 35% dextrose
volume prescribed	➡ 1000 ml
have %	➡ 50% dextrose

The formula is:

x ml / 35% = 1000 ml / 50%

The x equation is:

$$x \text{ ml} = 35\% \text{ times } \frac{1000 \text{ ml}}{50\%} = 35 \text{ times } 20 \text{ ml} = \textbf{700 ml}$$

➡ *1000 divided by 50 = 20*

700 ml of dextrose 1000 ml will give you the 350 g of dextrose you will need in your solution. However, you will still need to add sterile water qsad until you have a total solution of 1000 ml as ordered by the physician. (qsad means quantity needed to make total volume).

Total Volume	1000 ml
Dextrose 50% Solution	-700 ml
Sterile Water (qsad)	300 ml

Answer: You need to add 300 ml of sterile water to 700 ml of 50% dextrose to create 1000 ml of 35% dextrose.

qsad the quantity needed to make a prescribed amount.
milliequivalent (mEq) the unit of measure for electrolytes in a solution.

In order to calculate mEq for an electrolyte, the atomic weight and valence of the electrolyte must first be known. The weight is then divided by the valence.

MILLIEQUIVALENTS: —mEq

Electrolyte solutions are often used in hospitals. Electrolytes are substances which conduct an electrical current and are found in the body's blood, tissue fluids, and cells. Salts are electrolytes and saline solutions are commonly used electrolyte solutions.

COMMON ELECTROLYTES:

NaCl	Sodium Chloride
MgSO4	Magnesium Sulfate
KCl	Potassium Chloride
K Acetate	Potassium Acetate
Ca Gluconate	Calcium Gluconate
Na Acetate	Sodium Acetate

The concentration of electrolytes is expressed as milliequivalents (mEq) per milliliter or milliequivalents per liter.

A **milliequivalent** is a specific unit of measurement that cannot be converted into the metric system. A 0.9% solution of one electrolyte will have a different mEq value than a 0.9% solution of another because mEq values are different for different electrolytes. Milliequivalents are based on each electrolyte's atomic weight and electron properties known as **valence**.

EXAMPLE

A solution calls for 5 mEq of sodium that you have in a 1.04 mEq / ml solution of NaCl. How many ml of it do you need?

x ml/ 5 mEq = 1 ml/1.04 mEq

$$x \text{ ml} = 5 \text{ mEq times } \frac{1 \text{ ml}}{1.04 \text{ mEq}} = \frac{5 \text{ ml}}{1.04} = 4.8 \text{ ml}$$

Answer: 4.8 ml of the solution is needed.

COMMON SALINE SOLUTIONS:

0.9% NaCl	Normal Saline
0.45% NaCl	1/2 Normal Saline
0.2% NaCl	1/4 Normal Saline
3% NaCl	Hypertonic Saline

PERCENTS & SOLUTIONS (cont'd)

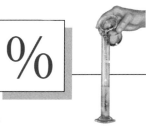

EXAMPLE—TOTAL PARENTERAL NUTRITION

A TPN order calls for the amounts on the left (including additives) to be made from the items on the right. The total volume is to be 1000 ml. How much of each ingredient do you need to prepare this TPN ?

TPN Order	On Hand
Aminosyn 4.25%	Aminosyn 8.5% 1000 ml
Dextrose 25%	Dextrose 70% 1000 ml

Additives:

KCl	20 mEq	KCl 2mEq / ml 10 ml
MVI	10 ml	MVI 10 ml
NaCl	24 mEq	NaCl 4.4mEq / ml 20 ml

Aminosyn

Using Percent Solutions Formula:

x ml / 4.25% = 1000 ml / 8.5%

x ml = 4.25% times $\dfrac{1000 \text{ ml}}{8.5\%}$ = 1000 ml times 0.5

➥ *4.25 divided by 8.5 = 0.5*

x ml = 500 ml

500 ml of aminosyn 8.5% is needed.

Dextrose

Using Percent Solutions Formula:

x ml/ 25% = 1000 ml / 70%

x ml = 25% times $\dfrac{1000 \text{ ml}}{70\%}$ = $\dfrac{25000 \text{ ml}}{70}$

x ml = 357.14 ml dextrose ➡ 357 ml

357 ml of dextrose 70% is needed.

Note: Generally, amounts less than 0.5 are rounded down and amounts greater than 0.5 are rounded up. However, some drugs may be rounded and others may not. You will need to know when you must be precise and when you may round for each drug.

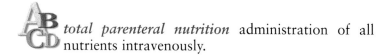 *total parenteral nutrition* administration of all nutrients intravenously.

KCl

Use a proportion equation:

$$x \text{ ml} / 20\text{mEq} = 1 \text{ ml}/ 2 \text{ mEq}$$

$$x \text{ ml} = 20 \text{ mEq times } \frac{1 \text{ ml}}{2 \text{mEq}} = 10 \text{ ml KCl}$$

10 ml KCl are needed.

MVI

Add the 10 ml MVI on hand.

NaCl

Use a proportion equation:

$$x \text{ ml} / 24 \text{ mEq} = 1 \text{ ml} / 4.4 \text{ mEq}$$

$$x \text{ ml} = 24 \text{ mEq times } \frac{1 \text{ ml}}{4.4 \text{ mEq}} = 5.45 \text{ ml}$$

5.45 ml of NaCl is needed.

Sterile Water

Add as needed (qsad) for a volume of 1000 ml.

Word Equation:

water needed = 1000 ml minus (other ingredients)

Other ingredients:

Aminosyn	500 ml
Dextrose	357 ml
KCl	10 ml
MVI	10 ml
NaCl	5.45 ml
total	882.45 ml

water needed = 1000 minus 882.45 = 117.55

117.55 ml sterile water is needed to fill the TPN order.

PERCENTS & SOLUTIONS
(cont'd)

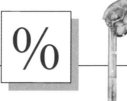

%

PERCENT SOLUTION FORMULA

$$\frac{x \text{ volume needed}}{\text{want \%}} = \frac{\text{volume prescribed}}{\text{have \%}}$$

PRACTICE PROBLEMS - TPN SOLUTIONS

A TPN order calls for the amounts on the left (including additives) to be made from the items on the right. The total volume is to be 250 ml. How much of each ingredient do you need to prepare this TPN ?

TPN Order	What you have
Aminosyn 2.5%	Aminosyn 8.5% 500 ml
Dextrose 7. 5%	Dextrose 50% 1000 ml

Additives:

KCl 4 mEq	KCl 2 mEq/ml 10 ml
Ca Gluconate 2 mEq	Ca Gluconate 4.4 mEq/ml 25 ml
Ped MVI 5 ml	Ped MVI 10 ml

Use the space to work out the answers.

1. **Aminosyn 8.5%**   Answer: _____ ml

2. **Dextrose 50%**   Answer:_____ ml

3. KCl 2 mEq/ml

Answer: _____ ml

4. Ca Gluconate 4.4 mEq/ml

Answer: _____ ml

5. Pediatric MVI 10 ml

Answer: _____ ml

6. Sterile Water (qs ad)

Answer: _____ ml

℞ *Answers for these problems can be found in the answer key beginning on page 347.*

CHILDREN'S DOSES

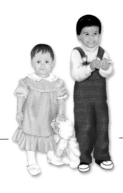

CALCULATION OF CHILDREN'S DOSES

The average doses in the U.S.P. (United States Pharmacopeia) and other drug reference sources are for adults. Doses for drugs that can be taken by a child are generally not given. When they are not, the adult dose needs to be lowered. One formula for this is:

CLARK'S RULE

$$\frac{\text{weight of child}}{150 \text{ lb}} \times \text{adult dose} = \text{dose for child}$$

150 lbs is considered an average weight for an adult. This is not a very precise way to calculate pediatric doses as there are many factors besides weight which may need to be taken into account: height, age, condition, etc. Another approach is based upon multiplying the adult dose by a ratio of the child's size to that of an average adult:

BODY SURFACE AREA FORMULA

$$\frac{\text{child bsa times adult dose}}{\text{average adult bsa}} = \text{child's dose}$$

The *body surface area* of a person is based on the person's height and weight. It is always given in square meters (m^2). 1.73 m^2 is commonly used as an average bsa for adults. A chart called a *nomogram* has been traditionally used to manually calculate bsa. Body surface area nomograms contain three columns of numbers: height, body surface, and weight. The bsa is identified by the intersection of a line drawn between the weight and height columns with the bsa column, which is in the middle. Now, bsa formulas are generally solved by computer. (There are a number that can be found on the Internet, for example.) For a comparison to the average bsa for adults (1.73 m^2), a bsa for a nine year old child that was 44" tall and weighing 50 lbs would be about .92 m^2.

Because of the many variables, however, conversion formulas for pediatric doses are not always appropriate and can lead to incorrect doses with some medications. **Although doses are generally given by the physician, pharmacy should always check children's doses to make sure they are appropriate by using a suitable drug information resource.** Children's doses are stated by kg of body weight (dose/kg). Since 1 kg = 2.2 lb, you can solve for the prescribed dose by using a proportion equation if you know the child's body weight. See the example at right.

body surface area a measure used for dosage that is calculated from the height and weight of a person and measured in square meters.

nomogram a chart showing relationships between measurements.

EXAMPLE—INFANT DOSE

An Antibiotic IV is prescribed for an infant. The dose is to be 15mg/kg twice a day. The baby weighs 12 lbs. How much drug is to be given for one dose? First you need to calculate the infant's weight in kilograms.

x kg / 12 lb = 1 kg / 2.2 lb

x kg = 12 lb times $\dfrac{1 \text{ kg}}{2.2 \text{ lb}} = \dfrac{12 \text{ kg}}{2.2} = 5.45$ kg

You can also easily solve this with a calculator:

➡ enter   12
➡ press   divide (/) key
➡ enter   2.2
➡ press   equal (=) key
➡ answer   5.45

You can solve the next part of this problem with a proportion equation or you can set up a simple word equation.

one dose = (amount of drug) times (number of kg of infant weight)

one dose = $\dfrac{15 \text{ mg}}{\text{kg}}$ times 5.45 kg

With a calculator:

➡ enter   15
➡ press   multiplication (*) key
➡ enter   5.45
➡ press   equal (=) key
➡ answer   81.75 mg

CALCULATIONS FOR BUSINESS

$

USUAL AND CUSTOMARY PRICE

The usual and customary price (U&C) is the lowest price charged if a patient pays cash, on that day, for that drug. Usual and customary prices are usually determined at the corporate level, although pharmacy prices are sometimes determined when the prescription is filled using a formula. Pharmacy computers are usually programmed to automatically calculate the usual and customary price when a prescription is filled.

> EXAMPLE:
>
> If prescription prices are determined using the following formula:
>
> average wholesale price (AWP) + professional fee = selling price of prescription
>
> and the professional fee is determined using the following chart:
>
> | AWP | Professional Fee |
> | --- | --- |
> | less than $20.00 | $4.00 |
> | $20.01 - $50.00 | $5.00 |
> | $50.01 and higher | $6.00 |
>
> and the AWP for 30 capsules of amoxicillin 250mg is $3.50, what will be the retail price of the prescription?
>
> Since the AWP for the prescription is less than $20.00, the professional fee is $4.00. Using the formula
>
> AWP + professional fee = selling price of prescription,
>
> $$\$3.50 + \$4.00 = \$7.50$$

Some pharmacies sell certain medications at a price lower than the acquisition cost. Therefore, the usual and customary price may be less than the average wholesale price (AWP) or less than the acquisition cost. Many third party plans reimburse the pharmacies based on the lowest amount: AWP, acquisition cost, or U&C, since the third parties do not want to pay more for a prescription than patient would pay by cash.

PRACTICE PROBLEMS -- USUAL AND CUSTOMARY

Calculate the retail price of the following prescriptions using the formula AWP + professional fee = retail price of prescription if the professional fee is determined using the chart in the example above:

1. Verapamil SR Tabs #30 AWP/100 $135.85   retail price _____

2. Glyburide 5 mg Tabs #30 AWP/1000 $480.15   retail price _____

3. Dexamethasone 4 mg Tabs #12 AWP/100 $62.50   retail price _____

4. Danazol 200 mg Caps #100 AWP/100 $322.38   retail price _____

5. Doxepin 150 mg Caps #30 AWP/100 $73.50   retail price _____

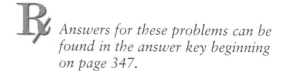

Answers for these problems can be found in the answer key beginning on page 347.

DISCOUNTS

Pharmacies sometimes give a 5 or 10% discount on the price of prescriptions to certain patients such as senior citizens that do not participate in third party programs. State pharmacy regulations or third party contractual agreements may prohibit discounting prescriptions that are covered by third party programs. Sometimes the discount is restricted to prescriptions purchased on certain days of the week.

EXAMPLE:

A senior citizen is paying for a prescription for amoxicillin 250 mg #30. The usual and customary price is $8.49; however this patient qualifies for a 10% discount. How much will the patient pay?

$$\$8.49 - 10\%(\$8.49) = \$8.49 - (0.1)(\$8.49) = \$8.49 - \$0.85$$
$$= \$7.64$$

PRACTICE PROBLEMS -- DISCOUNTS

Calculate how much the patient will pay for the following prescriptions if the patient qualifies for a 5% discount

1. Retail prescription price is $8.99   patient price after 5% discount _____

2. Retail prescription price is $18.41   patient price after 5% discount _____

3. Retail prescription price is $39.20   patient price after 5% discount _____

4. Retail prescription price is $99.90   patient price after 5% discount _____

5. Retail prescription price is $128.52   patient price after 5% discount _____

Calculate how much the patient will pay for the following prescriptions if the patient qualifies for a 10% discount

6. Retail prescription price is $8.99   patient price after 10% discount _____

7. Retail prescription price is $18.49   patient price after 10% discount _____

8. Retail prescription price is $39.30   patient price after 10% discount _____

9. Retail prescription price is $9.90   patient price after 10% discount _____

10. Retail prescription price is $180.55   patient price after 10% discount_____

CALCULATIONS FOR BUSINESS (cont'd)

$

GROSS PROFIT AND NET PROFIT

Gross Profit

The gross profit is the difference between the selling price and the acquisition cost. For cash prescriptions, the selling price is the usual and customary price for prescriptions paid by cash customers. To calculate gross profit, there is no consideration for any of the expenses associated with filling the prescription.

Gross profit = Selling price - acquisition cost

The gross profit can be expressed as a percent.

EXAMPLE:

A prescription for amoxicillin 250mg #30 has a usual and customary price of $8.49. The acquisition cost of amoxicillin 250mg #30 is $2.02. What is the gross profit?

Gross profit = Selling price - Acquisition cost

Gross profit = $8.49 - $2.02 = $6.47

Net Profit

The net profit is the difference between the selling price of the prescription and the sum of all the costs associated with filling the prescription. All the costs associated with filling the prescription include the cost of the medication, the cost of the container, the cost of the label, the cost of the bag, the cost of the labor to dispense the prescription, a portion of the rent, etc. For practical purposes, all the other costs can be grouped together and considered as a dispensing fee. Since the costs associated with operation of a pharmacy vary, the dispensing fee can vary.

Net profit = Selling price - Acquisition cost - Dispensing fee

or

Net profit = Gross profit - Dispensing fee

Net profit can also be expressed as a percent.

EXAMPLE:

A prescription for amoxicillin 250mg #30 has a usual and customary price of $8.49. The acquisition cost of amoxicillin 250mg #30 is $2.02. What is the net profit if the dispensing fee/professional fee is $5.50?

Net profit = Selling price - Acquisition cost - Dispensing fee

Net profit = $8.49 - $2.02 - $5.50 = $0.97

Answers for these problems can be found in the answer key beginning on page 347.

PRACTICE PROBLEMS -- GROSS PROFIT AND NET PROFIT

Use this table to determine the dispensing/professional fee

AWP	Professional Fee
less than $20.00	$4.00
$20.01 - $50.00	$5.00
$50.01 and higher	$6.00

and then calculate the gross profit and the net profit for the following prescriptions.

1. Zocor® 5 mg, 60 tablets

    acquisition cost = $85.47   AWP = $106.84   selling price = $109.93

    Gross profit = _____   **Net profit** = _____

2. Prilosec® 20 mg, 30 cap.

    acquisition cost = $99.20   AWP = $108.90   selling price = $116.38

    Gross profit = _____   **Net profit** = _____

3. Norvasc® 5 mg, 90 tablets

    acquisition cost = $97.92   AWP = $125.66   selling price = $117.82

    Gross profit = _____   **Net profit** = _____

4. Procardia® XL 30 mg, 100 tab.

    acquisition cost = $105.05   AWP = $131.31   selling price = $134.36

    Gross profit = _____   **Net profit** = _____

5. Vasotec® 10 mg, 100 tab.

    acquisition cost = $85.56   AWP = $102.94   selling price = $109.19

    Gross profit = _____   **Net profit** = _____

6. Relafen® 500 mg, 100 tab.

    acquisition cost = $88.88   AWP = $111.10   selling price = $120.27

    Gross profit = _____   **Net profit** = _____

7. Zoloft® 50 mg, 100 tab.

    acquisition cost = $172.44   AWP = $215.55   selling price = $226.50

    Gross profit = _____   **Net profit** = _____

8. Fosamax® 10 mg, 30 tablets

    acquisition cost = $50.91   AWP = $51.88   selling price = $57.62

    Gross profit = _____   **Net profit** = _____

9. Cardizem CD® 240 mg, 90 tablets

    acquisition cost = $154.10   AWP = $165.42   selling price = $179.69

    Gross profit = _____   **Net profit** = _____

10. Ticlid® 250 mg, 60 tablets

    acquisition cost = $99.44   AWP = $108.90   selling price = $122.07

    Gross profit = _____   **Net profit** = _____

REVIEW

ROMAN NUMERALS

When the second of two letters has a value equal to or larger than that of the first, their values are to be subtracted.

When the second of two letters has a value equal to or smaller than that of the first, their values are to be added.

CONDITIONS FOR USING RATIO AND PROPORTION

1. Three of the four values must be known.

2. Numerators must have the same units.

3. Denominators must have the same units.

STEPS FOR SOLVING PROPORTION PROBLEMS

1. Define the variable and correct ratios.

2. Set-up the proportion equation

3. Establish the x equation

4. Solve for x.

5. Express solution in correct units.

PERCENT SOLUTION FORMULA

$$\frac{x \text{ volume needed}}{\text{want \%}} = \frac{\text{volume prescribed}}{\text{have \%}}$$

CONVERSIONS

Liquid Metric

1 L	=	10 dl	=	1000 ml
1 dl	=	0.1 L	=	100 ml
1 ml	=	0.001 L	=	0.01 dl

Solid Metric

1 kg	=	1,000 g		
1 g	=	0.001 kg	=	1,000 mg
1 mg	=	0.001 g	=	1,000 mcg
1 mcg	=	0.001 mg		

Avoirdupois

1 lb	=	16 oz
1 oz	=	437.5 gr
1 gr	=	64.8 mg (.00648 g)

Apothecary

1 gal	=	4 qt
1 qt	=	2 pt
1 pt	=	16 fl oz
1 fl oz	=	8 fl dr
1 fl dr	=	60 m

Household

1 tsp	=	5 ml		
1 tbsp	=	3 tsp	=	15 ml
1 cup	=	8 fl oz		

Temperature

$9C = 5F - 160$

Conversions Between Systems

1 L	=	33.8 fl oz	1 lb	=	453.59 g
1 pt	=	473.167 ml	1 oz	=	28.35 g
1 fl oz	=	29.57 ml	1 g	=	15.43 gr
1 kg	=	2.2 lb	1 gr	=	64.8 mg

REVIEW

SELF TEST

CONVERT THE FOLLOWING.

the answer key begins on page 347

1. 500 g = _____ mg
2. 10 kg = _____ g
3. 250 ml = _____ L
4. 325 mg = _____ g
5. 120 mcg = _____ mg

6. 102 kg = _____ lb
7. 3.56 kg = _____ g
8. 473ml = _____ L
9. 145 lb = _____ kg
10. 30 kg = _____ mg

SOLVE THE FOLLOWING PROBLEMS IN THE SPACE PROVIDED.

1. Oral Polio Virus Vaccine (Poliovax®) should be stored in a temperature not to exceed 46 degrees Fahrenheit. What is this temperature in Centigrade?

2. A prescription reads for Erythromycin 150 mg every six hours for ten days. You have on hand Erythromycin 250 mg/5 ml. How much Erythromycin is needed for one dose?

3. You have an IV that needs $MgSO_4$ (Magnesium Sulfate) 10 mEq. You have on hand a bottle of $MgSO_4$ 4 mEq/ml. How much $MgSO_4$ do you need to inject into this IV bag?

4. You have an order for 20% Dextrose 500 ml. You have a 1000 ml bag of Dextrose 70%. How much of the Dextrose 70% do you need to use to make Dextrose 20% 500 ml? How much sterile water do you need?

R Answers for these problems can be found at the end of the text.

REVIEW

the answer key begins on page 347

CHOOSE THE CORRECT ANSWER:

1. A solution of Halperidol (Haldol®) contains 2 mg/ml of active ingredient. How many grams would be in 473 ml of this solution?

   a. 9.46 grams
   b. 0.946 grams
   c. 0.0946 grams
   d. 0.00946 grams

2 The physician orders Ferrous Sulfate 500 mg po qd x 30 days. You have on the shelf Ferrous Sulfate 220 mg/5 ml 473 ml. How many ml is required for one dose?

   a. 5.4 ml
   b. 8.4 ml
   c. 11.4 ml
   d. 13.4 ml

3. Using the information from the previous problem, approximately how many ml are required to completely fill this prescription?

   a. 162 ml
   b. 252 ml
   c. 342 ml
   d. 402 ml

4. The infusion rate of an IV is over twelve hours. The total volume is 800 ml. What would the infusion rate be in ml per minute?

   a. 66.6 ml / minute
   b. 6.6 ml / minute
   c. 0.6 ml / minute
   d. none of the above

5. You have a 70% solution of Dextrose 1000 ml. How many Kg of Dextrose is in 400 ml of this solution?

   a. 280 kg
   b. 28 kg
   c. 2.8 kg
   d. 0.28 kg

6. You receive an order for Vancomycin (Vancocin®) 10 mg/kg 500 ml to be infused over 90 minutes. The patient is five foot eleven inches tall and weighs 165 lb. What dose is needed for this patient?

   a. 750 mg
   b. 500 mg
   c. 250 mg
   d. 125 mg

7. The doctor orders Codeine gr $\frac{1}{4}$. How many milligrams is this equivalent to?

   a. 15 mg
   b. 30 mg
   c. 60 mg
   d. none of the above

8. You receive a prescription for Metronidazole (Flagyl®) 250 mg/5 ml po qid 240 ml. You find that you will have to compound this using 500 mg tablets. How many tablets will be needed to fill this order completely?

   a. 22 tablets
   b. 24 tablets
   c. 42 tablets
   d. 48 tablets

9. You are asked by the Pharmacist to add 45 mEq of Ca Gluconate in an IV bag of D5%W 1000 ml. You have a concentrated vial of Ca Gluconate 4.4 mEq/ml 50 ml. How many ml of this concentrated vial needs to be added to the IV bag?

   a. 1.2 ml
   b. 10.2 ml
   c. 0.12 ml
   d. 2.4 ml

ROUTES & FORMULATIONS

he way in which the body absorbs and distributes drugs varies with the route of administration.

Drugs are contained in products called **formulations**. There are many drug formulations and many different **routes** to administer them.

Routes of administration are classified as enteral or parenteral.

Enteral refers to anything involving the **alimentary tract**, i.e., from the mouth to the rectum. This tract is involved with digesting foods, absorbing nutrients, and eliminating unabsorbed wastes. There are four enteral routes of administration: oral, sublingual, buccal, and rectal.

Any route other than oral, sublingual, buccal, and rectal is considered a parenteral administration route.

The term **parenteral** means next to, or beside the enteral. It refers to any sites that are outside of or beside the alimentary tract.

For each route of administration, there are various formulations used to deliver the drug via that route.

Different dosage forms affect onset times, duration of action, or concentrations of a drug in the body. Some drugs are formulated in more than one dosage form with each form producing different characteristics in these areas. A consideration for selecting a particular route of administration or dosage form is the type of effect desired. A **local effect** occurs when the drug activity is at the site of administration (e.g., eyes, ears, nose, skin). A **systemic effect** occurs when the drug is introduced into the circulatory system by any route of administration and carried by the blood to the site of activity.

The prefix *intra* means into; so *intravenous* means into the venous (circulatory) system; *intraocular* means into the eye; and so forth. Other less commonly used parenteral routes include *intraarterial* (artery), *intracardiac* (heart), *intraspinal* (spinal cord), *intraosseous* (bone); *intraarticular* (joint), and *intrarespiratory* (lung); *intrathecal* (space under the arachnoid membrane of the brain or spinal chord).

FORMULATIONS

Enteral Route	Dosage Form
Oral	Tablets
	Capsules
	Bulk powders
	Solutions
	Suspensions
	Elixirs
	Syrups
Buccal	Tablets
	Solutions
Sublingual	Tablets
Rectal	Solutions
	Ointments
	Suppositories

Parenteral Route	Dosage Form
Intraocular	Solutions
	Suspensions
	Ointments
	Inserts
	Contact lenses
Intranasal	Solutions
	Suspensions
	Sprays
	Aerosols
	Inhalers
	Powders
Inhalation	Solutions
	Aerosols
	Powders
Intravenous	Solutions
Intramuscular	Suspensions
Intradermal	Emulsions
Dermal	Solutions
	Tinctures
	Collodions
	Liniments
	Suspensions
	Ointments
	Creams
	Gels

ROUTES

Enteral Routes are in red. Parenteral routes are in blue.
The term is followed by the organ(s) of absorption.

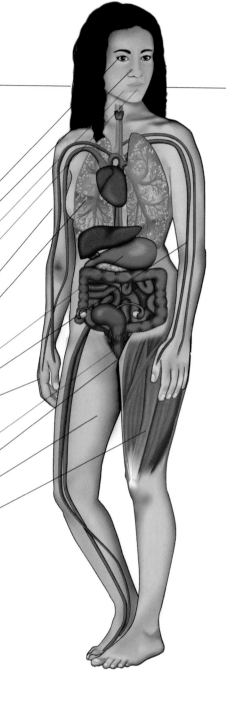

Intraocular	Eye
Intranasal	Nose
Buccal	Inside the cheek
Sublingual	Under the tongue
Dermal	Through or on the skin*
Inhalation	Lungs
Oral	Stomach and intestine
Intravenous	Venous circulatory system
Intradermal	Dermal layer of the skin*
Rectal	Rectum
Vaginal	Vagina
Subcutaneous	Subcutaneous layer of the skin*
Intramuscular	Muscle*

this route has various administration sites.

Parenteral Route	Dosage Form
Dermal (cont'd)	Lotions
	Pastes
	Plasters
	Powders
	Aerosols
	Transdermal patches
Subcutaneous	Solutions
	Suspensions
	Emulsions
	Implants
Vaginal	Solutions
	Ointments
	Creams

Parenteral Route	Dosage Form
Vaginal (cont'd)	Aerosol foams
	Powders
	Suppositories
	Tablets
	IUDs

ORAL FORMULATIONS

Oral administration is the most frequently used route of administration.

Oral dosage forms are easy to use, carry, and administer. The term used to specify oral administration is **peroral** or **PO** (per os). This indicates that the dosage form is to be swallowed and that absorption will occur primarily in the stomach and the intestine.

When formulations are orally administered, they enter the stomach, which is very acidic.

The stomach has a **pH** around 1-2. Certain drugs cannot be taken orally because they are degraded (chemically changed to a less effective form) or destroyed by stomach acid and intestinal enzymes. Additionally, the absorption of many drugs is affected by the presence of food in the stomach.

Drugs administered in liquid dosage forms generally reach the circulatory system faster than drugs formulated in solid dosage forms.

This is because the processes of **disintegration** and **dissolution** are not required. Oral liquids include solutions, suspensions, syrups, and elixirs. Solid oral dosage forms include tablets, capsules, and bulk powders.

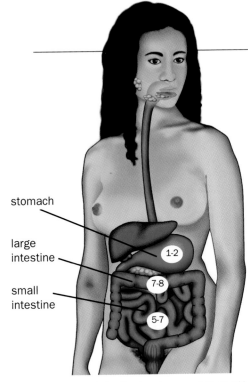

gastrointestinal organs and their pH

Gastrointestinal Action

The disintegration and dissolution of tablets, capsules, and powders generally begins in the stomach, but will continue to occur when the stomach content empties into the intestine. **Enteric coated** tablets are used when the drug can be degraded by the stomach acid. The enteric coating will not let the tablet disintegrate until it reaches the higher pHs of the intestine.

pH the pH scale measures the *acidity* or the opposite *(alkalinity)* of a substance. 7 is the neutral midpoint of the scale, values below which represent increasing acidity, and above which represent increasing alkalinity.

R Most oral dosage forms are intended for systemic effect, but not all. For example, antacids have a local effect confined to the gastrointestinal tract.

Inactive Ingredients

Oral formulations contain various ingredients beside the active drug. These include binders, lubricants, fillers, diluents, and disintegrants. They are added to help in the manufacture of the formulation and to help it disintegrate and dissolve when administered. A sample breakdown of ingredients is illustrated at right. (Note, however, that the breakdown for each formulation is different.)

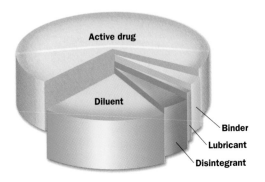

disintegration the breaking apart of a tablet into smaller pieces.

dissolution when the smaller pieces of a disintegrated tablet dissolve in solution.

SOLID FORMULATIONS

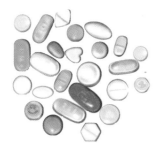

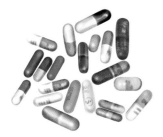

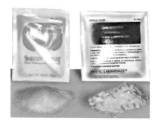

Tablets are hard formulations in which the drug and other ingredients are machine compressed under high pressure into a shape. Tablets vary in size, weight, hardness, thickness, and disintegration and dissolution characteristics depending upon their intended use. Most tablets are manufactured for oral use, and many are coated to give an identifying color or logo on the formulation. Sugar-coated tablets are coated with a sweet glaze. Film-coated tablets are coated with a non-sweet coating. Multiple compressed tablets contain one drug in an inner layer and another drug (or the same drug) compressed at a lower pressure over it as an outer layer. Repeat-action tablets initially release one dose of the drug and then release a second dose sometime later. Other popular tablets are chewable and effervescent.

Capsules contain the drug and the other ingredients packaged in a gelatin shell. There are several capsule sizes. The capsule size used in any formulation is based on the amount of material to be placed inside the capsule. The gelatin shell dissolves in the stomach and releases the contents of the capsule. The freed contents must still undergo disintegration and dissolution before the drug is absorbed into the circulatory system. There are some capsule formulations that contain liquid instead of powders inside the gelatin shell; these are called "soft" or "soft-gel" capsules. The active drug is already dissolved in the liquid.

Bulk powders (e.g., Goody's BC powders) contain the active drug in a small powder paper or foil envelope. The patient empties the envelope into a glass of water or juice and drinks the contents. Most of the drug and ingredients dissolve in the water before the patient takes it.

MODIFIED RELEASE FORMULATIONS

Several oral formulations release the drug so that a longer duration of action is achieved compared to a conventional tablet, capsule, or powder. These are called **modified release** products. A repeat action tablet is one example of this kind of formulation. The primary goal of these products is to reduce the number of doses a patient needs to take during a day (i.e., reduce the frequency of dosing). Some modified release products also control the blood concentrations of the drug better than conventional dosage forms.

Through the years, many terms have been used to identify these kinds of products. Some of these include sustained release (SR), sustained action (SA), extended release (ER or XR) prolonged action (PA), controlled release or continuous release (CR), time release (TR), and long acting (LA).

ORAL FORMULATIONS (cont'd)

LIQUID FORMULATIONS

Solutions

A **solution** is a clear liquid (not necessarily color-less) made up of one or more substances dissolved in a solvent. A **solvent** is a liquid that can dissolve another substance to form a solution. **Aqueous solutions** are the most common of the oral solutions. Aqueous means that water was used as the solvent. Although water is the most common solvent for oral solutions, alcohol, glycerin, propylene glycol (or combinations of these) can be used.

Syrups are concentrated or nearly saturated solutions of sucrose (i.e., sugar) in water. They are more viscous (thicker) than water, and contain less than 10% alcohol. Syrups containing flavoring agents are known as flavoring syrups (e.g., Wild Cherry Syrup), and medicinal syrups are those which contain drugs (e.g., Guaifenesin Syrup).

Nonaqueous solutions are those solutions which contain solvents other than water, either alone or in addition to water. Only a few nonaqueous solvents such as glycerin, alcohol, and propylene glycol can be used in oral solutions.

Elixirs are clear, sweetened, hydroalcoholic liquids intended for oral use. They can contain either alcohol soluble or water soluble drugs. Elixirs are usually less sweet and less viscous than syrups and are generally less effective in masking taste. Their alcohol content ranges from 5 - 40% (10 - 80 proof), though a few commercial elixirs contain no alcohol.

Spirits or essences are alcoholic or hydroalcoholic solutions of volatile substances (usually volatile oils) with alcohol contents ranging from 62 - 85% (124 - 170 proof). They are most frequently used as flavoring agents (e.g., Peppermint Spirit) but some spirits are used for their medicinal effect.

Tinctures are alcoholic or hydroalcoholic solutions of nonvolatile substances. Tinctures of potent drugs have 10 grams of the drug in each 100 ml of tincture; they are called 10% tinctures. Tincture of nonpotent tinctures generally have 20 grams of the drug per 100 ml of tincture.

Suspensions

Suspensions are formulations in which the drug does not completely dissolve in the liquid. The drug particles are suspended in the liquid. Since they are intended for oral administration, suspensions are sweetened and flavored.

The primary concern in formulating suspensions is that they tend to settle over time leading to a lack of dose uniformity. A well formulated suspension will remain suspended or settle very slowly, and can be easily redispersed with shaking.

Advantages of Solutions	**Disadvantages of Solutions**
➥ Completely homogenous doses	➥ Drugs and chemical are less stable in solutions than in dry forms
➥ Immediately available for absorption	➥ Some drugs are not soluble in solvents that are acceptable for therapeutic use
➥ For patients who cannot swallow tablets or capsules	➥ May require special additives or techniques to mask objectionable taste
➥ Doses can be easily adjusted	➥ More difficult to handle, transport, and store because of bulk and weight
	➥ Solutions in bulk containers require dosage measurement devices

Emulsions

It is well known that "oil and water don't mix." Yet, some formulations contain both aqueous and oleaginous (oil-based) components. These two non-mixable components can be formulated into a mix when an emulsifying agent (emulsifier) is used. Emulsifiers enable one of the components to be dispensed in the other in the form of tiny droplets or globules. If the oleaginous component is present as droplets, the emulsion is called an oil-in-water (o/w) emulsion. If the aqueous component is present as droplets, the emulsion is called a water-in-oil (w/o) emulsion.

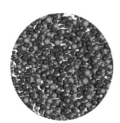

droplets in
an emulsion

Emulsions are used in many routes of administration. Oral administration can be used, but patients generally object to the oily feel of emulsions in the mouth. But some times, emulsions are the formulation of choice to mask the taste of a very bitter drug or when the oral solubility or bioavailability of a drug is to be dramatically increased. More typically, emulsions are used for topical administration as creams, lotions, or ointment bases.

Emulsions are physically unstable and tend to separate into two distinct phases over time. **Creaming** occurs when dispersed droplets merge and rise to the top or fall to the bottom of the emulsion. A creamed emulsion can be easily redispersed by shaking. **Coalescence** (breaking or cracking) is the irreversible separation of the dispersed phase.

Gels

Gels are made using substances called **gelling agents** that increase the viscosity (or thickness) of the medium in which they are placed.

There are many gelling agents. Some of the common ones are acacia, alginic acid, Carbopols® (now known as carbomers), gelatin, methylcellulose, tragacanth, and xanthan gum. Though each gelling agent has some unique properties, there are some generalizations that can be made.

➡ Most gelling agents require 12 - 24 hours to reach maximum viscosity and clarity.

➡ Gelling agents are used in concentrations of 0.5% up to 10% depending on the agent.

➡ It is easier to add the active drug before the gel is formed if the drug doesn't interfere with the gel formation.

➡ Only Carbopol® 934P, methylcellulose, hydroxypropylmethylcellulose, and sodium carboxymethylcellulose are recommended for oral administration.

Advantages of Suspensions	Disadvantages of Suspensions
➡ Can orally administer drugs that are insoluble in acceptable solvents	➡ Tend to settle over time leading to a lack of dose uniformity
➡ Can be taken or administered to patients who cannot swallow tablets or capsules	➡ Unpleasant oral texture
➡ Masks objectionable taste of some drugs	
➡ Drugs are chemically more stable than in solution	

SUBLINGUAL & BUCCAL

The mouth is the route of administration for certain drugs where a rapid action is desired.

Formulations used in the mouth are generally fast dissolving uncoated tablets which contain highly **water soluble** drugs. These tablets are placed under the tongue (**sublingual** administration). When the drug is released from the tablet, it is quickly absorbed into the circulatory system since the membranes lining the mouth are very thin and there is an rich blood supply to the mouth.

Nitroglycerin is the best known example of a sublingual tablet formulation.

Nitroglycerin is sublingually administered since it is degraded in the stomach and intestine. Nitroglycerin is also available in a translingual aerosol that permits a patient to spray droplets of nitroglycerin under the tongue. There are also some steroid sex hormones that are sublingually administered.

Sublingual administration has certain limitations.

For various reasons (including the condition of the mouth, the patient, etc.), other routes of administration are considered more convenient for many drugs that would otherwise be candidates for sublingual administration. An additional consideration is that holding a drug in the mouth for almost any period of time is unpleasant since most drugs have a bitter taste.

The buccal cavity is also in the mouth and refers to the insides of the cheek.

Buccal tablets are placed in the pouch between the cheeks and the teeth to dissolve. Like the sublingual administration route, the buccal cavity allows for rapid absorption of drugs and bypasses first-pass metabolism in the liver.

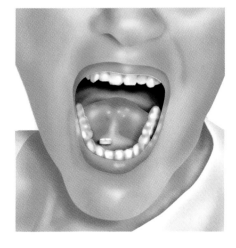

Using Sublingual Tablets

Sublingual tablets are highly water soluble, so patients should first take a sip of water to wet their mouth if it is dry.

The tablet is then placed far under the tongue and the mouth is closed and must remain closed until the tablet dissolves and is absorbed. No food or beverages should be placed in the mouth until the drug is fully absorbed.

 Like many medical terms, *sub, trans, and lingua* are Latin words. They mean under, across or over, and tongue respectively.

water soluble the property of a substance being able to dissolve in water.

RECTAL

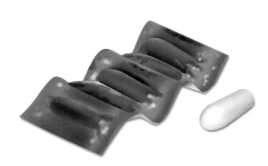

suppositories

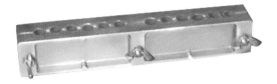

mold used for making suppositories

Enemas

Enemas create an urge to defecate due to the injection of fluid into the rectum. A cleansing enema injects water or a cleansing solution. A retention enema injects an oil that is held in the rectum to soften the stool. Frequent use of enemas is discouraged as it can can have significant adverse effects.

Drugs are administered via the rectum either for a local effect or to avoid degradation caused by oral administration.

Local effects may include the soothing of inflamed hemorrhoidal tissues or promoting laxation. Rectal administration for systemic activity is preferred when the drug is destroyed by stomach acid or intestinal enzymes, or if oral administration is unavailable (if the patient is vomiting, unconscious, or incapable of swallowing oral formulations). Rectal administration is used to achieve a variety of systemic effects including asthma control, antinausea, motion sickness, and anti-infective therapy.

The most common rectal administration forms are suppositories, solutions, and ointments.

Suppositories are semisolid dosage forms that dissolve or melt when inserted into the rectum. Suppositories are manufactured in a variety of shapes and are used in other routes of administration such as vaginal or urethral. Most rectal solutions are used as enemas or cleansing solutions. Ointments are intended to be spread around the anal opening and are most often used to treat inflamed hemorrhoidal tissues.

Rectal dosage forms have certain significant disadvantages.

They are not preferred by most patients. They are inconvenient. Moreover, rectal absorption of most drugs is frequently erratic and unpredictable.

 hemorrhoid painful swollen veins in the anal/rectal area, generally caused by strained bowel movements from hard stools.

PARENTERAL ROUTES

Parenteral routes of administration are used for a variety of reasons.

If an orally administered drug is poorly absorbed, or is degraded by stomach acid or intestinal enzymes, then a parenteral route may be indicated. Some parenteral routes are also preferred when a rapid drug response is desired, as in an emergency situation. Parenteral routes of administration are also useful when a patient is uncooperative, unconscious, or otherwise unable to take a drug by an enteral route.

There are disadvantages of formulations given by parenteral routes.

One is cost. Many parenterals are more expensive than enteral route formulations. Another is that many parenterals require skilled personnel to administer them. A third disadvantage is that once a parenteral drug is administered, it is most difficult to remove the dose if there is an adverse or toxic reaction. Finally, some types of parenteral administration have risks associated with invading the body with a needle (e.g., infection, thrombus, etc.).

Several parenteral routes require a needle and some type of propelling device (syringe, pump) to administer a drug.

These routes of administration are the intravenous, intramuscular, intradermal, and subcutaneous. These injectable routes have several characteristics in common. The formulations that can be used with injectables are limited to solutions, suspensions, and emulsions. Any other dosage formulation cannot pass through the syringe. These formulations must be **sterile** (bacteria-free) since they are placed in direct contact with the internal body fluids or tissues where infection can easily occur. The pH of the formulation must also be carefully maintained. This is commonly done by adding ingredients to the formulation to create a **buffer system**. A fourth characteristic is that limited volumes of formulation can be injected. Too great an injection volume can cause pain and cell death (**necrosis**).

PARENTERALS

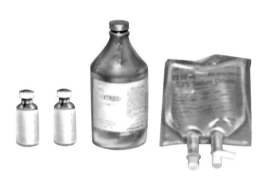

Which Parenteral?

Besides meaning any route of administration other than enteral, "parenteral" is commonly used to describe drugs administered through syringes. It is also used to describe the various bottles, vials, and bags used in preparing and delivering solutions for intravenous administration. It is possible to say that parenterals are prepared and parenterally administered at parenteral sites. As a result, extreme care must be taken when using the word parenteral so that the intended meaning is clear to all.

Route of Administration	Needle Gauge	Needle Length
Intravenous	16 - 20	1 - 1.5"
Intramuscular	19 - 22	1 - 1.5"
Subcutaneous	24 - 27	3/8 - 1"
Intradermal	25 - 26	3/8"

Syringe needle recommendations for injectable routes of administration *sterile* a sterile condition is one which is free of *all* microorganisms, both harmful and harmless.

buffer system ingredients in a formulation designed to control the pH.

necrosis the death of cells.

ROUTES

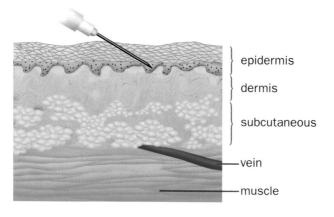

epidermis
dermis
subcutaneous
vein
muscle

Intradermal

Intradermal injections are administered into the top layer of the skin at a slight angle using short needles.

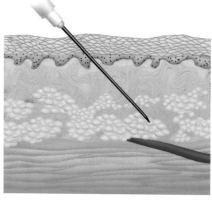

Subcutaneous

Subcutaneous injections are administered to the subcutaneous tissue of the skin using 3/8 inch to 1 inch needles.

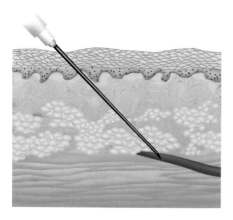

Intravenous

Intravenous injections are administered directly into veins.

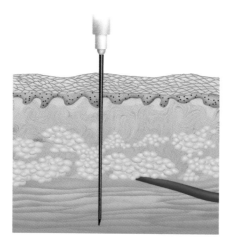

Intramuscular

Intramuscular injections are administered into muscle tissue using 1 to 1.5 inch needles.

INTRAVENOUS FORMULATIONS

Intravenous dosage forms are administered directly into a vein and therefore the circulating blood.

It takes about 20 seconds for intravenously administered drugs to circulate throughout the body. Solutions are the most common intravenously administered formulations. Most solutions are **aqueous**, but they may also have glycols, alcohols, or other nonaqueous solvents in them.

Injectable suspensions are difficult to formulate because they must possess suitable syringeability and injectability.

Syringeability refers to the ease with which the suspension can be drawn from a container into a syringe. **Injectability** refers to the properties of the suspension while being injected, such as flow evenness, freedom from clogging, etc.

Emulsions are formulations that contain both aqueous and nonaqueous (oil) components.

Fat emulsions in total parenteral nutrition (TPN) solutions are used to provide triglycerides, fatty acids, and calories for patients who cannot absorb them from the gastrointestinal tract.

Dry powder formulations are also manufactured for intravenous use, but they must be reconstituted with a suitable diluent to make a liquid formulation.

Powders are used for drugs which are not stable in liquid form. They are reconstituted just prior to use with a solvent called a **diluent**. The most common diluents are Sterile Water for Injection USP, Bacteriostatic Water for Injection USP, Sodium Chloride Injection USP, and Ringer's Injection USP. A drug product's package insert will indicate the appropriate diluent to use.

COMPLICATIONS

There are a number of complications that can occur from intravenous administration. Some have already been mentioned: sterility, excessive volumes, maintaining pH. Additional complications are thrombosis, phlebitis, air emboli, and particulate material.

➡ **Thrombus** (blood clot) formation can result from many factors: extremes in solution pH, particulate material, irritant properties of the drug, needle or catheter trauma, and selection of too small a vein for the volume of solution injected.

➡ **Phlebitis,** or inflammation of the vein, can be caused by the same factors that cause thrombosis.

➡ **Air emboli** occur when air is introduced into the vein. The human body is generally not harmed by very small amounts of air injected into the venous system, but *excess air injected into the veins can be fatal,* and it is necessary to remove all air bubbles from formulation and administration sets before use.

➡ **Particulate material** can include small pieces of glass that chip from the product's vial or rubber that comes from the rubber closure in the vials. Although great care is taken to eliminate the presence of particulate material, a final filter in the administration line just before entering the venous system is an important precaution.

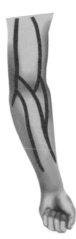
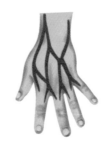
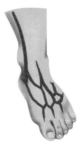

Intravenous Sites

Several sites on the body are used to intravenously administer drugs: the veins of the antecubital area (in front of the elbow), the back of the hand, and some of the larger veins in the foot. On some occasions, a vein must be exposed by a surgical cut.

aqueous water based.

diluent a solvent that dissolves a freeze-dried powder or dilutes a solution.

infusion the gradual injection of an intravenous solution (usually over more than 30 minutes) into a patient.

DEVICES

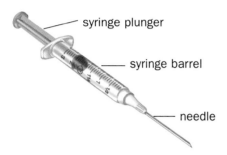

syringe plunger

syringe barrel

needle

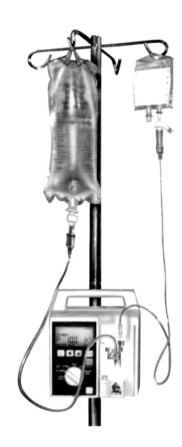

a solution bag and a minibag connected to an infusion pump

Syringes

Simple syringe and needle setups can be used to inject formulations over a short period of time (generally up to 2 minutes). There are a variety of syringe sizes and needle sizes; syringe size is selected based on the volume of the formulation to inject. The needle size is generally based on the route of administration being used (IV, IM, SC, ID). Some products come from the manufacturer with syringes and needles already assembled and prefilled.

Infusion

Infusion is the gradual intravenous injection of a volume of fluid into a patient. The infusion solution is generally a large volume (500 ml to 1,000 ml) of electrolyte solution such as D5W (dextrose 5% in water) or 1/2NS (one-half normal saline, 0.45% sodium chloride in water). It is intravenously infused at a rate of 2 ml to 3 ml per minute.

The solution bag has two ports: an administration set port and a medication port. The administration set provides the connection between the fluid bag and the needle in the patient. The administration set may also be connected to an infusion pump to control the flow rate. A simple syringe and needle may be used to inject a drug through the medication port into the solution bag. Sometimes a second small plastic bag containing the drug can be piggybacked onto the administration set or through an infusion pump.

Infusion Pumps

Administration devices that were dependent upon gravity have been shown to have a variable delivery rate. To ensure a constant delivery rate, controlled rate infusion pumps are used. Beginning in the late 1980s, patients were allowed to operate these pumps for occasional self administration of analgesics. The term patient controlled analgesia (PCA) was coined to describe this. PCA devices can provide on-demand dosing or a constant infusion rate of drug.

INTRAMUSCULAR

Drugs are often given by the intramuscular route to patients unable to take them by oral administration.

This route is also used for drugs that are poorly absorbed from the gastrointestinal tract. It is generally considered less hazardous and easier to use than the intravenous route. However, patients generally experience more pain from intramuscular administration than intravenous administration.

Intramuscular (IM) injections are made into the muscle fibers that are under the subcutaneous layer of the skin.

Needles used for the injections are generally 1 inch to 1.5 inches long, and are generally 19 to 22 gauge in size. The principal sites of injection are the **gluteal maximus** (buttocks), **deltoid** (upper arm), and **vastus lateralis** (thigh) muscles. When giving intramuscular injections into the gluteus maximus, one must be aware of the thickness of gluteal fat, particularly in female patients and an appropriate size needle must be used. Otherwise, the injection will not reach the muscle.

The site of injection should be as far as possible from major nerves and blood vessels to avoid nerve damage and accidental intravenous administration.

Injuries that can occur following intramuscular injection are abscesses, cysts, embolism, hematoma, skin sloughing, and scar formation. To avoid injury when a series of injections are given, the injection site is changed or rotated. Generally only limited volumes can be given by intramuscular injection: 2 ml in the deltoid and thigh muscles, and up to 5 ml in the gluteus maximus.

Intramuscular injections generally result in lower but longer lasting blood concentrations than with intravenous administration.

Part of the reason is that intramuscular injections have an absorption step which delays the time to peak concentrations. Also, when a formulation is injected, a **depot** forms inside the muscle tissue where the drug deposits. Absorption from this depot is dependent on many factors such as muscle exercise, particle size of the drug, and the salt form of the drug used in the formulation.

FORMULATIONS

Drugs for intramuscular injection are formulated as:

➡ solutions;

➡ suspensions;

➡ **colloids** in aqueous and oleaginous (oil-based) solvents;

➡ oil-in-water **emulsions;**

➡ water-in-oil emulsions.

Colloids and suspensions both contain insoluble particles in solution, but the particles in colloids are about 100 times smaller than those in suspensions.

Emulsions are mixtures of two liquids, generally oil and water, which are not miscible in each other. One liquid is spread through the other by mixing or shaking, and the use of a stabilizing substance called an **emulsifier** helps keep the mixture together.

Different salt forms of the drug may also be used to take advantage of a slower dissolution rate or a lower solubility.

All these things can be varied to achieve the desired absorption rate. In general, aqueous solutions have a faster absorption rate than oleagineous solutions. Both of these have a faster absorption rate than colloids or suspensions.

depot the area in the muscle where the formulation is injected during an intramuscular injection.

colloids particles up to a hundred times smaller than that those in suspensions that are, however, likewise suspended in a solution.

emulsions mixture of two liquids that do not dissolve into each other in which one liquid is spread through the other by mixing and using a stabilizer called an emulsifier.

INJECTION SITES

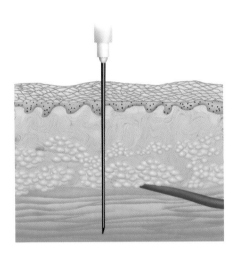

When administering intramuscular injections, it is necessary to adjust for any layers of body fat (especially in the gluteal area) and to use a size of needle that will penetrate to the muscle.

Z-Tract Injection

This is a technique used for medications that stain the skin (e.g., iron dextran injection) or irritate tissues (e.g., diazepam). The skin is pulled to one side prior to injection. Then the needle is inserted and the injection is performed. Once the needle is removed, the skin is released so that the injection points in the skin and muscle are no longer aligned. This keeps the drug from entering the subcutaneous tissue and staining or irritating the skin. A Z-track injection is generally 2 to 3 inches deep.

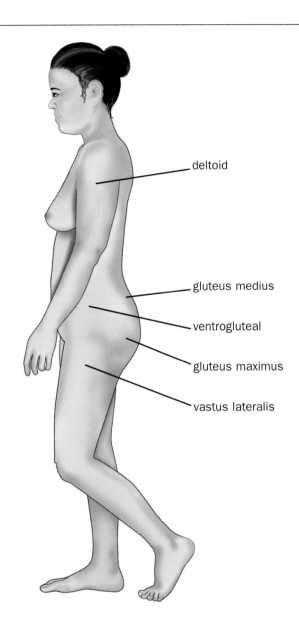

- deltoid
- gluteus medius
- ventrogluteal
- gluteus maximus
- vastus lateralis

 Intramuscular injections are generally more painful than intravenous injections.

SUBCUTANEOUS

The subcutaneous (SC, SQ) route is a versatile route of administration that can be used for both short term and very long term therapies. The injection of a drug or the implantation of a device beneath the surface of the skin is made in the loose tissues of the upper arm, the front of the thigh, and the lower portion of the abdomen. The upper back also can be used as a site of subcutaneous administration. The site of injection is usually rotated when injections are given frequently. The maximum amount of medication that can be subcutaneously injected is about 2 ml. Needles are generally 3/8 to 1 inch in length and 24 to 27 gauge.

Absorption of drugs from the subcutaneous tissue is influenced by the same factors that determine the rate of absorption from intramuscular sites.

However, there are fewer blood vessels in the subcutaneous tissue than in muscle, and absorption may be slower than with intramuscular administration. On the other hand, absorption after subcutaneous administration is generally more rapid and predictable than with oral administration. There are several ways to change the absorption rate. Using heat, or massaging the site have been found to increase absorption rates of many drugs. Also, there are various co-administered drugs which have been shown to increase absorption rate. By contrast, epinephrine decreases blood flow, which in turn decreases the absorption rate.

Many different solution and suspension formulations are given subcutaneously, but insulin is the most important drug routinely administered by this route.

Insulin comes in many different formulations each having a characteristic rate of absorption. The rate is controlled by the same factors used for intramuscular formulations: slowly soluble salt forms, suspensions versus solutions, differences in particle size, viscosity (thickness) of the injection form, etc.

In spite of the advantages of this route of administration, there are some precautions to observe.

Drugs which are irritating or in very **viscous** (thick) suspensions may produce serious adverse effects (including abscesses and necrosis) and be painful to the patient.

INJECTION SITES

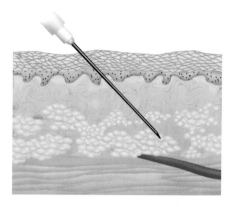

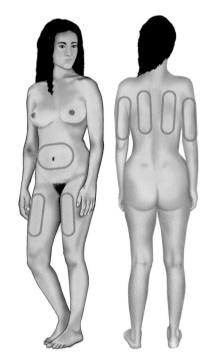

Subcutaneous injection sites are:

➥ lower abdomen;

➥ front of thigh;

➥ upper back;

➥ back of upper arm.

 viscosity the thickness of a liquid. A measure of a liquid's resistance to flow.

INTRADERMAL

Intradermal injections involve small volumes that are injected into the top layer of skin.

They are used for diagnostic reasons, desensitization, or immunization. Their effects are generally local rather than systemic.

An intradermal injection forms a *wheal*, or raised blister-like area, from which the drug will slowly be absorbed into the dermis.

The dermis is the layer of the skin just beneath the epidermis. It contains more blood vessels than the epidermis but fewer than most other injection sites. As a result, absorption is gradual.

The usual site for intradermal injections is the rear of the forearm.

Needles are generally 3/8 inches long and 25 to 26 gauge. For this route of administration, 0.1 ml of solution is the maximum volume that can be administered.

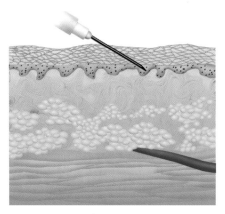

cross-section of an intradermal injection

ABCD *biocompatibility* not irritating; does not promote infection or abscess.

wheal a raised blister-like area on the skin caused by an intradermal injection.

IMPLANTS

One of the most popular ways to achieve very long term drug release is to place the drug in a delivery system or device that is implanted into the body tissue. The subcutaneous tissue is the ideal tissue for implantation of such devices. Implantation generally requires a surgical procedure or a specialized injection device. The fact that the device will be in constant contact with the subcutaneous tissue requires that the device materials be **biocompatible** (i.e., not irritating) and won't promote infection or sterile abscess. An advantage of the subcutaneous tissue for the site of implantation is that the device can be easily removed if necessary.

There are many devices that are used in subcutaneous implantation. Norplant® are silicone rods that provide contraception for up to five years. Viadur™ Duros® implants are made of titanium alloy and are capable of delivering a drug for up to 1 year. Other devices include degradable microspheres, vapor pressure devices for morphine delivery, osmotic pressure devices for insulin delivery, and magnetically activated pellets.

Sometimes ports and pumps are placed in subcutaneous tissue and an attached delivery catheter is placed in a vein, cavity, artery, or CNS system. This allows for the injection of intravenous fluids, total parenteral nutrition (TPN) solutions, chemotherapy agents, or antibiotics.

a Norplant® implant

OPHTHALMIC FORMULATIONS

Drugs are administered to the eye for local treatment of various eye conditions and for anesthesia.

Formulations that are used include aqueous solutions, aqueous suspensions, ointments, and implants. *Every ophthalmic product must be manufactured to be sterile in its final container.* Also, because of the sensitivity of the eye, various elements of the formulation, including pH and viscosity, must be carefully controlled.

A major problem of ophthalmic administration is the immediate loss of a dose by natural spillage from the eye.

The normal volume of tears in the eye is estimated to be 7 microliters, and if blinking occurs, the eye can hold up to 10 microliters without spillage. The normal commercial eyedropper dispenses 50 microliters of solution. As a result, *more than half of a dose will be lost from the eye by overflow.* The ideal volume of drug solution to administer would be 5 to 10 microliters. However, microliter dosing eye droppers are not generally available to patients.

Other problems include lacrimal (tear) drainage and very rapid absorption by the eyelid lining.

Tears that wash the eyeball flow from the **lacrimal gland** across the eye and drain into the **lacrimal canalicula** (tear ducts). In man, the rate of tear production is approximately 2 microliters per minute, and so the entire tear volume in the eye turns over every 2 to 3 minutes. This rapid washing and turnover accounts for loss of an ophthalmic dose in a relatively short period of time. It can also cause systemic absorption because the drug drains into the lacrimal sac and is then emptied into the gastrointestinal tract. A similar and frequently occurring problem is caused by absorption of the drug into the **conjunctiva** (eyelid lining). The drug is then rapidly carried away from the eye by the circulatory system.

OPHTHALMIC ADMINISTRATION

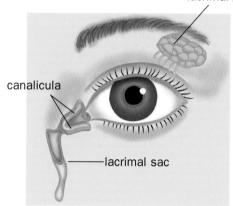

anatomy of the eye

Administration Considerations

➡ The eye is very sensitive, requiring careful formulation for sterility, pH, viscosity, etc. to avoid irritation.

➡ The eye only holds a very small volume of liquid (7-10 microliters), so most eyedropper doses are lost through overflow.

➡ Systemic absorption can occur from drainage through the tear ducts or absorption through the eyelid.

 Ophthalmic administration is used to deliver a drug on the eye, into the eye, or onto the conjunctiva. Drug penetration into the eye (**transcorneal transport**) is not considered an effective process as it is estimated that only one-tenth of a dose penetrates into the eye.

 ophthalmic related to the eye.

lacrimal gland the gland that produces tears for the eye.

lacrimal canalicula the tear ducts.

conjunctiva the eyelid lining.

transcorneal transport drug transfer into the eye.

Most ophthalmic solutions and suspensions are dispensed in eye dropper bottles.

Because of the problems of this route, patients must be shown how to properly instill the drops in their eyes, and every effort should be made to emphasize the need for instilling only one drop, not two or three.

To maintain longer contact between the drug and the surrounding tissue, suspensions, ointments, and inserts have been developed.

Ophthalmic suspensions are aqueous, with the particle size kept to a minimum to prevent irritation of the eye. Ointments tend to keep the drug in contact with the eye longer than suspensions. Most ophthalmic ointment bases are a mixture of mineral oil and white petrolatum and have a melting point close to body temperature. But ointments tend to blur patient vision as they remain viscous and are not removed easily by the tear fluid. Therefore, ointments are generally used at night as additional therapy to eye drops used during the day.

There are three types of devices commonly used to deliver ophthalmic dosages: hydrogel (soft) contact lenses, non-erodible inserts, and soluble inserts.

Hydrogel contact lenses are placed in a solution containing a drug such as an antibiotic, and the lenses absorb some of the drug solution. The lenses are then placed in the eye and the drug will release from the lenses over a period of time. Ocusert® is a non-erodible ocular insert designed to deliver pilocarpine at a controlled rate for up to 7 days. The insert is placed between the eyeball and the lower eyelid. With the Ocusert®, patients use a fraction of the amount of pilocarpine they would with drop therapy. The biggest disadvantage of the insert is its tendency to float on the eyeball, particularly in the morning after waking. Soluble ophthalmic drug inserts are dried solutions that have been fashioned into a film or rod. These solid inserts are placed between the eyeball and the lower eyelid, and as they absorb tears, they slowly erode away. Lacrisert® is a soluble insert used in the treatment of moderate to severe dry eye syndrome.

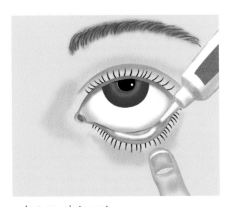

using an eye dropper

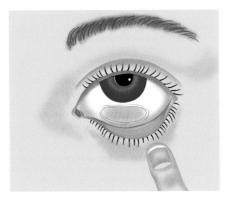

using an ointment

Ocusert®

Ophthalmic ointment tubes are typically small, holding approximately 3.5 g of ointment and fitted with narrow gauge tips which permit the extrusion of narrow bands of ointment.

INTRANASAL FORMULATIONS

The adult nasal cavity has a capacity of about 20 ml, a very large surface area for absorption, and a very rich blood supply.

The formulations used for intranasal administration are primarily used for their decongestant activity on the **nasal mucosa**, the cellular lining of the nose. The drugs that are typically used are decongestants, antihistamines, and corticosteroids.

The intranasal absorption of some drugs produces blood concentrations similar to when the drug is intravenously administered.

Because of this, intranasal administration is being investigated as a possible route of administration for insulin in the treatment of diabetes mellitus and for glucagon in the treatment of hypoglycemia. Intranasal administration also serves as a possible alternate route for drugs that are seriously degraded or poorly absorbed using oral administration.

Intranasal formulations include solutions, suspensions, sprays, aerosols, and inhalers.

Each product is formulated so it will not irritate the mucosa. Generally solutions or suspensions are administered by drops or as a fine mist from a nasal spray or aerosol container. Nasal sprays are preferred to drops because drops are more likely to drain into the back of the mouth and throat and be swallowed. Spray plastic bottles are common devices used to administer nasal mists. Glass containers with a metered actuator are gradually replacing the plastic spray bottles.

If the drug is sufficiently volatile, it can be administered in a nasal inhaler.

The **nasal inhaler** is a cylindrical tube with a cap that contains fibrous material impregnated with a volatile drug. The cap is removed and the inhaler tip is placed just inside the nostril. As the patient inhales, air is pulled through the tube and the vaporized drug is pulled into the nasal cavity.

DEVICES

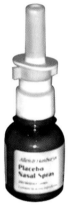

nasal spray

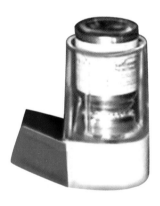

nasal aerosol

 nasal mucosa the cellular lining of the nose.

nasal cavity the cavity behind the nose and above the roof of the mouth that filters air and moves mucous and inhaled contaminants outward and away from the lungs.

nasal inhaler a device which contains a drug that is vaporized by inhalation.

USING A NASAL SPRAY

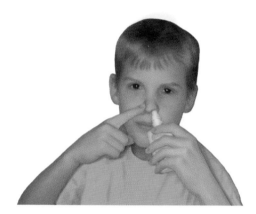

using a nasal spray

How to Use Intranasal Sprays or Pumps

1. Blow your nose gently to clear the nostrils.

2. Wash your hands with soap and warm water.

3. Hold your head in an upright position.

4. Close one nostril with one finger.

5. With the mouth closed, insert the tip of the spray or pump into the open nostril. Breath in through the nostril while quickly and firmly squeezing the spray container or activating the pump.

6. Hold your breath for a few seconds, and then breathe out through your mouth.

7. Repeat this procedure for the other nostril only if directed to do so.

8. Rinse the spray or pump tip with hot water, and replace the cap tightly on the container.

9. Wash your hands.

There are three ways a dosage can be lost following nasal administration.

The nasal lining contains enzymes which can metabolize and degrade some drugs. In addition, normal mucous flow, which protects the lungs by moving mucus and inhaled contaminants away from the lungs and out the nostril, will carry the drug with it as well. Finally, nasal administration often causes amounts of the drug to be swallowed. In some cases, enough drug will be swallowed to be equal to an oral dose. This may lead to a systemic effect from the drug even though it is intranasally administered.

Intranasal dosage forms should not be used for prolonged periods.

This may lead to chronic swelling (edema) of the nasal mucosa which aggravates the symptoms the dosage forms were intended to relieve. As a result, intranasal administration should be for short periods of time (no longer than 3 to 5 days). Patients should be advised not to exceed the recommended dosage and frequency of use.

Ways Intranasal Dosage Is Lost

✔ enzymes in the mucosa metabolize certain drugs;

✔ normal mucous flow removes drug;

✔ amounts of the drug are swallowed.

 Because it can lead to irritation and swelling, intranasal administration is generally kept to limited volumes for short periods of time.

INHALATION FORMULATIONS

Inhalation dosage forms are intended to deliver drugs to the pulmonary system (lungs).

The lungs have a large surface area for absorption and a rich blood supply. This route avoids the problems of degradation and poor absorption found with the oral route. However, there is enough inconsistency in the absorption of drugs from the lungs that this route is not considered an alternative to intravenous administration.

Gaseous or volatile anesthetics are the most important drugs administered via this route.

Other drugs administered affect lung function, act as bronchodilators, or treat allergic symptoms. Examples of drugs administered by this route are adrenocorticoid steroids (beclomethasone), bronchodilators (isoproterenol, metaproterenol, albuterol), and antiallergics (cromolyn sodium).

Most of the inhalation dosage forms are aerosols that depend on the power of compressed or liquefied gas to expel the drug from the container.

Aerosols are easy to use, and have no danger of contamination. However, they are not very effective in delivering a drug to the respiratory tract. This is not due to poor aerosol design, but to the physical barriers of the airway and lungs that any inhalation dosage form must overcome to be effective.

Particle size is the critical factor with these dosage forms.

Large particles (about 20 microns) hit in the back of the mouth and throat and are eventually swallowed rather than inhaled. Particles from 1 to 10 microns reach the bronchioles. Smaller particles (0.6 micron) penetrate to the **alveolar sacs** of the lungs where absorption is rapid, but retention is limited since a large fraction of the dose is exhaled. The particles that reach the alveolar sacs and remain there are responsible for providing systemic effects. Breathing patterns and the depth of breathing also play important roles in the delivery of drugs into the lung by inhalation aerosols.

ABSORPTION

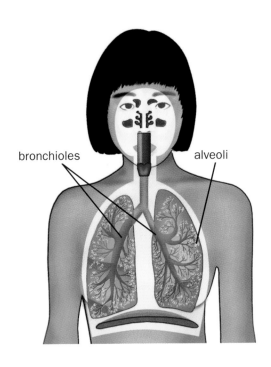

bronchioles   alveoli

For an inhalation dosage to reach the alveoli of the lungs, it has to pass through a series of twists, turns, and increasingly smaller passageways. When the drug reaches the alveoli, it will be absorbed directly into the circulatory system. Because of the difficult route from the mouth to the alveoli, varying amounts of inhaled drug are lost along the way.

inspiration breathing in.

alveolar sacs (alveoli) the small sacs of specialized tissue that transfer oxygen out of inspired air into the blood and carbon dioxide out of the blood and into the air for exhalation.

DEVICES

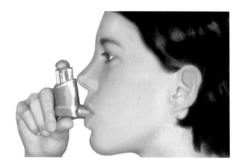

using an aerosol (MDI)

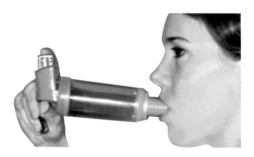

using an aerosol (MDI) with spacer

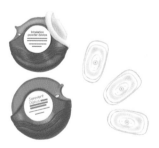

Diskus®

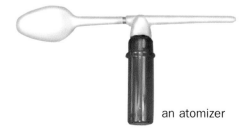

an atomizer

Metered Dose Inhalers (MDI's)

Aerosols to administer drugs by inhalation use special metering valves that deliver a fixed dose when the aerosol is activated. These are called "metered dose inhalers." The amount of drug released with each activation is regulated by a valve that has a fixed capacity or fixed dimensions.

Adapters and Spacers

Coordination is required on the part of the patient between breathing in (**inspiration**) and activation of the aerosol. Extender devices or spacers have been developed to assist patients who cannot coordinate these two processes. The spacer goes between the aerosol's mouthpiece and the patient's mouth. The spacer allows the patient to separate activation of the aerosol from inhalation by 3 to 5 seconds.

Dry Powder Inhalers

Some drugs are administered in powder form using a special inhalation device. The device automatically releases the drug when the user inhales. The powdered drug is supplied in hard gelatin capsules, cartridges, or disks (e.g., Diskus®).

Atomizers and Nebulizers

Atomizers are devices which break a liquid up into a spray. One type of atomizer uses a squeeze bulb to blow air across a liquid solution causing the liquid to vaporize. As the liquid vaporizes, the air stream created by the bulb also carries the spray out of the device and into the mouth. A nebulizer contains an atomizing unit inside a chamber. When the rubber bulb is squeezed, the drug solution is drawn up the dip tube and aerosolized by the passing air stream.

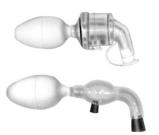

nebulizers

DERMAL FORMULATIONS

The skin is the largest and heaviest organ in the body and accounts for about 17% of a person's weight.

It forms a barrier that protects the underlying organ systems from trauma, temperature, humidity, harmful penetrations, moisture, radiation, and microorganisms. Dosage forms that are applied to the skin are called dermal dosage forms.

Most dermal dosage forms are used for local effects on or within the skin.

Dermal formulations are used as protectants, lubricants, emollients, or drying agents, or for the specific effect of the drug present. Examples of treatments using dermal formulations include minor skin infections, itching, burns, diaper rash, insect stings and bites, athlete's foot, corns, calluses, warts, dandruff, acne, psoriasis, and eczema. Some dermal formulations promote **percutaneous absorption** (i.e., absorption through the skin).

Dermal administration has a number of advantages.

It provides an ease of administration not found in other routes, and usage by patients is generally good. It can also provide continuous drug delivery. In addition, dermal formulations can be easily removed if necessary. The major disadvantage of this route of administration is that the amount of drug that can be absorbed will be limited to about 2 mg/day. This is often a significant limitation if the route is being considered for systemic therapy.

Basic rules of percutaneous absorption:
➡ More drug is absorbed when the formulation is applied to a larger surface area.
➡ Formulations or dressings that increase the hydration of the skin generally improve absorption.
➡ The greater the amount of rubbing in (inunction) of the formulation, the greater the absorption.
➡ The longer the formulation remains in contact with the skin, the greater will be the absorption.

---

 percutaneous absorption the absorption of drugs through the skin, often for a systemic effect.

hydrates absorbs water.

stratum corneum the outermost cell layer of the epidermis.

THE SKIN

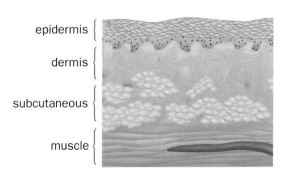

epidermis {
dermis {
subcutaneous {
muscle {

The skin is composed of three layers of tissue:
➡ epidermis;
➡ dermis;
➡ subcutaneous tissue.

The skin is generally 3 - 5 millimeters thick, though it is thicker in the palms and soles of the feet and thinner in the eyelids and genitals. Within the skin are several other structures: hair follicles, sebaceous glands, sweat glands, and nails.

The outer layer of epidermis is called the **stratum corneum**. In normal skin, this layer is continually replaced by new cells from underneath. The turnover time from cell development to shedding of the dead cells (sloughing) is about 21 days.

The stratum corneum is a barrier to drug penetration. It is about 10 micrometers thick, but can swell to approximately three times that by absorbing as much as five times its weight in water. When the stratum corneum absorbs water (**hydrates**), it becomes easier for drugs to penetrate. For that reason, certain dressings are designed to do this. Also, some skin conditions such as eczema and psoriasis cause the stratum corneum to hydrate and increase the absorption of some drugs.

FORMULATIONS

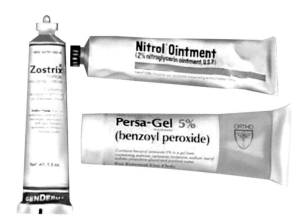

Ointments, Creams, Gels, and Lotions

Ointments, creams, gels, and lotions are the most popular dermal formulations. Physically, they appear to be very similar in consistency and texture, but there are differences. **Ointments** have drugs that have been incorporated into a base. There are several different types of bases ranging from petrolatum to polyethylene glycols. **Creams** are semisolid emulsions, and are less viscous and lighter in texture than ointments. Creams have an added feature in that they "vanish" or disappear with rubbing. **Gels** are dispersions of solid drugs in a jelly-like vehicle. **Lotions** are suspensions of solid drugs in an aqueous vehicle.

Solutions, Tinctures, Collodions, and Liniments

Dermal **solutions** and **tinctures** are generally used as anti-infective agents. Both are generally dispensed in small volumes, and should be packaged in containers that are convenient to use. Dropper bottles (glass bottles with an applicator tip) are most often used. Examples of solutions and tinctures are Coal Tar Solution, Hydrogen Peroxide, Povidone Iodine Tincture, and Compound Benzoin Tincture.

Collodions are liquid preparations of pyroxylin dissolved in a solvent mixture of alcohol and ether. Pyroxylin looks like raw cotton and is slowly but completely soluble in the solvent mixture. When applied to the skin, the solvent rapidly evaporates, leaving a protective film on the skin that contains a thin layer of the drug. **Liniments** are alcoholic or oleaginous solutions generally applied by rubbing.

Pastes, Powders, Plasters

Pastes are generally used for their protective action and for their ability to absorb secretions from skin lesions. Pastes contain more solid material than ointments, and are stiffer and less penetrating. Medicinal **powders** are a mixture of drug and an inert (inactive) base such as talcum or corn starch. Powders have different dusting and covering capability. **Plasters** are solid or semisolid adhesive masses that are spread on a suitable backing material. They provide prolonged contact at the site of application. Some of the common backing materials used are paper, cotton, felt, linen, muslin, silk, and moleskin. The backing is cut into different shapes appropriate to cover the affected area.

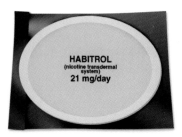

Transdermal Patches, Tapes, and Gauzes

Transdermal systems (patches, tapes, and gauzes) *deliver drugs through the skin for a systemic effect.* The systems can be divided into two kinds: those that control the rate of drug delivery to the skin, and those that allow the skin to control the rate of drug absorption. The first type is for potent drugs that must have their absorption rate controlled by a device. The second type is for less potent drugs. The largest problems with transdermal patches are skin sensitivity experienced by some patients, and technical difficulties associated with the adhesiveness of the systems to different skin types and under various conditions.

Aerosols

Percutaneous aerosols are generally used to apply anesthetic and antibiotic dosages for local effect.

VAGINAL FORMULATIONS

Vaginal administration has many of the same characteristics found with other parenteral routes of administration.

It avoids the degradation that occurs with oral administration; doses can be retrieved if necessary; and it has the potential of providing long term drug absorption. However, vaginal administration leads to variable absorption since the vagina is a physiologically and anatomically dynamic organ with pH and absorption characteristics changing over time. Another disadvantage of this route is that administration of a formulation during menstruation could predispose the patient to **Toxic Shock Syndrome.** There is also a tendency of some dosage forms to be expelled after insertion into the vagina.

Formulations for this route of administration are solutions, powders for solutions, ointments, creams, aerosol foams, suppositories, tablets, and IUDs.

Powders are used to prepare solutions for vaginal douches used to cleanse the vagina. The powders are supplied either as bulk or unit dose packages and are dissolved in a prescribed amount of water prior to use. Most douche powders are used for their hygienic effects, but a few contain antibiotics.

Vaginal administration gives the opportunity for long term administration.

This potential has been explored in the area of contraception protection using **intrauterine devices (IUDs)**. The first IUD was developed in 1970 and was effective for 21 days. The vaginal ring was worn until the onset of menstruation, removed during menstruation, and then reinserted for another 21 days. Several IUDs have been marketed since that time, including the Progestasert®.

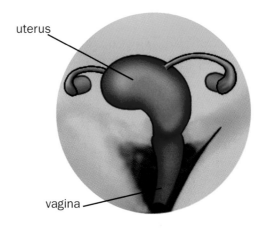

uterus

vagina

The Vagina

The vagina is a cylinder-like organ that leads from the cervix and uterus to an external opening. It is used for intercourse, releases menstrual fluids, and is the lower portion of the birth canal.

Toxic Shock Syndrome (TSS)

Toxic shock syndrome is a rare and potentially fatal disease that results from a severe bacterial infection of the blood. In women, it can be caused when bacteria natural to the vagina move into the bloodstream. Though primarily associated with the use of super-absorbency tampons, it has also been associated with various vaginal dosage forms. Its symptoms include a high fever, nausea, skin rash, faintness, and muscle ache. It is treated with antibiotics and other medicines.

Suppositories

Vaginal suppositories are employed as **contraceptives**, feminine hygiene antiseptics, bacterial antibiotics, or to restore the vaginal mucosa. Vaginal suppositories are inserted high in the vaginal tract with the 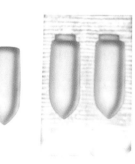 aid of a special applicator. The suppositories are usually globe, egg, or cone-shaped and weigh about 5 grams.

Suppositories are made from a variety of bases. Glycerinated gelatin (glycerin and gelatin) is excellent for prolonged local effects since it softens slowly. Polyethylene glycols dissolve when inserted into a body cavity, so the base does not need to be formulated to melt at body temperature. This allows convenient storage without refrigeration.

Of these suppository bases, glycerinated gelatin, is the preferred base for vaginal suppositories. It dissolves slowly in mucous secretions (generally in about 30 minutes) to provide prolonged release of the active drug. Glycerinated gelatin suppositories are made of 70 parts glycerin, 20 parts gelatin, and 10 parts water. They are translucent, resilient, and have a soft, rubbery texture.

Ointments, Creams, and Aerosol Foams

Vaginal ointments, creams, and aerosol foams typically contain antibiotics, estrogenic hormonal substances, and contraceptive agents.

Creams and foams are placed in a special applicator tube, and the tube is then inserted high in the vaginal tract. The applicator plunger is depressed and the formulation is deposited.

IUD

The Progestasert® IUD (intrauterine device) releases an average of 60 micrograms of progesterone per day for a period of one year. This IUD is replaced annually to maintain contraception. ParaGard® is an IUD that releases copper ions to prevent contraception. It has been shown to be effective for several years.

Tablets

Vaginal tablets, also called inserts, have the same activity and are inserted in the same manner as vaginal suppositories. Patients should be instructed to dip the tablet into water before insertion. Also, because tablets are generally used at bedtime and can be messy if the formulation is an oleaginous base, it should be recommended to patients that they wear a sanitary napkin to protect nightwear and bed linens. These same instructions should be given to patients receiving vaginal suppositories.

contraceptive device or formulation designed to prevent pregnancy.

intrauterine device (IUD) an intrauterine contraceptive device that is placed in the uterus for a prolonged period of time.

REVIEW

KEY CONCEPTS

ROUTES AND FORMULATIONS

✔ The way in which the body absorbs and distributes drugs varies with the route of administration.

✔ Enteral refers to anything involving the tract from the mouth to the rectum. There are four enteral routes: oral, sublingual, buccal, and rectal. Oral administration is the most frequently used.

✔ Parenteral refers to anything next to or beside the enteral route. Some parenteral routes use formulations that are injected. Other parenteral formulations do not require injection.

✔ A local effect occurs when the drug activity is at the site of administration (e.g., eyes, ears, nose, skin). A systemic effect occurs when the drug is introduced into the circulatory system.

ENTERAL ROUTES AND FORMULATIONS

✔ Oral administration is the most frequently used route of administration.

✔ Drugs administered in liquid dosage forms generally reach the circulatory system faster than drugs formulated in solid dosage forms.

✔ The primary goal of modified release dosage forms is to reduce the number of doses a patient must take per day.

✔ The mouth has two enteral routes of administration: sublingual (under the tongue) and buccal (in the cheek pouch).

✔ Rectal administration is used for both systemic and local effects. Suppositories, ointments, and solutions are common dosage forms.

PARENTERAL ROUTES AND FORMULATIONS

✔ Any route other than oral, sublingual, buccal, and rectal is considered a parenteral administration route. These routes are often preferred when oral administration causes drug degradation or when a rapid drug response is desired, as in an emergency situation.

✔ The parenteral routes requiring injection for administration are intravenous, intramuscular, intradermal, and subcutaneous. Solutions must be sterile (bacteria-free), have an appropriate pH, and be free of particulate material.

✔ Intramuscular injections generally result in lower but longer lasting blood concentrations than with intravenous administration.

✔ The subcutaneous (SC, SQ) route can be used for both short term and very long term therapies. Insulin is the most important drug routinely administered by this route.

✔ Intradermal administration is used for diagnostics, desensitization, and immunization.

✔ Ophthalmic administration can lead to a significant loss of the dose due to spillage and drainage.

✔ Inhalation dosage forms deliver drugs to the lungs. MDIs, dry powder inhalers, and nebulizers are common devices used to administer drug formulations.

✔ Dermal formulations vary from gels and lotions to aerosols, ointments, and pastes. Transdermal patches are also common dosage forms.

✔ Vaginal dosage forms (e.g., suppositories, tablets, solutions) are most often used for local effect. However, long term systemic effects can be achieved with IUDs.

SELF TEST

MATCH THE TERMS.   *answers can be checked in the glossary*

aqueous

buffer system

degradation

emulsions

hydrates

local effect

nasal inhaler

nasal mucosa

ophthalmic

percutaneous

solvent

sterile

sublingual

systemic effect

viscosity

water soluble

- a condition which is free of all microorganisms.
- a device which contains a drug that is vaporized by inhalation.
- a liquid that dissolves another substance in it.
- absorbs water.
- ingredients in a formulation designed to control the pH.
- mixture of two liquids that are not miscible in each other.
- the absorption of drugs through the skin, often for a systemic effect.
- related to the eye.
- the cellular lining of the nose.
- the change of a drug to a less effective or ineffective form.
- the property of a substance being able to dissolve in water.
- a measure of a liquid's thickness or resistance to flow.
- under the tongue.
- water based.
- when a drug is introduced into the circulatory system.
- when drug activity is at the site of administration.

CHOOSE THE BEST ANSWER.   *the answer key begins on page 347*

1. Which of the pH values listed below indicates a substance may be alkaline?
   a. pH 1-2
   b. pH 3-4
   c. pH 5-6
   d. pH 7-8

2. The stomach has a pH of around
   a. 3-4.
   b. 7.
   c. 5-6.
   d. 1-2.

3. Which of the following routes is least likely to give a systemic effect?
   a. oral
   b. sublingual
   c. rectal
   d. intradermal

4. _____ tablets have a sweet glaze and _____ tablets have a non-sweet coating.
   a. Film-coated, multiple compressed
   b. Sugar-coated, controlled release
   c. Sugar-coated, multiple compressed
   d. Sugar-coated, film-coated

REVIEW

5. Solutions are generally not used with the _____ route of administration.
   a. sublingual
   b. rectal
   c. intranasal
   d. vaginal

6. Which is not an oral liquid formulation?
   a. syrup
   b. gel
   c. tablet
   d. emulsion

7. The best known example of a sublingual tablet formulation is
   a. hydrochlorothiazide.
   b. nitroglycerin.
   c. digoxin.
   d. codeine.

8. Which is a parenteral route of administration?
   a. oral
   b. vaginal
   c. sublingual
   d. rectal

9. _____ are painful swollen veins.
   a. TSS
   b. IUD
   c. Emboli
   d. Hemorrhoids

10. _____ injections are administered into the top layer of the skin at a slight angle using short needles.
    a. IUD
    b. Z-Tract
    c. TSS
    d. Intradermal

11. _____ injections are administered to the subcutaneous tissue of the skin using 3/8 to 1 inch needles.
    a. Subcutaneous
    b. Intramuscular
    c. Intravenous
    d. Transdermal

12. _____ injections are administered into muscle tissue using 1 to 1 1/2 inch needles.
    a. Subcutaneous
    b. Transdermal
    c. Intravenous
    d. Intramuscular

13. A/an _____, also known as a blood clot, is a complication that can occur from intravenous administration.
    a. phlebitis
    b. thrombus
    c. air embolus
    d. ingestion

14. _____ can occur if air is introduced into a vein and can be fatal.
    a. Phlebitis
    b. Air emboli
    c. Thrombus
    d. Toxic shock

15. Needle sizes of _____ are commonly used for intravenous injections.
    a. 16 G to 20 G
    b. 25 G to 27 G
    c. 20 G to 25 G
    d. 22 G to 24 G

16. Needles for intramuscular injections are generally _____ G and _____ inches long.
    a. 19 to 22, 1 to 1.5
    b. 23 to 25, 1 to 1.5
    c. 25 to 27, 3/8 to 1
    d. 19 to 22, 3/8

17. _____ injections are generally more painful than _____ injections.
    a. Intravenous, intramuscular
    b. Intramuscular, intravenous

18. Needles for subcutaneous injection are generally _____ and _____.
    a. 3/8 to 1 inch; 18 G to 20 G
    b. 1 to 1.5 inches; 24 G to 27 G
    c. 3/8 to 1 inch; 24 G to 27 G
    d. 1 to 1.5 inches; 18 G to 20 G

19. The usual site for intradermal injections is
    a. the stomach.
    b. the rear of the forearm.
    c. the buttocks.
    d. the thigh.

20. Needles for intradermal injections are generally _____ and _____.
    a. 1 inch; 18 G to 20 G
    b. 3/8 inch; 25 G to 26 G
    c. 1.5 inches; 18 G to 20 G
    d. 3 inches; 16 G to 20 G

21. A raised blister-like area on the skin caused from an intradermal injection is called a/an
    a. IUD.
    b. TSS.
    c. wheal.
    d. phlebitis.

22. The average tear volume in the eye is 10 microliters. The average drop size for an eyedropper is _____ microliters.
    a. 50
    b. 25
    c. 10
    d. 7

23. Which ophthalmic formulation will maintain the drug in contact with the eye the longest?
    a. solution
    b. suspension
    c. gel
    d. ointment

24. Which pathway would the use of a metered dose inhaler (MDI) follow?
    a. mouth, trachea, alveoli, bronchioles
    b. mouth, bronchioles, trachea, alveoli
    c. mouth, trachea, bronchioles, alveoli
    d. bronchioles, alveoli, nasal cavity, trachea

25. The Norplant® device is made of cylindrical silicone rods that slowly release progesterone to provide contraception for up to 5 years. The rods are _____ implants.
    a. intradermal
    b. subcutaneous
    c. intramuscular
    d. intrathecal

PARENTERALS

In parenteral therapy, there are special requirements for how formulations are made and packaged and how they are administered.

Parenterals have been administered in institutional settings for decades. In the past two decades, their use outside of the institution has grown dramatically. Agencies such as home care companies, outpatient clinics, and community pharmacies are providing the services and skills for patients and caregivers to administer these formulations.

Parenterals are packaged as two general types of products: *large volume parenteral* (LVP) solutions and *small volume parenteral* (SVP) solutions.

LVP solutions are typically bags or bottles containing larger volumes of intravenous solutions. Common uses of LVP solutions without additives include correction of electrolyte and fluid balance disturbances, nutrition, and vehicles for administering other drugs.

SVP solutions are generally contained in ampules, piggyback bags, prefilled syringes, and vials.

Their contents are withdrawn by syringe and can be added to a LVP solution or injected directly into the patient.

Inspections

Parenteral solutions should always be visually inspected before use. Formulated or admixed solutions should be inspected after compounding. Visual inspection can show two of the six characteristics of parenteral solutions: particulate material and stability. (Lack of stability is indicated by precipitation or crystallization in the solution). Inspection is generally performed against a brightly lit white background.

Visual inspection cannot reveal anything about the sterility, pH, osmolarity, presence of pyrogens, or chemical degradation of the drug. Special equipment and skilled personnel are needed to determine these factors. Since sterility cannot be determined visually, good aseptic technique must be used when dealing with parenteral solutions.

CHARACTERISTICS

Because intravenous products are administered directly into the bloodstream, there are a number of special considerations and precautions that must be taken.

✔ **Solutions for injection must be sterile –i.e., free from bacteria and other microorganisms.**

Techniques that maintain sterile conditions and prevent contamination must be followed. These are called **aseptic techniques.**

✔ **Solutions must be free of all visible particulate material.**

Examples of such contaminants are glass, rubber cores from vial closures, cloth or cotton fibers, metal, and plastic. Undissolved particles of an active drug will be present in intravenous suspensions, but no contaminants should be present.

✔ **All parenteral solutions must be pyrogen-free.**

Intravenous solutions can cause **pyretic** (fever) reactions if they contain pyrogens. **Pyrogens** are chemicals that are produced by microorganisms. They are soluble in water and are not removed by sterilizing or filtering the solution.

✔ **The solution must be stable for its intended use.**

Most admixtures are prepared hours in advance of when they are to be administered. So the stability of a particular drug in a particular intravenous solution must be considered in the admixture preparation. This information is generally available in a number of reference sources.

✔ **The pH of intravenous solution should not vary significantly from physiological pH, about 7.4.**

Sometimes, other factors may be more important, such as when acidic or alkaline solutions are needed to increase drug solubility or used as a therapeutic treatment themselves.

✔ **Intravenous solutions should be formulated to have an osmotic pressure similar to that of blood.**

Osmotic pressure is the characteristic of a solution determined by the number of dissolved particles in it. Osmolarity is a unit of measure of osmotic pressure and is expressed in terms of osmoles (Osmol) or milliosmoles (mOsmol) per liter.

Blood has an osmolarity of approximately 300 mOsmol per liter. Both 0.9% sodium chloride solution and 5% dextrose solution have a similar osmolarity. When a solution has an osmolarity equivalent to that of blood, it is called **isotonic.**

Intravenous solutions that have greater osmolarity than blood are called **hypertonic**, and those with lower osmolarity, **hypotonic.** Both hypertonic and hypotonic solutions may cause damage to red blood cells, pain, and tissue irritation. However, it is at times necessary to administer such solutions. In these cases, the solutions are usually given slowly through large, free flowing veins to minimize the reactions.

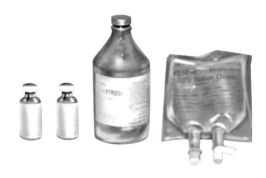

Parenteral Routes

Principles discussed in this chapter pertain to drugs administered via the following routes of administration:

➡ intravenous
➡ intramuscular
➡ intradermal
➡ subcutaneous
➡ epidural
➡ intrathecal
➡ intranasal
➡ inhalation
➡ ophthalmic

 aseptic techniques techniques or methods that maintain the sterile condition of products.

pyrogens chemicals produced by microorganisms that can cause *pyretic* (fever) reactions in patients.

osmotic pressure a characteristic of a solution determined by the number of dissolved particles in it.

isotonic when a solution has an osmolarity equivalent to that of blood.

hypertonic when a solution has a greater osmolarity than that of blood.

hypotonic when a solution has a lesser osmolarity than that of blood.

LVP SOLUTIONS

Large volume parenteral (LVP) solutions are intravenous solutions packaged in containers holding 100 ml or more.

There are three types of containers: glass bottle with an air vent tube, glass bottle without an air vent tube, and plastic bags. The most common sizes are 100, 250, 500, and 1,000 ml. The top of the LVP solution container is hung on an administration pole. At the other end of the container are two ports of about the same length. One is the administration set port, and the other is the medication port. Graduation marks to indicate the volume of solution in the container are on its front. They are marked at 25 ml to 100 ml intervals depending on the overall size of the container.

The administration set port has a plastic cover on it to maintain the sterility of the bag.

The cover is easily removed. Solution will not drip out of the bag through this port because of a plastic diaphragm inside the port. When the spike of the administration set is inserted into the port, the diaphragm is punctured, and the solution will flow out of the bag into the administration set. This inner diaphragm cannot be resealed once punctured.

The medication port is covered by a protective rubber tip.

Drugs are added to the LVP solution through this port using a needle and syringe. There is an inner plastic diaphragm about one half inch inside the port, just like the administration set port. This inner diaphragm is also not self-sealing when punctured by a needle, but the protective rubber tip prevents solutions from leaking from the bag once the diaphragm is punctured.

ADMINISTRATION

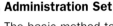

Administration Set

The basic method to administer a LVP solution is to use an administration set. The set contains a spiked plastic device to pierce the administration set port on the LVP container.

This connects to a **volume control** or **drip chamber** that may be used to set the **flow rate** (the rate ordered by the physician at which the solution is to be administered to the patient, generally measured in ml/hour). A clamp pinching the tubing may also be used to regulate flow or the flow may be controlled using an infusion pump. The line then leads to a rubber injection port with a needle that is placed in the patient.

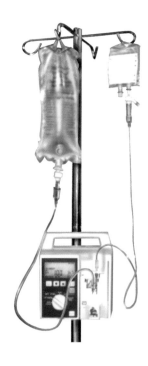

Piggybacks

Medications are often administered with piggybacks, which are small volumes of fluid (usually 50 - 100 ml) infused into the administration set of an LVP solution. Piggybacks are typically infused over a period of thirty to sixty minutes. Some medications are also administered directly into a volume control chamber.

 flow rate the rate (in ml/hour or ml/minute) at which the solution is administered to the patient.

piggybacks small volume solutions added to an LVP.

DEVICES

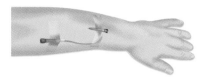

Heparin Lock

In some instances, a patient may not have a primary LVP solution, yet must receive piggyback medications. This is done through a heparin lock, which is a short piece of tubing attached to a needle or intravenous catheter. When the tubing is not being used for the piggyback, heparin is used to fill the tubing. Heparin prevents blood from clotting in the tube.

Other Devices

Infusion pumps, syringe pumps, and **ambulatory pumps** are devices used to administer LVP solutions and control flow rates.

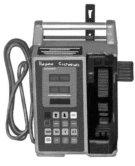

Administration sets are threaded through infusion pumps, and the pumps control the flow rate. Syringe pumps expel solutions from a syringe into an administration set such as a heparin lock. An ambulatory pump is about the size of a hand. It allows patients to have some freedom of movement compared to being restricted to an infusion pump attached to an administration pole. All of these devices have made the infusion process much more accurate and easier to administer and have been a major factor in the growth of home infusion care.

Plastic bags have advantages not found with glass bottles.

They do not break. They weigh less. They take up less storage space, and they take up much less disposal space. The plastic bag system is not vented to outside air. It collapses as the solution is administered, so a vacuum is not created inside.

Some drugs and solutions may not be used with plastic because they interact with it.

In these cases, glass IV bottles are used. They are packaged with a vacuum, sealed by a solid rubber closure, and the closure is held in place by an aluminum band. Graduation marks are along the sides of the bottle and are usually spaced every 25 ml to 50 ml. The solution bottle is hung on an administration pole in an inverted position using the aluminum or plastic band on the bottom of the bottle.

Solutions flow from the glass containers to the patient through a special administration set.

For solutions to flow out of a glass container, air must be able to enter the container to relieve the vacuum as the solution leaves. Some bottles have air tubes built into the rubber closure for this. Some bottles do not, in which case a special administration set with a filtered airway in the spike must be used.

Common LVP Solutions

Many intravenous solutions are commercially available. Four solutions are commonly used either as LVP solutions or as the primary part of an admixture solution:

➡ sodium chloride solution;
➡ dextrose solution;
➡ Ringer's solution;
➡ Lactated Ringer's solution.

Various combinations of different strengths of sodium chloride and dextrose solutions are also available, e.g., 5% dextrose and 0.45% sodium chloride, or 5% dextrose and 0.2% sodium chloride.

 heparin lock an injection device used when a primary LVP solution is not available.

infusion the slow continuous introduction of a solution into the blood stream.

SVP SOLUTIONS

Small volume parenteral (SVP) solutions are packaged products that are either directly administered to a patient or added to another parenteral formulation.

When a drug is added to a parenteral solution, the drug is referred to as the **additive**, and the final mixture is referred to as the **admixture**. SVP solutions are supplied in prefilled syringes, ampules, glass or plastic vials sealed with a rubber closure, or plastic minibags. Powdered drugs are supplied in vials that must be reconstituted (dissolved in a suitable solvent) before being added to the intravenous solution.

Ampules are elongated sealed glass containers with a neck that must be snapped off.

Most ampules are weakened around the base of the neck for easy breaking. These will have a colored band around the base of the neck. Some ampules, however, must first be scored and weakened with a file or the top may shatter. Once an ampule is opened, it becomes an open-system container.

Minibags are made of the same plastic materials as LVPs and contain the same types of solutions found in LVPs.

Minibags are just smaller in size since they contain only 50 - 100 ml of solution.

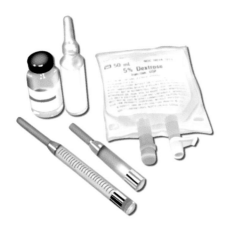

small volume parenterals

ADDING SVPs TO LVPs

Generally the LVP solution is used as a continuous infusion because of its large volume and slow infusion rate. SVP solutions can be introduced into the on-going LVP infusion by injecting the SVP into the medication port of the container or the volume control chamber of the administration set. However, most often the SVP is put into a minibag and used as a piggyback on the LVP.

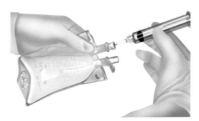

Using a Needle and Syringe to Add a SVP to a LVP:

1. Remove the protective covering from the LVP package.

2. Assemble the needle and syringe.

3. If the drug in the SVP is in powder form, reconstitute it with the recommended diluent.

4. Swab the SVP and medication port of the LVP with an alcohol swab.

5. Draw the necessary volume of drug solution into the syringe from the SVP.

6. Insert the needle into the medication port and through the inner diaphragm. The medication port should be fully extended to minimize the chance of going through the side of the port.

7. Inject the SVP solution into the LVP.

8. Remove the needle from the LVP.

9. Shake and inspect the admixture.

Note: This procedure will be done in a laminar flow hood.

READY-TO-MIX SYSTEMS

Ready-to-mix systems consist of a specially designed minibag with an adapter for attaching a drug vial. The admixing takes place just prior to administration. The major advantages of ready-to-mix systems include a significant reduction in waste and lower potential for medication error because the drug vial remains attached to the minibag and can be rechecked if necessary. However, the systems do cost more, and there is the potential that the system will not be properly activated so that the patient receives only the diluent or a partial dose.

Ready-to-Mix Systems

Add-Vantage®

Add-a-Vial®

Mini-Bag Plus®

CRIS® Controlled Release Infusion System

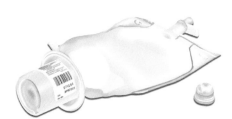

the Add-Vantage® system

Drugs and other additives can be packaged in glass or plastic vials.

The drugs or other additives may be either in liquid form or as **lyophilized** (freeze dried) powders. Powders must be reconstituted with a suitable solvent (**diluent**) before use. Vials have a rubber stopper through which a needle is inserted to withdraw or add to the contents. Before withdrawing solution from a vial, an equal volume of air is usually drawn up in the syringe and injected into the vial. This pressurizes the vial and helps in withdrawing solution from the vial. Some medications are packaged under pressure or can produce gas (and pressure) upon reconstitution. In such cases, air is not injected into the vial before withdrawing the solution.

Vials may be prepared for single dose or multidose use.

Single dose vials do not contain preservatives and should be discarded after one use. Multidose vials contain a preservative to inhibit bacterial contamination once the vial has been used. Also, the rubber closure will reseal on a multidose vial. These vials can be used for a number of doses of variable volume.

There are two varieties of prefilled syringes.

One type, a cartridge type package, is a single syringe and needle unit which is to be placed in a special holder before use. Once the syringe and needle unit is used, it is discarded but the holder can be used again with a new unit. Another type of prefilled syringe consists of a glass tube closed at both ends with rubber stoppers. The prefilled tube is placed into a specially designed syringe that has a needle attached to it. After using this type of prefilled syringe, all of the pieces are discarded.

additive a drug that is added to a parenteral solution.

admixture the resulting solution when a drug is added to a parenteral solution.

lyophilized freeze-dried.

diluent a solvent that dissolves a lypholized powder or dilutes a solution.

SYRINGES & NEEDLES

The basic parts of a syringe are the barrel, plunger, and tip.

The barrel is a tube that is open at one end and tapers into a hollow tip at the other end. The plunger is a piston-type rod with a slightly cone-shaped stopper that passes inside the barrel of the syringe. The tip of the syringe provides the point of attachment for a needle. The volume of solution inside a syringe is indicated by graduation lines on the barrel. Graduation lines may be in milliliters or fractions of a milliliter, depending on the capacity of the syringe. The larger the capacity, the larger the interval between graduation lines.

There are several common types of syringe tips.

Slip-Tip® tips allow the needle to be held on the syringe by friction. The needle is reasonably secure, but it may slip off if not properly attached or if considerable pressure is used. **Luer-Lok®** tips have a collar with grooves that lock the needle in place. **Eccentric** tips, which are off-center, are used when the needle must be parallel to the plane of injection such as in an intradermal injection. **Oral syringes** have tips larger than a Slip-Tip®. Needles will not fit on oral syringes. Therefore, they are used to administer liquids by routes other than parenteral administration.

Syringes come in sizes ranging from 1 to 60 ml.

As a rule, the correct syringe size is the next size larger than the volume to be measured. For example, a 3 ml syringe should be selected to measure 2.3 ml, or a 5 ml syringe to measure 3.8 ml. In this way, the graduation marks on the syringe will be in the smallest possible increments for the volume measured. Syringes should not be filled to capacity because the plunger can be easily dislodged.

SYRINGES

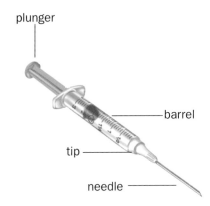

plunger

barrel

tip

needle

A syringe with graduation marks

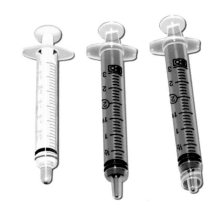

Different syringe tips

Drawing Liquids into the Syringe

Liquids are drawn into the syringe by pulling back on the plunger. The tip of the syringe must be fully submerged in the liquid to prevent air from being drawn into the syringe. Generally, an excess of solution is drawn into the syringe so that any air bubbles may be expelled by holding the syringe tip up, tapping the syringe until the air bubbles rise into the hub, and depressing the plunger to expel the air. This ensures that the hub will be completely filled with solution and the volume of delivery will be accurate.

Measuring Volume

The volume of solution in a syringe is measured to the edge of the plunger's stopper while the syringe is held upright and all the air has been removed from the syringe.

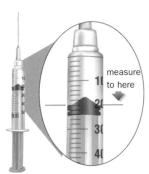

measure to here

Disposable needles should always be used when preparing admixtures as they are presterilized and individually wrapped to maintain sterility.

NEEDLES

Parts

A needle has three parts: the **hub**, the **shaft**, and the **bevel**. The hub is at one end of the needle and is the part that attaches to the syringe. It is designed for quick and easy attachment and removal. The shaft is the long, slender stem of the needle that is angled at one end to form a point called the "bevel." The hollow bore of the needle shaft is known as the **lumen**.

Sizes

Needle sizes are indicated by length and **gauge**. The length of a needle is measured in inches from where the shaft meets the hub to the tip of the bevel. Needle lengths range from 3/8 inch to three and a half inches. Some special use needles are even longer. The gauge of a needle, used to designate the size of the lumen, ranges from 27 (the smallest) to 13 (the largest). *In other words, the higher the gauge number, the smaller is the lumen.* The hubs are color-coded for each gauge size.

Needle sizes are chosen based on both the viscosity (thickness) of the parenteral solution and the type of rubber closure in the container. Needles with relatively small lumens can be used for most solutions. However, some viscous solutions require needles with larger lumens. One problem is that larger needles are more likely to damage the rubber closures of solution containers, causing particles to fall into the container and contaminate the solution. This is called "**coring**." Therefore, small gauge needles are used if the rubber closure can be easily cored, regardless of the solution viscosity.

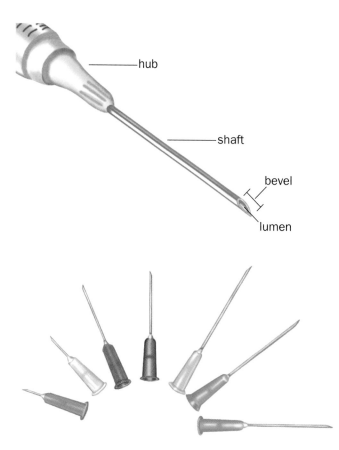

Different size needles

 Slip-Tip®, Luer-Lok®, eccentric, oral different types of syringe tips.

hub the part of the needle that attaches to the syringe.

shaft the stem of the needle that provides the overall length of the needle.

bevel an angled surface at the tip of a needle.

gauge a measurement — with needles, the higher the gauge, the smaller the lumen.

lumen the hollow center of a needle.

coring when a needle damages the rubber closure of a parenteral container causing fragments of the closure to fall into the container and contaminate its contents.

FILTERS

Filters are used to remove particulate materials or microorganisms from solutions.

They can be attached to the end of a syringe, to the end of an administration set, or they can be part of the needle. They are divided into two basic groups: depth filters and membrane filters. **Depth filters** work by trapping particle as solution moves through twisting channels. A **membrane filter** consists of many small pores of a uniform size that retain particles larger than the pores. Filters have a wide range of pore sizes. Common ones are 0.22, 0.45, 1, 5, or 10 mm (microns).

Filters can be found in a variety of packaging.

Membrane filters often are packaged in a round plastic holder that can be attached easily to the end of a syringe. Some filters are attached to administration sets and serve as "final filters," filtering the solution immediately before it enters the patient's vein. Some administration sets have filters that are already built into the set. Filters also can be placed inside of needles; these are called *filter needles*. Double ended filter needles comprise a simple unit that has a filter between two needles. This allows the transfer of solution directly from one container to another container and eliminates the need for using a syringe to transfer the solution. Filters also are supplied as single units to be used in specialized filtration apparatus.

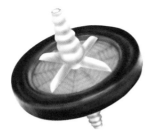

Membrane Filters

A membrane filter similar to the one above is often placed between the syringe and needle before the medication is introduced into a LVP or SVP container. Double ended filter needles are also used to transfer solutions from a vial directly into a bottle or bag. This eliminates the need of using a syringe.

MEMBRANE FILTERS

Membrane filters are intended to filter a solution only as it is expelled from a syringe. A common scenario would be to transfer a reconstituted powder drug solution into a LVP or SVP following these steps:

1. A needle is attached to the syringe.

2. The reconstituted powder drug solution is pulled into the syringe.

3. Air bubbles are removed from the syringe.

4. The needle is removed from the syringe.

5. A membrane filter is then attached to the syringe.

6. Another needle is placed on the end of the filter.

7. Air is eliminated from the filter chamber by holding the syringe in a vertical position so that the needle is pointing upward. The air in the filter chamber is then expelled by slowly pushing in the plunger. Air must be expelled before the filter becomes wet or the air will not pass through the filter. Do not pull back on the plunger when the membrane filter is being used because the filter may rupture.

8. Once air has been expelled, the needle is introduced into the final LVP or SVP container and pressure is slowly and continuously applied to push the solution through the filter into the container.

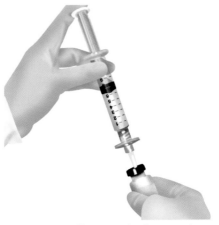

A membrane filter attached to a syringe and needle

DEPTH FILTERS

Depth filters are constructed of randomly oriented fibers or particles (e.g., diatomaceous earth, porcelain, asbestos) that have been pressed, wound, or otherwise bonded together to form a tortuous pathway for solution flow.

The depth filter is rigid enough so the solution may be filtered either as it is pulled into or expelled from the syringe, but not both ways in the same procedure. If a drug solution is to be filtered as the solution is pulled into a syringe, the following steps are used:

1. The filter needle is attached to the syringe.

2. The solution is pulled into the syringe.

3. The filter needle is removed.

4. A new needle is attached to the syringe.

5. The solution is expelled from the syringe.

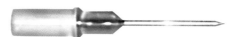

The depth filter is inside the hub of this filter needle.

FINAL FILTERS

A filter that filters a solution immediately before it enters the patient's vein is called a **final filter**. Some administration sets contain final filters as part of the set. Some filters are designed to be attached to administration sets and serve as final filters.

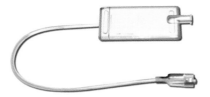

A Pall® final filter

membrane filter a filter that filters solution as the solution is expelled from the syringe.

depth filter a filter that can filter solutions being drawn into or expelled from a syringe, but not both ways in the same procedure.

final filter a filter that filters solution immediately before it enters a patient's vein.

LAMINAR FLOW HOODS

Microorganisms invisible to the eye are present in dust and particulate matter in natural air and on most surfaces, even those that appear clean.

Unless aseptic techniques are used to prepare parenteral solutions, contamination can easily occur from the environment in which the product is being prepared or from the person preparing it.

The best way to reduce the environmental risk is to use a laminar flow hood which establishes and maintains an ultraclean work area.

Room air is drawn into a horizontal hood and passed through a prefilter to remove relatively large contaminants such as dust and lint. The air is then channeled through a high efficiency particulate air (**HEPA**) filter that removes particles larger than 0.3 μm (microns).[*] The purified air then flows over the work surface at a uniform velocity (i.e., **laminar flow**) of 80 - 100 ft./min. The constant flow of air from the hood prevents room air from entering the work area and removes contaminants introduced into the work area by material or personnel.

The surfaces of the hood's work area are clean, not sterile.

Therefore, it is necessary to use techniques which maintain the sterility of all sterile items. These are called **aseptic techniques.** They apply to the technician, the laminar flow hood, and all substances and materials involved in the procedure.

[*] Laminar flow hoods used in preparing parenteral formulations must be Class 100 (less than 100 particles of 0.5 micon size per cubic foot).

ABCD *aseptic techniques* methods or techniques that maintain the sterility of sterile items.

laminar flow continuous movement at a uniform rate in one direction.

HEPA filter a high efficiency particulate air filter.

Types of Laminar Flow Hoods
Because **horizontal laminar flow hoods** blow air toward the operator, **vertical flow hoods** are preferred when protection for both the personnel and the environment is desired. A vertical flow hood functions by passing air through a HEPA filter and directing it down toward the work area. As the air passes through the work surface, it is redirected to the outside air through the back of the hood.

ASEPTIC TECHNIQUES FOR WORKING IN LAMINAR FLOW HOODS

Positioning of material and working inside a hood aseptically requires training, practice, and attention to details.

- ✔ **Never sneeze, cough, or talk directly into a hood.**
- ✔ **Close doors or windows.** Breezes can disrupt the air flow enough to contaminate the work area.
- ✔ **Perform all work at least 6 inches inside the hood** to derive the benefits of the laminar air flow. Laminar flow air begins to mix with outside air near the edge of the hood.
- ✔ **Maintain a direct, open path between the filter and the area inside the hood.**
- ✔ **Place nonsterile objects, such as solution containers or your hands, downstream from sterile ones.** Particles blown off these objects can contaminate anything downstream from them.
- ✔ **Do not put large objects at the back of the work area next to the filter.** They will disrupt air flow.

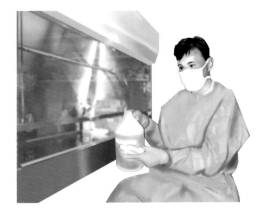

Laminar flow hoods do not provide a sterile environment. They provide an ultraclean work area.

LAMINAR AIR FLOW

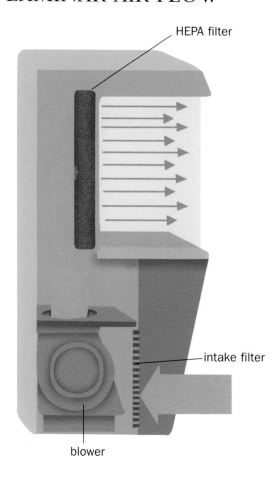

HEPA filter

intake filter

blower

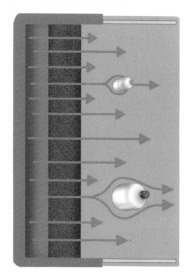

view from above

The illustration at left shows how a horizontal laminar air flow hood draws in air through its filters and channels it outward in over the work surface.

The illustration above shows how air is channeled around objects on the work surface. Note that there is a "dead" area (sometimes called "zone of turbulence") behind the large container.

BIOLOGICAL SAFETY HOODS

Biological safety hoods protect both personnel and the environment from contamination. They are used when preparing hazardous drugs. A biological safety cabinet functions by passing air through a HEPA filter and directing it down toward the work area. As the air approaches the work surface, it is pulled through vents at the front, back, and sides of the hood. A major portion of the air is recirculated back into the cabinet and a minor portion passes through a secondary HEPA filter and is exhausted into the room. Biological safety hoods are not the same as vertical laminar flow hoods.

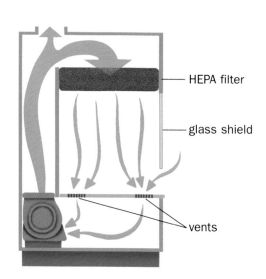

HEPA filter

glass shield

vents

ASEPTIC TECHNIQUES

Personnel involved with admixing parenteral solutions must use good aseptic techniques.

Aseptic techniques are the sum total of methods and manipulations required to minimize the contamination of sterile products. Contamination can be from microorganisms and/or particulate material. Working in a laminar flow hood does not, by itself, guarantee aseptic technique. The guidelines on these pages must also be followed, along with any facility and manufacturer guidelines that apply.

Turn On Flow Hood

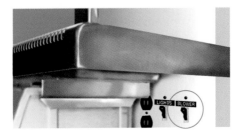

✔ Turn the laminar flow hood on and let it operate for at least 30 minutes before use in order to produce an ultraclean environment. Maintain a designated "clean" area around the hood.

Clothing and Barriers

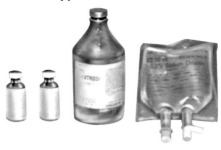

✔ Wear clean lint-free garments or barrier clothing, including gowns, hair covers, and a mask.

✔ Wear sterile gloves.

✔ Follow facility or manufacturer guidelines for putting on and removing barrier clothing. Unless barriers are put on properly, they can easily become contaminated.

Cleaning Laminar Flow Hoods

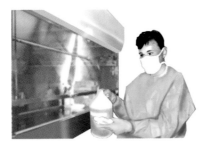

✔ Clean the inside of the hood with a suitable disinfectant. First clean the metal pole used to hang the containers.

✔ Then the sides of the hood are cleaned using up and down motions moving from the back of the hood toward the front.

✔ Then the bottom of the hood is cleaned using side-to-side motions moving from the back of the hood toward the front.

Collect Supplies

✔ Assemble all necessary supplies checking each for expiration dates and particulate material.

✔ Plastic solution containers should be squeezed to check for leaks.

✔ Use only presterilized needles, syringes, and filters. Check the protective covering of each to verify they are intact.

✔ Remove dust coverings before placing supplies in the hood.

Wash hands

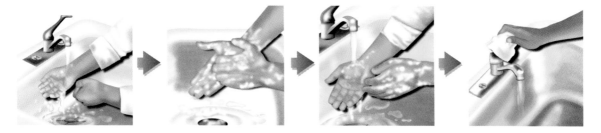

✔ Remove all jewelry.

✔ Stand far enough away from the sink so clothing does not come in contact with it.

✔ Turn on water. Wet hands and forearms thoroughly. Keep hands pointed downward.

✔ Scrub hands vigorously with an antibacterial soap.

✔ Work soap under fingernails by rubbing them against the palm of the other hand.

✔ Interlace the fingers and scrub the spaces between the fingers.

✔ Wash wrists and arms up to the elbows.

✔ Thoroughly rinse the soap from hands and arms.

✔ Dry hands and forearms thoroughly using a nonshedding paper towel.

✔ Use a dry paper towel to turn off the water faucet.

✔ After hands are washed, avoid touching clothes, face, hair, or any other potentially contaminated object in the area.

Position Supplies in Hood

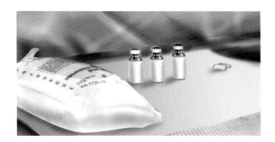

✔ Place supplies in the hood with smaller supplies closer to the HEPA filter and larger supplies further away from the filter.

✔ Space supplies to maximize laminar flow.

Sterilize Puncture Surfaces

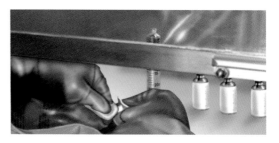

✔ Swab all surfaces that require entry (puncture) with an alcohol wipe. Avoid excess alcohol or lint that might be carried into the solution.

 Sterile supplies often have instructions for use as well as expiration dates. Always follow such instructions along with any facility or manufacturer instructions.

WORKING WITH VIALS

There are two types of parenteral vials that are used in making admixtures.

One contains the drug already in the solution. The other contains a powder that must be dissolved in a diluent to make a solution. In either case, a needle will be used to penetrate the closure in the vial.

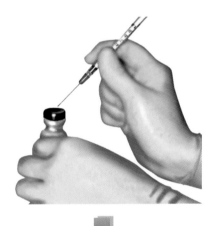

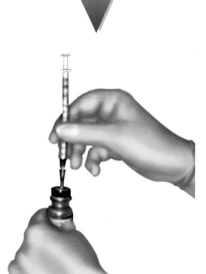

PREVENTING CORING

There is the potential of "coring" when pushing a needle through the rubber stopper of a vial or medication port.

As the needle penetrates the stopper, it can cut small pieces from the stopper which can fall into the vial. To prevent coring, follow these steps:

✔ Place the vial on a flat surface and position the needle point on the surface of the rubber closure so that the bevel is facing upward and the needle is at about a 45 to 60 degree angle to the closure surface.

✔ Put downward pressure on the needle while gradually bringing the needle up to an upright position. Just before penetration is complete, the needle should be at a vertical (90 degree) angle.

 coring when a needle damages the rubber closure of a parenteral container causing fragments of the closure to fall into the container and contaminate its contents.

VIALS CONTAINING SOLUTIONS

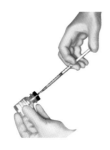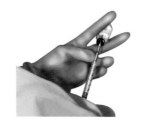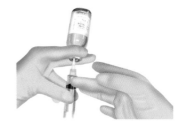

✔ Draw into the syringe a volume of air equal to the volume of drug to be withdrawn. This will pressurize the vial and help in withdrawing the solution.

✔ Penetrate the vial without coring and inject the air.

✔ Turn the vial upside down. Using one hand to hold the vial and the barrel of the syringe, pull back on the plunger with the other hand to fill the syringe. Fill the syringe with a slight excess of solution.

✔ Tap the syringe to allow air bubbles to come to the top of the syringe. Press the plunger to push air and excess solution into the vial.

✔ Transfer the solution into the final container, again minimizing coring.

VIALS CONTAINING LYPHOLIZED POWDER

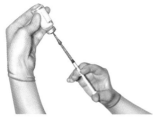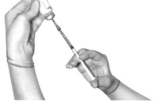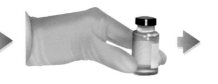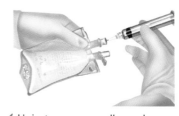

✔ Determine the correct volume of diluent and withdraw it from its vial following the steps outlined above for vials containing solutions.

✔ Transfer the diluent into the vial containing powder.

✔ Once the diluent is added, remove a volume of air into the syringe that is slightly more than the volume of diluent added. This will create a slight negative pressure in the vial and lowers the chance that aerosol droplets will be sprayed when the needle is withdrawn.

✔ After withdrawing the needle, swirl the vial until the drug is dissolved.

✔ Using a new needle and syringe, use the steps outlined above for vials containing solutions to withdraw the correct volume of reconstituted drug solution into the syringe.

✔ Transfer the reconstituted solution to the final container, again making sure to minimize coring.

WORKING WITH AMPULES

Ampules are always broken open at the neck.

Ampules have a colored stripe around the neck if they are pre-scored to indicate the neck has been weakened by the manufacturer to facilitate opening. Some ampules are not pre-scored by the manufacturer, and the neck must first be weakened (scored) with a fine file.

TO OPEN AN AMPULE

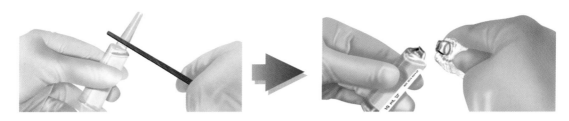

- ✔ If the ampule is not pre-scored, use a fine file to lightly score the neck at its narrowest point. Do not file all the way through the glass.
- ✔ Hold the ampule upright and tap the top to settle the solution into the ampule.
- ✔ Swab the neck of the ampule with an alcohol swab.

- ✔ Wrap a gauze pad around the neck of the ampule. This will help protect fingers if the ampule shatters and will reduce the possibility of splinters becoming airborne.
- ✔ Grasp the top of the ampule with the thumb and index finger of one hand. Grasp the bottom of the ampule with the other hand.
- ✔ Quickly snap the ampule moving your hands outward and away. Do not open the ampule toward the HEPA filter or any other sterile supplies in the hood. If the ampule does not snap easily, rotate it slightly and try again.
- ✔ Inspect the opened ampule for glass particles that may have fallen inside, and use a filter needle if necessary when withdrawing the solution.

 ampules sealed glass containers with an elongated neck that must be snapped off.

sharps needles, jagged glass or metal objects, or any items that might puncture or cut the skin.

TRANSFERRING SOLUTION

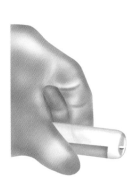 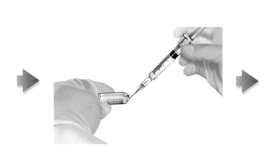 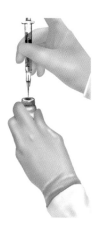

✔ Hold the ampule down at about a 20 degree angle.

✔ Attach a filter needle to a syringe.

✔ Insert the filter needle into the ampule. Avoid touching the opening of the ampule with the needle point.

✔ Position the needle on the shoulder area of the ampule. Place its beveled edge against the side of the ampule to avoid pulling glass particles into the syringe.

✔ Withdraw solution into the syringe but keep needle submerged to avoid withdrawing air into the syringe.

✔ Withdraw needle from ampule and remove all air bubbles from the syringe.

✔ Exchange the filter needle for a new filter needle or membrane filter and transfer the solution into the final container.

DISPOSAL

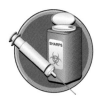

Discarded gloves, needles, syringes, ampules, vials, and prefilled syringes used in preparing parenterals pose a source of contamination and must be disposed of properly. In many health care facilities and other locations, such disposal containers often have a label that says **"Sharps"** on it, indicating objects that might puncture or cut the skin of anyone who handles them.

✔ Always separate sharps from other refuse for disposal.

✔ Receptacles that are easy to identify and are leakproof, punctureproof, and sealable should be used exclusively for this type of hazardous waste.

✔ Needles should not be clipped or recapped in order to prevent aerosolization or accidental needle sticks.

✔ Excess solutions should be returned to their original vial, an empty vial, or some other suitable, closed container before disposal.

SPECIAL SOLUTIONS

TOTAL PARENTERAL NUTRITION SOLUTIONS

Total parenteral nutrition (TPN) solutions are complex admixtures used to provide nutritional support to patients who are unable to take in adequate nutrients through their digestive tract. These admixtures are composed of dextrose, fat, protein, electrolytes, vitamins, and trace elements. They are hypertonic solutions.

Base parenteral nutrition solutions are available in 2,000 and 3,000 ml sizes. The base solution consists of:

➡ an amino acid solution (a source of protein);
➡ a dextrose solution (a source of carbohydrate calories).

These solutions, sometimes referred to as macronutrients, make up most of the volume of a parenteral nutrition solution. Several electrolytes, trace elements, and multiple vitamins (together referred to as micronutrients) may be added to the base solution to meet individual patient requirements. Common electrolyte additives include sodium chloride (or acetate), potassium chloride (or acetate), calcium gluconate, magnesium sulfate, and sodium (or potassium) phosphate. Multiple vitamin preparations containing both water soluble and fat soluble vitamins are usually added on a daily basis. A trace element product containing zinc, copper, manganese, selenium, and chromium may be added.

Intravenous fat (lipid) emulsion can be added as a source of essential fatty acids and a concentrated source of calories. Fat provides nine calories per gram, compared to 3.4 calories per gram provided by dextrose. Intravenous fat emulsion may be admixed into the total parenteral nutrition solution or piggybacked into the administration line. When intravenous fat emulsion is admixed with a TPN solution, the resulting solution is referred to as a **total nutrient admixture (TNA)**.

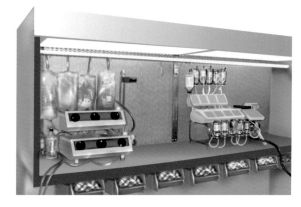

TPN preparation system

Administration

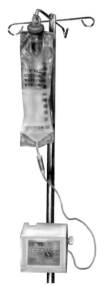

TPN solutions are generally (though not always) administered via the subclavian vein under the collar bone over 8 to 24 hours. Slow administration using this vein minimizes the adverse effects that may occur with such a hypertonic solution. The subclavian vein is large and close to the heart, so the solution is diluted rapidly by the large volume of blood in the heart.

To assure their accurate delivery, nutrition solutions are almost always administered with an intravenous infusion pump. Parenteral nutrition solutions are commonly administered through an in-line filter in the administration set positioned as close to the patient as possible. However, intravenous fat emulsion, either alone or as part of a TNA solution, can be administered through an in-line filter only if it has a pore size of 1.2 micron or larger. An alternative is to piggyback the intravenous fat emulsion into the administration set below the in-line filter.

peritoneal dialysis solution a solution placed in and removed from the peritoneal cavity to remove toxic substances.

irrigation solution large volume splash solutions used during surgical or urologic procedures to bathe and moisten body tissues.

DIALYSIS SOLUTIONS

Dialysis refers to the passage of small particles through membranes. This is caused by **osmosis,** the action in which a drug in a solution of a higher concentration will move through a permeable membrane (one that can be penetrated) to a solution of a lower concentration. This principle is the basis for another type of special solution.

Peritoneal dialysis solutions are used by patients who have compromised kidney function. The solution is administered directly into the peritoneal cavity (the cavity between the abdominal lining and the internal organs) to remove toxic substances, excess body waste, and serum electrolytes through osmosis. *These solutions are hypertonic to blood so the water will not move into the circulatory system. But the toxic substances will move into the dialysis solution.*

Peritoneal solutions are administered several times a day. The solution is permitted to flow into the abdominal cavity, and then remains in the cavity for 30 to 90 minutes. It is then drained by a siphon tube into discharge bottles. This procedure is repeated many times a day and may use up to 50 liters of solution. For this reason, peritoneal dialysis solutions are supplied in containers larger than 1,000 ml capacity.

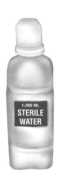

IRRIGATION SOLUTIONS

Irrigation solutions are not administered directly into the venous system but are subject to the same stringent controls as intravenous fluids. They are packaged in containers that are larger than 1,000 ml capacity and are designed to empty rapidly. **Surgical irrigation Solutions** (splash solutions) are used to:

➼ bathe and moisten body tissues;
➼ moisten dressings;
➼ wash instruments.

They are typically Sodium Chloride for Irrigation or Sterile Water for Irrigation.

Urologic Irrigation Solutions are used during operations to:

➼ maintain tissue integrity,
➼ remove blood to maintain a clear field of vision.

Glycerine Irrigation and 3% Sorbital Irrigation Solutions are commonly used because they are non-hemolytic (i.e., do not damage blood cells).

 osmosis the action in which drug in a higher concentration solution passes through a permeable membrane to a lower concentration solution.

dialysis movement of particles in a solution through permeable membranes.

UNITS OF MEASUREMENT

There are different ways to express the concentration of a drug in a parenteral solution.

Each method of expressing the concentration is related to a particular property of the solution. The common concentrations and their units are listed on these pages.

MOLARITY

Molarity is an expression of the number of moles of a drug in a volume of solution. A mole is the number of grams numerically equal to the **molecular weight** of the drug. The molecular weight is the sum of the atomic weights of all the atoms that make up the drug molecule. Potassium chloride (KCl) has a molecular weight of 74.6. So, one mole of potassium chloride is 74.6 grams.

Molarity concentrations are expressed as mole/liter (written as mol/L, or M). A 1M solution of potassium chloride contains 74.6 grams of the drug in 1000 ml (1 liter) of solution.

Some molarity concentrations are expressed as millimoles per liter (written as mM/L). A millimole is one-thousandth of a mole.

Salt Forms

Drugs come in different salt forms for a variety of reasons, and the salt form and **"waters of hydration"** must be factored into determining the molecular weight of a drug. For example, chloride comes as the sodium salt, the potassium salt, and the calcium salt.

Waters of hydration are water molecules that can attach to drug molecules. Calcium chloride ($CaCl_2$) exists in three different forms, **anhydrous** (no waters), dihydrate (2 associated waters), and hexahydrate (six waters of hydration). *The dihydrate form is the one used in making parenteral solutions.*

OSMOLES

Another expression for an amount of drug is the osmole (Osmol). An osmole is equal to the molecular weight of the drug divided by the number of **ions** formed when a drug dissolves in solution.

$$\text{osmole} = \frac{\textbf{molecular weight}}{\textbf{\# of ions}}$$

For example, potassium chloride forms two ions when it dissolves in solutions. Therefore, 1 Osmol of potassium chloride would be its molecular weight (74.6 grams) divided by two: 37.3 grams. Anhydrous calcium chloride forms three ions when it dissolves in solution: one calcium ion and two chloride ions. 1 Osmol would be its molecular weight (111.0 grams) divided by three: 37.0 grams.

Most drug solution concentrations are expressed as Osmol/liter (written as Osmol/L). Some concentrations are expressed as mOsmol/L. A milliosmole is one-thousandth of an osmole.

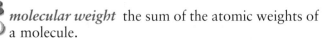

molecular weight the sum of the atomic weights of a molecule.

ion molecular particles that carry electric charges.

anhydrous without water molecules.

waters of hydration water molecules that attach to drug molecules.

equivalent weight a drug's molecular weight divided by its valence, a common measure of electrolyte concentration.

valence the number of positive or negative charges on an ion.

EQUIVALENTS

Another expression for an amount of drug is the **equivalent weight (Eq)**. It is used to describe concentrations of electrolytes such as potassium chloride, sodium chloride, sodium acetate, etc.

When an electrolyte dissolves in solution, it divides into **ions,** particles which carry electric charges that can be positive or negative. The number of positive *or* negative charges (but not both added together) is called the **valence** of the ions. It indicates the ions' ability to combine with other atoms or molecules.

An equivalent weight is equal to the molecular weight of the drug divided by the valence of the ions that form when the drug is dissolved.

$$\text{equivalent weight} = \frac{\text{molecular weight}}{\text{valence}}$$

Equivalent concentrations are expressed as an equivalent weight per liter (written as Eq/L). Equivalent concentrations are also expressed as milliequivalents per liter (written as mEq/L). A milliequivalent is one-thousandth of an equivalent weight.

EXAMPLE

Potassium chloride (KCl) splits into one potassium ion (K^+) and one chloride ion (Cl^-).

➡ KCl's valence is 1 since there is either one positive charge on the potassium ion or one negative charge on the chloride ion.

➡ The equivalent weight of KCL is 74.6 grams divided by one: 74.6 grams.

EXAMPLE

Anhydrous calcium chloride ($CaCl_2$, 111.0 grams) splits into one calcium ion having two positive charges (++) and two chloride ions, each having one negative charge (-).

➡ Its valence is 2.
➡ The equivalent weight of $CaCl_2$ is 111.0 grams divided by two: 55.5 grams.

PERCENTAGE WEIGHT PER VOLUME

Percentage concentrations refer to the drug's weight per 100 ml if the drug is a solid, or the drug's volume per 100 ml if the drug is a liquid.

$$\text{solid: } \% = \frac{\text{weight (gm)}}{\text{100 ml}}$$

$$\text{liquid: } \% = \frac{\text{volume (ml)}}{\text{100 ml}}$$

For example, a 5% dextrose solution contains 5 grams of dextrose (a solid) in 100 ml of solution. A 5% acetic acid solution (common household vinegar) contains 5 ml of acetic acid (a liquid) per 100 ml of solution.

Percentage concentrations are applied to other formulations besides parenteral solutions. A 10% zinc oxide ointment would have 10 grams of zinc oxide (a solid) in 100 grams of ointment.

INTERNATIONAL UNITS

Because the potency and purity of drugs from biological sources vary depending on the source, they are measured by **units of activity** rather than by weight. Units may be abbreviated as IU, or U, and are expressed for example as 2,000 U, 1,000,000 U, etc. Drugs commonly measured in international units include penicillin, insulin, heparin, and some vitamins.

REVIEW

KEY CONCEPTS

PARENTERALS

✔ Parenterals are packaged as two types of products: large volume parenteral (LVP) solutions and small volume parenteral (SVP) solutions.

✔ Solutions for injection must be sterile, free of all visible particulate material, pyrogen-free, stable for their intended use, have a pH around 7.4, and in most (but not all) cases isotonic.

LVP SOLUTIONS

✔ The flow rate is the rate at which the solution is administered to the patient.

✔ Infusion pumps, syringe pumps, and ambulatory pumps are devices used to administer LVP solutions and control flow rates.

SVP SOLUTIONS

✔ When a drug is added to a parenteral solution, the drug is referred to as the additive, and the final mixture is referred to as the admixture.

SYRINGES AND NEEDLES

✔ Syringes come in sizes ranging from 1 to 60 ml. As a rule, a syringe size is used that is one size larger than the volume to be measured.

✔ Needle sizes are indicated by length and gauge. The higher the gauge number, the smaller is the lumen (the hollow bore of the needle shaft). Large needles may be needed with highly viscous solutions but are more likely to cause coring.

FILTERS

✔ Syringe filters are often used to remove particulate materials from solutions, and sometimes to remove microorganisms.

LAMINAR FLOW HOODS

✔ A laminar flow hood establishes and maintains an ultraclean work area for the preparation of admixtures.

ASEPTIC TECHNIQUES

✔ Aseptic techniques maintain the sterility of all sterile items and are used in preparing admixtures.

WORKING WITH VIALS

✔ There is the potential of coring the rubber stopper of a vial.

WORKING WITH AMPULES

✔ Ampules may be manufactured with pre-scored necks, or they may have to be scored with a file.

SPECIAL SOLUTIONS

✔ Parenteral nutrition solutions are complex admixtures composed of dextrose, fat, protein, electrolytes, vitamins, and trace elements. They are hypertonic solutions. Most of the volume of TPN solutions is made up of macronutrients: amino acid solution (a source of protein) and a dextrose solution (a source of carbohydrate calories).

UNITS OF MEASUREMENT

✔ Equivalent (Eq/L) or milliequivalent (mEq/L) concentrations are commonly used to describe concentrations of electrolytes in solution.

✔ Percentage concentrations refer to the drug's weight per 100 ml if the drug is a solid, or the drug's volume per 100 ml if the drug is a liquid.

SELF TEST

MATCH THE TERMS.

answers can be checked in the glossary

admixture

aseptic techniques

bevel

dialysis

diluent

gauge

HEPA filter

hypertonic

hypotonic

ion

isotonic

osmolarity

pyrogens

- • a characteristic of a solution determined by the number of dissolved particles in it.
- • when a solution has a lesser osmolarity than that of blood.
- • a high efficiency particulate air filter.
- • a solvent that dissolves a lypholized powder or dilutes a solution.
- • a needle measurement: the higher the _____, the smaller the lumen.
- • when a solution has an osmolarity equivalent to that of blood.
- • an angled surface, at the tip of a needle.
- • chemicals produced by microorganisms that can cause fever reactions in patients.
- • molecular particles that carry electric charges.
- • movement of particles in a solution through permeable membranes.
- • techniques or methods that maintain sterility of sterile products.
- • the resulting solution when a drug is added to a parenteral solution.
- • when a solution has a greater osmolarity than that of blood.

CHOOSE THE BEST ANSWER.

the answer key begins on page 347

1. An intravenous solution that is formulated to have an osmolarity equivalent to that of blood is _____ to it.
   a. isotonic
   b. hypotonic
   c. hypertonic
   d. none of the above

2. Intravenous products are administered into the
   a. skin.
   b. muscle.
   c. lungs.
   d. blood.

3. Visual inspection of parenteral solutions against a brightly lit background can show the presence of _____ and _____.
   a. particle contamination, precipitation
   b. pH, precipitation
   c. chemical degradation of a drug, osmolarity
   d. pyrogens, precipitation

4. The pH of an intravenous solution should be about
   a. 1.0.
   b. 2.4.
   c. 7.4.
   d. 9.4.

REVIEW

5. Aseptic techniques are methods used to maintain
   a. pH.
   b. sterility of sterile products.
   c. osmotic pressure.
   d. pyrogens.

6. When a solution is free from soluble products produced by microorganisms it is said to be
   a. sterile.
   b. pyrogen free.
   c. isotonic.
   d. particle free.

7. Large volume parenterals (LVPs) are packaged in containers holding _____ or more.
   a. 5 ml
   b. 10 ml
   c. 100 ml
   d. 2,000 ml

8. The medication port on an administration set is covered by a _____ tip.
   a. plastic
   b. rubber
   c. aluminum
   d. cotton

9. Heparin is used in a heparin lock to
   a. improve the visibility of particle contamination.
   b. maintain the flow rate.
   c. maintain the pH.
   d. keep blood from clotting in the device.

10. Glass LVP solution bottles are
    a. used when drugs or solutions interact with plastic.
    b. the most common type of LVP container.
    c. not sterile.
    d. made of unbreakable glass.

11. LVPs usually have _____ infusion rates.
    a. lyophilized
    b. rapid
    c. slow
    d. instantaneous

12. Small volume parenteral solutions generally will contain not more than ___ of solution.
    a. 5 ml
    b. 25 ml
    c. 100 ml
    d. 500 ml

13. Single-dose vials
    a. can be reused within 48 hours if refrigerated.
    b. do not contain preservatives.
    c. contain preservatives.
    d. can be reused within 24 hours if refrigerated.

14. You are to use 2.4 ml of diluent to reconstitute a vial of medication. What size of syringe should be used?
    a. 20 ml
    b. 10 ml
    c. 5 ml
    d. 3 ml

15. Of the following needles, which size of needle is most likely to cause coring?
    a. 13 G
    b. 16 G
    c. 20 G
    d. 23 G

16. _____ tips allow the needle to be held by friction and _____ tips have a collar with grooves that lock the needle in place.
    a. Slip-Lok®, Luer-Lok®
    b. Eccentric, Luer-Lok®
    c. Slip-Lok®, eccentric
    d. Luer-Lok®, oral

17. The hollow center of a needle is the
    a. gauge.
    b. hub.
    c. lumen.
    d. bevel.

18. Which type of filter is constructed of fibers or particles pressed together to form a tortuous pathway?
    a. depth
    b. membrane
    c. final
    d. sterilization

19. Why is air generally injected into a vial before a volume of solution is removed?
    a. keeps the drug dissolved in the solution
    b. provides a negative pressure in the vial so the solution will not spray when the needle is removed
    c. helps withdraw the solution by pressurizing the vial
    d. prevents the vial closure from coring

20. When using the laminar flow hood, a technician should work inside the hood at least
    a. two inches.
    b. four inches.
    c. six inches.
    d. eight inches.

21. Laminar flow hoods provide a _____ work area.
    a. sterile
    b. stable
    c. zone of turbulence
    d. ultraclean

22. In horizontal laminar flow hoods, air blows
    a. down toward the work area.
    b. away from the operator.
    c. toward the operator.
    d. up toward the HEPA filter.

23. In laminar flow, the air flows in _____ direction(s).
    a. four
    b. three
    c. two
    d. one

24. A laminar flow hood should be turned on for _____ minutes before use in order to produce a particle free environment.
    a. 5
    b. 15
    c. 30
    d. 60

25. Solutions containing dextrose, fatty acids, amino acids and other micronutrients are called _____ solutions.
    a. TPN
    b. TNA
    c. peritoneal
    d. splash

COMPOUNDING

Extemporaneous compounding is the on-demand preparation of a drug product according to a physician's prescription, formula, or recipe.

Compounding has always been a component of Pharmacy. There is an art involved in using raw ingredients to formulate a drug product that meets the special needs of particular patients. It requires specialized knowledge of the physical and chemical properties of drugs and their vehicles. It also requires proper training and skill. This chapter will focus on the terminology, equipment, and basic principles of extemporaneous compounding.

There are various aspects of compounding.

It can mean the preparation of suspensions, dermatologicals, and suppositories; the conversion of one dosage form into another; the preparation of select dosage forms from bulk chemicals; the preparation of intravenous admixtures, parenteral nutrition solutions, and pediatric dosage forms from adult dosage forms; the preparation of radioactive isotopes; or the preparation of cassettes, syringes, and other devices for administering drugs in the home setting.

The demand for pharmaceutical compounding has grown substantially.

Reasons for this include the growth of home health care, the unavailability of certain drug products, orphan drugs, veterinary compounding, and biotechnology derived drug products. Newly evolving dosage forms and therapies also suggest that compounding will become more common in pharmacy practice.

Technicians, under pharmacist supervision, are increasingly involved in compounding.

Specific responsibilities will vary from environment to environment. Therefore, it is necessary to know and understand the specific responsibilities and requirements that apply to your job.

SPECIAL NEEDS

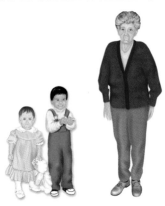

Compounding is done for many special reasons, including:

➡ Pediatric patients requiring diluted adult strengths of drugs;

➡ patients needing an oral solution or suspension of a product that is only available in another form;

➡ patients with sensitivity to dyes, preservatives, or flavoring agents found in commercial formulations;

➡ dermatological formulations with fortified (strengthened) or diluted concentrations of commercially available products;

➡ specialized dosages for therapeutic drug monitoring;

➡ care for hospice patients in pain management;

➡ compounding for animals.

COMPOUNDING AND MANUFACTURING

There are many guidelines that have been published by governmental agencies and professional organizations that pertain to compounding in Pharmacy. The guidelines address topics ranging from the definition of compounding to specifications for compounding equipment. For example, the National Association of Boards of Pharmacy (NABP) has defined compounding and manufacturing in their *Good Compounding Practices Applicable to State Licensed Pharmacies* as follows:

Compounding is defined as "the preparation, mixing, assembling, packaging, or labeling of a drug or device (i) as the result of a practitioner's prescription drug order or initiative based on the practitioner-patient-pharmacist relationship in the course of professional practice, or (ii) for the purpose of, or as an incident to, research, teaching, or chemical analysis and not for sale or dispensing. Compounding also includes the preparation of drugs or devices in anticipation of prescription drug orders based on routine, regularly observed prescribing patterns."

Manufacturing is defined as "the production, preparation, propagation, conversion, or processing of a drug or device, either directly or indirectly, by extraction from substances of natural origin or independently by means of chemical or biological synthesis, and includes any packaging or repackaging of the substance(s) or labeling or relabeling of its container, and the promotion and marketing of such drugs or devices. Manufacturing also includes the preparation and promotion of commercially available products from bulk compounds for resale by pharmacies, practitioners, or other persons."

Two prominent professional organizations are the National Association of Boards of Pharmacy (NABP) and the American Society of Health-System Pharmacists (ASHP). Each of these organizations has published statements that compounding is an integral part of Pharmacy. NABP's document titled *Model Rules for Pharmaceutical Care* states that "Each pharmacy shall be of sufficient size to allow for the safe and proper storage of prescription drugs and the compounding and/or preparation of prescription drug orders." ASHP's guidelines titled *Minimum Standard for Pharmacies in Hospitals* states that "Drug formulations, dosage forms, strengths and packaging that are not available commercially but are needed for patient care shall be prepared by appropriately trained personnel in accordance with applicable practice standards and regulations (e.g., FDA, State Board of Pharmacy). Adequate quality assurance procedures shall exist for these operations."

Accuracy and Stability In Compounding

Different dosage units of the same manufactured product must essentially have the same content and characteristics, and they are tested to confirm this. However, there is no such testing or proof for extemporaneously compounded products. As a result, compounding accuracy and the stability of the compounded product are important issues. The USP defines **stability** of dosage forms as the chemical and physical integrity of the dosage unit, and when appropriate, the ability of the unit to maintain protection against microbiological contamination.

The supervising pharmacist must determine that a product can be accurately compounded and *will be stable for its expected use. Accuracy is then essential* in all weighing, measurements, and other activities in the compounding process.

COMPOUNDING GUIDELINES

Additional Guidelines on Performing Compounding in a Pharmacy

In addition to the mandate documents, the NABP and ASHP have published the following guidelines on how to perform compounding in pharmacy.

➡ *Good Compounding Practices Applicable to State Licensed Pharmacies* (NABP)
➡ *Model Rules for Sterile Pharmaceuticals* (NABP)
➡ *Technical Assistance Bulletin on Compounding Nonsterile Products in Pharmacies* (ASHP)
➡ *Technical Assistance Bulletin on Quality Assurance for Pharmacy – Prepared Sterile Products* (ASHP)

These documents should be reviewed and understood thoroughly by any personnel that will be involved in compounding in a pharmacy. A brief summary of some of the key points in these documents is given below.

Personnel

The guidelines give the responsibility and authority for the management of the compounding area to the pharmacist. The guidelines outline the duties of the pharmacist and the pharmacist's responsibilities for other personnel in the compounding area. These guidelines also list the qualifications a pharmacist must have to compound and recommends further training and continuing education responsibilities. The appropriate clothing to be worn by pharmacy personnel is also given.

Facilities and Equipment

The guidelines go into great detail about the physical design and maintenance of the compounding area. They specify that the compounding area, either non-sterile or sterile, should be a designated area away from the "routine dispensing and counseling functions and high traffic areas" of the pharmacy. The guidelines also recommend compounding equipment that should be in the compounding area.

Ingredient Standards

Raw chemicals are supplied in many levels of purity. The table below summarizes some of the different purity classifications applied to chemicals (from least pure to most pure). It is desired that USP or NF grade be the "lowest" grade of purity used in compounding and that if that grade is not available, then a "higher" grade of purity can be used if deemed acceptable by the pharmacist.

Grade of Chemical	Description
Technical (commercial)	Commercial or industrial quality, generally of indeterminate quality
CP (chemically pure)	More refined than technical grade, but still of unknown quality; only partial analytical information available
USP/NF	Meets standards set by the USP/NF
FCC	Meets specifications of Food Chemical Codex
ACS reagent	High purity; meets specifications of the Reagent Chemicals Committee of the American Chemical Society
AR (analytical reagent)	Very high purity
HPLC	Very high purity; used in high pressure chromatography
Spectroscopic grade	Very high purity
Primary standard	Highest purity; used in standard solutions for analytical purposes

ABCD *formulation record* formulas and procedures (i.e., recipes) for what should happen when a formulation is compounded.

compounding record a record of what actually happened when the formulation was compounded.

Packaging and Storage

The pharmacist is responsible for the appropriate packaging of compounded formulations and for the storage of all ingredients, drugs, supplies, and formulations in the compounding area. The appropriate container will depend on the physical and chemical properties of the compounded formulation and its intended use.

Packaging materials should not chemically react with any drug or ingredient in the formulation. Other packaging considerations include its strength, visibility, moisture protection, ease of use, and cost.

Materials used in compounding should be stored according to the manufacturers' labeling or USP/NF requirements. Materials should be marked with the date of receipt and the date the container is opened, and the materials should be rotated to use the oldest stock first. Materials should not be used beyond their expiration date. Materials that specify storage temperatures use the definitions listed in the table below.

Documentation and Record Keeping

Documentation and record keeping provide information that is directly applicable to the formulation being compounded. They provide a basis for professional judgement and for legal liability. They also provide for consistency when formulations are compounded over and over again. And if there is a problem in the formulation, they provide a mechanism to systematically review procedures and ingredients.

The guidelines recommend that four sets of records be kept in the compounding area:

➡ a formulation record (compounding formulas and procedures, a master sheet, a "recipe") – what should happen when the formulation is compounded;

➡ a compounding record – what actually happened when the formulation was compounded;

➡ standard operating procedures (SOPs) for equipment maintenance, equipment calibration, handling and disposal of supplies, etc.;

➡ ingredients records with certificates of purity and MSDSs (Material Safety Data Sheets).

Sample document templates for each of these types of records are in the companion *Workbook and Certification Review* accompanying this text.

Storage Temperature Definitions

Freezer	-20°C to -10°C
Protect from Freezing	Store above 0°C
Cold	Any temperature not exceeding 8°C
Refrigerator	Between 2°C and 8°C
Cool	Between 8°C and 15°C
Room Temperature	Temperature in the work area
Controlled Room Temperature	Thermostatically controlled at 20°C to 25°C
Warm	Between 30°C and 40°C
Excessive Heat	Any temperature above 40°C

EQUIPMENT

Each individual compounded prescription can be viewed as a four step process: measure, mix, mold, and package.

Not all steps are needed in every compounded prescription, but they indicate the type of equipment necessary for compounding.

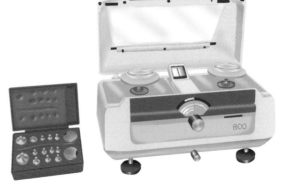

To Measure

Balance, weights, weighing containers, volumetric glassware (graduates, pipets, flasks, syringes, buret).

To Mix

Beakers, Erlenmeyer flasks, spatulas, funnels, sieves, mortar and pestle.

To Mold

Hot plates, suppository molds, capsule shells, ointment slabs.

To Package

Prescription bottles, capsule vials, suppository boxes, ointment jars.

Degree of Error

Class A prescription balances can weigh as little as 120 mg of material with a 5% error. 5% is generally considered an acceptable error in most pharmaceutical processes.

Small Quantities

When a prescription calls for less than 120 mg of an ingredient, a precise amount of the drug (greater than 120 mg) is mixed with an inert (inactive) powder so that a fraction of the resulting mix weighing at least 120 mg will contain the amount of drug needed. This fraction of the mixed powders is called an **aliquot.**

Balance

A balance is used to determine the weight of a powder, dosage form, liquid, etc. Most pharmacies have a **Class A prescription balance**. The Class A balance is a 2 pan torsion type balance which uses both internal and external weights. The balance has a rider which adds the internal weights to the right hand pan. The rider is always calibrated in the metric system (grams), though some riders also have calibration marks in the apothecary system (grains).

Sensitivity

Class A balances have a sensitivity requirement of up to 6 mg. The **sensitivity** of a balance is the amount of weight that will move the balance pointer one division mark on the marker plate.

Capacity

Class A balances have a minimum weighable quantity of 120 mg and most have a maximum weighable quantity of 60 grams, though some will weigh up to 120 grams.

Weights

A proper set of metric weights is essential for prescription compounding. These are usually brass cylindrical weights ranging from 1 gram to 50 gram and fractional weights of 10 mg to 500 mg. Weights should be stored in their box. They must be handled with forceps (not with fingers!) to prevent soiling and erosion of the weights.

calibrate to set, mark, or check the graduations of a measuring device.

aliquot a portion of a mixture.

trituration the process of grinding powders to reduce particle size.

sensitivity the amount of weight that will move the balance pointer one division mark on the marker plate.

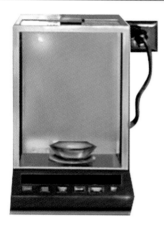

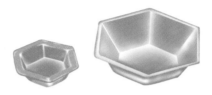

Electronic or Analytical balance

A method for weighing quantities smaller than 120 mg with acceptable accuracy is to use either an electronic or analytical balance. Electronic balances come in a variety of sizes and shapes. Most are top-loading balances and have sensitivities around 1 mg. Analytical balances may be found in some pharmacies, but are generally found in research laboratories. They have extremely high sensitivities and are designed to weigh milligram and microgram quantities of materials.

Weighing Papers or Weighing Boats

Weighing papers or weighing boats should always be placed on the balance pans before any weighing is done. These protect the pans from damage and also provide a convenient way to transfer the weighed material from the balance to another vessel. Weighing papers are made of nonabsorbable glassine paper and weighing boats are made of polystyrene. When using weighing papers, the paper should be diagonally creased from each corner and then flattened and placed on the pans. This ensures a collection trough in the paper. New weighing papers or weighing boats should be used with each new drug weighing to prevent contamination.

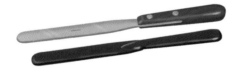

Spatulas

Spatulas are used to transfer solid ingredients. They are also used as the mixing instruments in semisolid dosage forms such as ointments and creams. Spatulas are available in a variety of sizes and are made of stainless steel, hard rubber, or plastic. Stainless steel spatulas can be corroded with certain materials such as iodine and in these cases, the rubber or plastic spatulas should be used. Always check that spatulas are clean before use.

Mortars and Pestles

Mortars and pestles are made of three types of materials: glass, wedgwood, and porcelain. Wedgwood and porcelain mortars are earthenware, relatively coarse in texture, and are used to 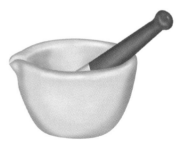 grind crystals and large particles into fine powders. The process of grinding powders to reduce the particle size is call **tritura-tion**. Glass mortars and pestles are preferable for mixing liquids and semisolid dosage forms.

USING A BALANCE

In order to obtain an accurate weight of components on the prescription balance, appropriate techniques must be used. The following steps should always be taken to insure accuracy.

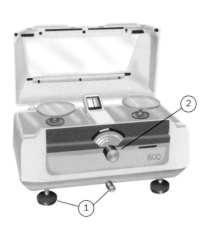

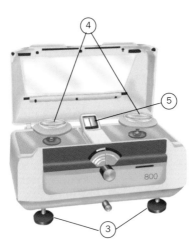

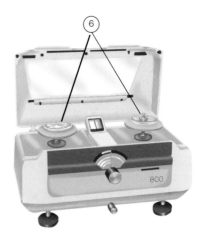

1. Lock the balance by turning the arrest knob. *Level the balance front to back* by turning the leveling screw feet all the way into the balance and then moving them the same direction until the 4 sides of the balance are equidistant from the benchtop. For balances with leveling bubbles, move the leveling screw feet until the bubble is in the middle of the tube.

2. Set the internal weights to zero. This is done by turning the calibrated dial (i.e., rider) to zero.

3. Unlock the balance and *level it left to right* by adjusting the leveling screw feet if needed. To shift the pointer left, grasp both screw feet between thumbs and forefingers and rotate so that the thumbs move inward. To shift the pointer to the right, rotate both screw feet so that the thumbs move outward. Continue adjusting the screw feet slowly until the pointer rests at the center of the marker plate.

4. Lock the balance. Place a weighing boat or glassine paper on each weighing pan. (If using weighing papers, fold diagonally and then gently flatten.)

5. Unlock the balance by releasing the arrest knob. If the pointer does not rest at the center of the marker plate, then level the balance from left to right to account for weight differences between the weigh boats or papers.

6. Lock the balance and place the required weights in the boat on the right pan. Place the material to be weighed in the boat on the left pan.

arrest knob the knob on a balance that prevents any movement of the balance pans.

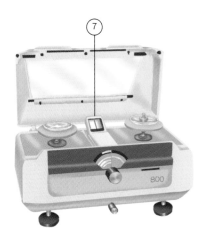

7. Unlock the balance and note the shift of the pointer on the marker plate. If the pointer shifts left, too much of the drug is on the pan and a portion should be removed. If it shifts right, there is too little drug and more should be added.

8. Once you have made an accurate measurement, double check to make sure that you have weighed the correct substance (check the label) and that you have used the correct weights (internal and external).

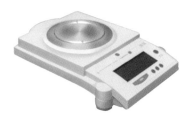

an electronic balance

Basic Guidelines for Using a Balance

There are some general rules about using a balance that help to maintain the balance in top condition.

✔ Always use the balance on a level surface and in a draft free area.

✔ Always cover both pans with weighing papers or use weighing boats. These protect the pans from abrasions, eliminate the need for repeated washing, and reduce loss of drug to porous surfaces.

✔ A clean paper or boat should be used for each new ingredient to prevent cross contamination of components.

✔ The balance must be readjusted after a new weighing paper or boat has been placed on each pan. Weighing papers taken from the same box can vary in weight by as much as 65 mg. Larger weighing boats can vary as much as 200 mg.

✔ Always arrest the balance before adding or removing weight from either pan. Although the balance is noted for its durability, repeated jarring of the balance will ultimately damage the working mechanism of the balance and reduce its accuracy.

✔ Use a spatula to add or remove ingredients from the balance. Do not pour ingredients out of the bottle.

✔ Always clean the balance, close the lid, and arrest the pans before storing the balance between uses.

Using an Electronic Balance

Electronic balances have digital displays and may have internal calibration capabilities. These may either be top-loading or encased to protect the balance from dust and drafts. To use an electronic balance, follow these guidelines:

✔ Always use the balance on a level surface in a draft free area.

✔ If the balance has a level bubble, make sure the bubble is inside the bulls eye and make adjustments in the leveling feet as needed.

✔ Place a weighing boat or a single sheet of weighing paper on the pan.

✔ When the balance has determined the final weight, press the tare bar to compensate for the weight of the weighing boat.

✔ As ingredients are added or removed from the weighing boat, the digital display will show the weight of the ingredient in the boat. Make sure the balance has determined the final weight before adding or removing any ingredient.

VOLUMETRIC EQUIPMENT

In compounding, liquid drugs, solvents, or additives are measured in volumetric glassware or plasticware.

Volumetric means "measures volume." Common volumetric vessels are pipets, cylindrical and conical graduates, burets, syringes, and volumetric flasks. The volume capacity is etched on the vessel wall, and some devices will have graduation marks to measure partial volume.

Volumetric vessels are either "to deliver" (TD) or "to contain" (TC).

"To deliver" means that the vessel must be completely emptied to dispense the needed volume. Single volume pipets, syringes, droppers and some calibrated pipets are TD vessels. "To contain" means that the vessel does not need to be completely emptied to dispense the needed volume. Volumetric flasks and cylindrical and conical graduated cylinders and some calibrated pipets are TC vessels.

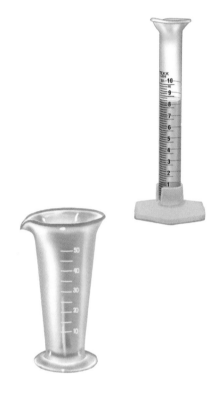

Graduated Cylinders

Graduated cylinders, both cylindrical and cone shaped, are used for measuring and transferring liquids. Cylindrical graduates are the preferred device because they are more accurate. Graduated cylinders are available in sizes ranging from 5 ml to 4,000 ml. When selecting a graduated cylinder, always choose the smallest one capable of containing the volume to be measured. Avoid measurements of volumes that are below 20 percent of the capacity of the graduated cylinder because the accuracy is unacceptable. For example, a 100 ml graduated cylinder cannot accurately measure volumes below 20 ml. When measuring small volumes, such as 20 ml and less, it is often preferable to use a syringe or pipet.

Volumetric Flasks

Volumetric flasks have slender necks and wide bulb-like bases. Volumetric flasks are single volume glassware and come in sizes ranging from 5 ml to 4,000 ml. There is a calibration mark etched on the neck of the flask. When the flask is filled to that mark, the flask contains that volume. Volumetric flasks are hard to use if dissolving solids in liquid because of the narrowness of the neck. If solids are to be dissolved in the flask, it is best to partially fill the flask with liquid, dissolve, and then fill the flask with more liquid to the calibration mark.

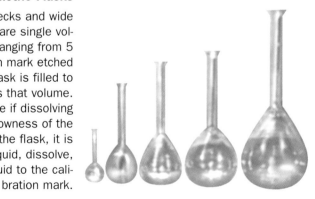

volumetric measures volume. Volumetric vessels are either TD (to deliver) or TC (to contain).

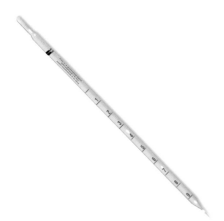

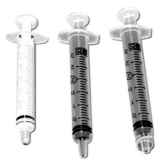

Pipets

Pipets are thin glass tubes recommended for the delivery of all volumes less than 5 ml and required for delivering volumes less than 1 ml (in the absence of an appropriate syringe). A rubber pipet bulb is used to draw liquid into the pipet. There are two basic types of pipets:

➥ The single volume or transfer pipet is the most accurate and simplest to use, but is limited to the measurement of a single fixed volume. They are normally used for the accurate transfer of 1.0, 2.0, 5.0, 10.0, and 25.0 ml of liquid.

➥ The calibrated pipet has several calibration marks from a point near the tip to the capacity of the pipet. It can deliver multiple volumes of liquid with good precision.

➥ A micropipet is a type of pipet with two parts, a handpiece and a disposal tip. The handle section usually has a turn screw that adjusts the volume of liquid drawn into the pipet tip. Each micropipet is calibrated for a range of volumes such as 1-20, 1-100, 1-200 or 1-1000 microliters. When determining which range to use, select the smallest range that will accommodate the volume of liquid to be measured.

Syringes

Syringes come in sizes from 0.5 ml to 60 ml and in a variety of materials and styles. For most compounding tasks involving small volumes, a disposable hypodermic syringe or an oral syringe made of plastic is used. Syringes have graduation marks on the barrel for measuring partial volumes. As when selecting a graduated cylinder, choose the smallest syringe capable of containing the volume to be measured.

 Erlenmeyer flasks (right), beakers, and prescription bottles, regardless of markings, are *not volumetric glassware*, but are simply containers for storing and mixing liquids. The designated volume is only the *approximate* capacity of the vessel.

LIQUID MEASUREMENT

Selecting a Liquid Measuring Device

✔ *Always use the smallest device (graduated cylinder, pipet, syringe) that will accommodate the desired volume of liquid.* This will minimize the potential for errors of measurement associated with misreading the scale.

✔ Use a calibrated pipet, micropipet, or syringe to measure/deliver volumes less than 1 ml.

✔ Remember that oily and viscous liquids will be difficult to remove from graduated cylinders and pipets, and at best require long drainage time. Consider using a syringe instead, or measuring by weight rather than volume.

✔ Never use prescription bottles, non-volumetric flasks, beakers, or household teaspoons as measurement devices.

✔ Liquids have a **meniscus** when they are poured into containers. The surface of the liquid curves downward toward the center. If the container is very narrow, the meniscus can be quite large. When reading a volume of a liquid against a graduation mark, *hold the measuring device so the meniscus is at eye level and read the mark at the bottom of the meniscus.* Viewing the level from above will create the incorrect impression that there is more volume in the measuring device.

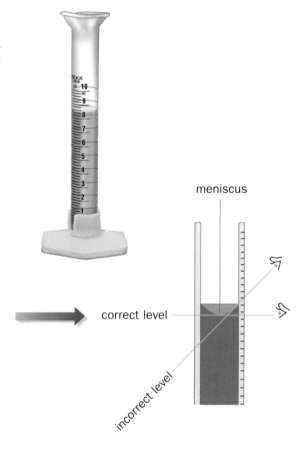

meniscus

correct level

incorrect level

Droppers

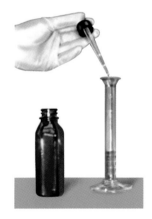

Medicine droppers can be used to deliver small doses of liquid medication. But the medicine dropper must first be calibrated because the drop size will vary from dropper to dropper and from liquid to liquid. Personal factors can also contribute to the inaccuracy of droppers. Two individuals dispensing the same liquid from identical droppers may produce drops of different sizes because of variations in the pressure, speed of dropping, and the angle at which the dropper is held.

To calibrate a medicine dropper, slowly drop the drug formulation into a small cylindrical graduate (10 ml), and count the number of drops needed to add several milliliters (ml) to the graduated cylinder. Calculate the average number of drops per ml. Some commercially produced medications are packaged with a marked dropper which has already been calibrated for that preparation.

Graduated Cylinders

Cylindrical graduates are more accurate than conical graduates. The following steps will help to maximize accuracy when using either a cylindrical or conical graduate.

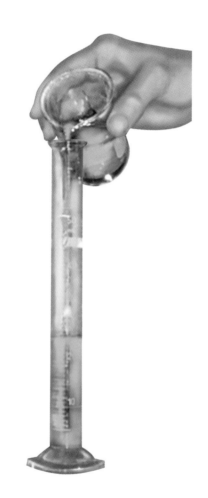

1. Either place the graduated cylinder on a flat surface that will allow you to view it at eye level or hold the graduated cylinder by the base with the left hand (for a right handed person) and elevated so that the desired mark is at eye level.

2. Hold the solution container with the right hand and pour the liquid to be measured into the center of the graduated cylinder. This will avoid the error resulting from liquid adhering to the wall of the graduated cylinder (especially viscous liquids).

3. As the surface of the liquid approaches the desired mark, decrease the pouring rate or use a dropper or pipet to bring the level to final volume. The final volume should be determined by aligning the bottom of the meniscus with the desired graduation mark.

4. Transfer the liquid from the graduated cylinder to the appropriate vessel or container, allowing about 15 seconds for aqueous and hydroalcoholic liquids to drain. Approximately 60 seconds (or more) will be required for more viscous liquids such as syrups, glycerin, propylene glycol, and mineral oil.

Special Precautions When Using Graduated Cylinders

✔ While graduated cylinders are volumetric devices, they are not mixing devices. They should not be used as the container to dissolve solids in liquids. A solution should be prepared in a beaker or flask, and then placed in the graduated cylinder for final volume adjustments.

✔ Do not assume that the final volume of a prescription will be the sum of the individual volumes of ingredients. This is particularly important with the admixture of aqueous and nonaqueous solutions such as alcohol and water. When these solutions are mixed, the total volume is less than the sum of the two volumes.

 meniscus the curved surface of a column of liquid.

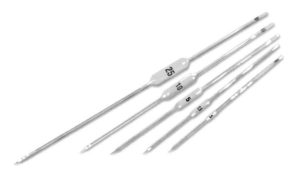

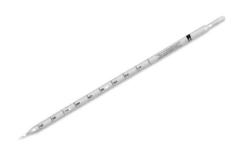

Single Volume Pipets

Single volume pipets have only one graduation mark, and that is the indicated volume of the pipet (e.g., 5 ml, 10 ml, etc.). As a result, the pipet is filled, and then emptied. There is no partial filling done with a single volume pipet. The steps in using a single volume pipet are:

1. Using a rubber bulb for suction, draw the liquid into the pipet until it is above the graduation mark.

2. Remove the pipet from the solution.

3. Wipe the end of the pipet with a tissue or Kimwipe.

4. While holding the pipet in a vertical position, release the pressure inside the bulb and allow the liquid to flow into a waste beaker until the bottom of the meniscus coincides with the graduation mark. Droplets which remain suspended from the tip of the pipet can be removed by touching the pipet to the inside of the waste beaker.

5. Allow the pipet to drain for 30 seconds (or up to 3 minutes for viscous liquids) while touching the tip of the pipet to the inner side of the receiving vessel.

Calibrated Pipets

The calibrated pipet is filled and emptied the same way as a single volume pipet. However, it has multiple graduation marks that allow partial volumes to be transferred by noting the meniscus level before and after delivery. For example, you can deliver 1.50 ml of a liquid by filling the pipet to 8.50 ml and then allowing it to drain until the meniscus reaches 7.00 ml. A second delivery could be made by allowing the meniscus to reach 5.50 ml. The final graduation of the pipet is usually some distance above the pipet tip so that delivery is performed from graduation to graduation and not from graduation to tip as with the single volume pipet.

From a practical standpoint, *the calibrated pipet is the preferred pipet for compounding.* Just about any prescription requiring small volumes can be compounded with just three basic sizes of pipets: a 1 ml pipet subdivided in 1/100 ml graduations, a 2 ml pipet subdivided in 1/10 ml graduations, and a 5 ml pipet subdivided in 1/10 ml graduations.

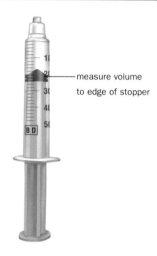

measure volume
to edge of stopper

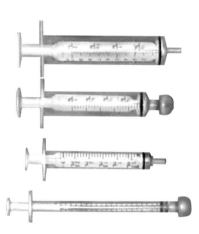

Syringes

Syringes come in a variety of sizes ranging from 0.5 ml (calibrated in 0.01 ml graduations) to 60 ml (calibrated in 2 ml graduations). Syringes may be used to deliver a wide range of liquid volumes with a high degree of accuracy. Measurements made with syringes are more accurate and precise than those made with cylindrical graduates. They are especially useful for measuring and delivering viscous liquids. Besides being easy to use, plastic disposable syringes are unbreakable and economical. Like graduated cylinders and pipets, select a syringe that equals or barely exceeds the volume to be measured.

Liquids are pulled into the syringe by pulling back on the plunger. The tip of the syringe must be fully submerged in the liquid to prevent drawing air into the syringe. Generally, an excess of solution is drawn into the syringe so that any air bubbles may be expelled by holding the syringe tip up, tapping the syringe until the air bubbles rise into the hub, and depressing the plunger to expel the air. This ensures that the hub will be completely filled with solution and the volume of delivery will be accurate.

Oral Syringes

Oral syringes are available for accurately administering liquid medication to the patient. They are especially useful when administering non-standard doses. Oral syringes have tips that are larger than tips on hypodermic syringes so needles can't be placed on these syringes. After the dose is drawn into the syringe, a cap is placed on the tip to prevent leakage and prevent contamination.

Oral syringes can be used with a device called an Adapt-a-Cap®. Adapt-a-Caps® do not work with hypodermic syringes (i.e., Slip-Tip® or Luer-Lok®). The cap portion of the Adapt-a-Cap® screws onto the bottle containing the liquid, and the oral syringe is fitted into the other side of the cap. When the bottle is inverted, liquid can be withdrawn by pulling back on the syringe plunger. When the required volume has been withdrawn, the bottle is righted, and the syringe is removed from the Adapt-a-Cap®.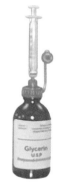

MIXING SOLIDS AND SEMISOLIDS

Mixing Powders

When mixing two powders of unequal quantity, a technique called **geometric dilution** is used. The smaller amount of powder is diluted in steps by additions of the larger amount of powder. If the two powders are just mixed together without this technique, a homogenous (fully and evenly combined) mixture will not result.

To correctly mix the powders, the smaller amount of powder is first triturated with an approximate equal portion of the larger amount of powder in a mortar. This first triturate is then mixed with an approximate equal portion of the larger amount of powder, and these are again triturated in the mortar. This dilution process is continued until all of the two powders have been mixed in the mortar.

Spatulation mixes powders using a spatula. The mixing can be done in a mortar, on an ointment slab, or in a plastic bag.

When powders are triturated together in a mortar with a pestle, the overall size of the particles is reduced. With spatulation, there is no particle size reduction so the powders must be of fine particle size and of uniform size before the process begins. There is also no pressure applied to the mixture when it is blended so the resulting blend is light and "fluffy."

This method is used when mixing eutectic compounds. Eutectic compounds liquefy when they are brought together. First the compounds should be mixed with a "carrier" powder (i.e., magnesium oxide, calcium carbonate, starch, lactose) and then blended by spatulation. Some eutectic compounds are aspirin, salicylic acid, camphor, benzocaine, and lidocaine.

Ointment Slabs

Some ointments and creams are prepared on ointment slabs which are porcelain or ground glass plates, often square or rectangular, that provide a hard nonabsorbable surface for mixing compounds. Spatulas are used to mix the ingredients of the formulation. Many times drugs are **levigated** prior to being incorporated into an ointment to reduce the grittiness of the final formulation.

GEOMETRIC DILUTION

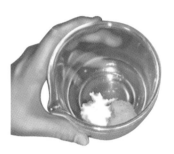

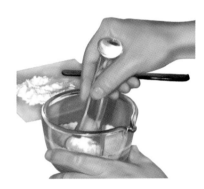

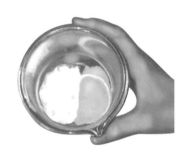

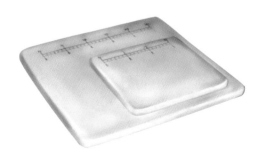

geometric dilution a technique for mixing two powders of unequal quantity.
spatulation mixing powders with a spatula.
levigation triturating a powder drug with a solvent in which it is insoluble to reduce its particle size.

Levigation

Levigation is a technique used to reduce the particle size of a powder drug by triturating it with a solvent in which the drug is insoluble. This is generally done before the drug is incorporated into a formulation such as a suspension, an ointment, a suppository base, etc. For example, hydrocortisone (used in ointments) is levigated with glycerin before being incorporated into an ointment base. This reduces the size of the hydrocortisone particles so the resulting ointment will be smooth, not gritty. Levigation can be done with a mortar and pestle or on an ointment slab.

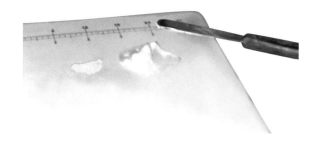

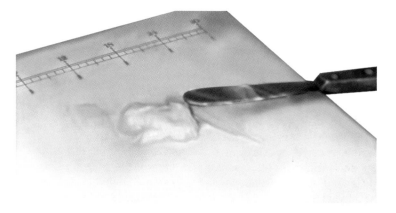

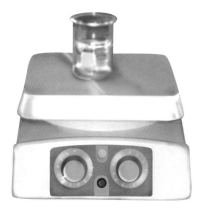

Hot Plates

Sometimes solids are mixed by melting them together in a beaker on a hotplate. The hotplate needs to be a special low temperature (25°C to 120°C) hotplate, and not a standard laboratory type hotplate; those hotplates heat at 125°C to 150°C at their lowest setting. If a low temperature hotplate is not available, a water bath or steam bath will suffice. Most solids and semisolids used in pharmaceutical compounding will completely melt by 70°C. The melt is removed from the hotplate and allowed to cool to room temperature with constant stirring using a stirring rod, spatula, or magnetic stirring bar. Forced cooling in cold water, ice water, or ice will change the consistency and texture of the final product.

COMPOUNDING PRINCIPLES FOR DOSAGE FORMS

Aqueous Solutions

Solutions are probably the most commonly compounded products. Solutions are clear liquids (but not necessarily colorless liquids) in which the drug is completely dissolved. The simplest compounded solution is the addition of a drug in liquid form to a liquid vehicle. This involves the careful measurement of the drug using graduated cylinders or syringes, and then diluting the drug to the final volume. The resulting mixture should be thoroughly shaken or stirred to ensure adequate mixing. Purified water is the most common solvent for pharmaceutical solutions, but combinations of ethanol, glycerin, propylene glycol, or a variety of syrups may be used, depending on the product requirements.

When solids are to be dissolved in solution, they must be carefully weighed using a prescription balance. Most solids dissolve easily in a solvent. However, some may need to be triturated first to reduce the particle size and increase the dissolution rate. Others require that the solvent be heated (but not overheated, since some drugs decompose at higher temperatures). Some drugs require vigorous shaking, stirring, or **sonication** (the application of sound waves using sonic mixing equipment) to affect dissolution.

The solubility of the drug must be known before attempting to dissolve it in a solution. If a drug is not soluble in a vehicle, then no amount of mixing will help.

The solubility of a drug in a solvent may be described in a variety of ways. References generally express the solubility in terms of the volume of solvent required to dissolve one gram of the drug. A small distinction, but an important one, needs to be made about these solubility values. The solubilities are given as grams of solute per milliliter of solvent, not per milliliter of final solution. If the concentration is going to be close to the solubility, this distinction may be relevant. Solubilities may also be expressed in more subjective terms such as those given in the table below.

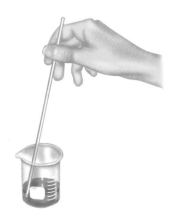

Most solutions require thorough shaking or stirring for adequate mixing.

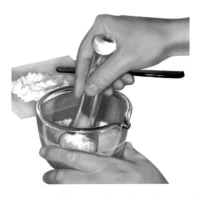

Some solids need to be triturated before mixing in a solution.

Descriptive Terms	Parts of Solvent Needed for 1 Part Solute
Very soluble	< 1
Freely soluble	1 - 10
Soluble	10 - 30
Sparingly soluble	30 - 100
Slightly soluble	100 - 1,000
Very slightly soluble	1,000 - 10,000
Practically insoluble or insoluble	> 10,000

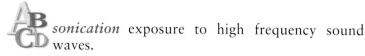

sonication exposure to high frequency sound waves.

Syrups

A syrup is a concentrated or nearly saturated solution of sucrose in water. Syrups containing flavoring agents are known as flavoring syrups (e.g., Cherry Syrup, Acacia Syrup, etc.); medicinal syrups are those which contain drugs (e.g., Guaifenesin Syrup).

When a reduction in calories or sucrose properties is desired, syrups can be prepared from sugars other than sucrose (e.g., glucose, fructose), non-sugar polyols (e.g., sorbitol, glycerin, propylene glycol, mannitol), or other non-nutritive artificial sweeteners (e.g., aspartame, saccharin). Non-nutritive sweeteners do not produce the same viscosity as with sugars and polyols, so viscosity enhancers such as methylcellulose are added. Polyols, though less sweet than sucrose, produce good viscosity and have some preservative and solvent qualities. A 70% sorbitol solution is a commercially available syrup vehicle.

Syrups are primarily made by two methods, with or without heat. Using heat is a faster method, but it cannot be used with heat sensitive ingredients. When using heat, the temperature must be carefully controlled to avoid overheating sucrose and making the syrup darker in color and more likely to ferment. When making syrups without heat, stirring or shaking generally provides the energy to produce the solution. In this case, a vessel that is about twice as large as the final volume of the product is needed to provide room for adequate mixing.

Nonaqueous Solutions

Nonaqueous solutions are those that contain solvents other than water, either alone or in addition to water. There are several types of nonaqueous solutions:

- ➡ elixir
- ➡ tincture
- ➡ spirit
- ➡ fluid extracts
- ➡ glycerates
- ➡ collodions
- ➡ liniments
- ➡ oleaginous solutions

Elixirs, collodions, and oleaginous solutions are the most commonly compounded nonaqueous solutions. Elixirs are clear, sweetened, hydroalcoholic liquids intended for oral use. Oleaginous solutions (e.g., corn oil, peanut oil, mineral oil) can be used for oral, topical, or parenteral administration. Collodions are limited to topical application. Because elixirs are hydroalcoholic solutions, they can be used to dissolve either alcohol soluble or water soluble drugs. Collodions and oleaginous solutions would be suitable for more lipophilic ingredients.

When compounding these formulations, separately dissolve the alcohol soluble ingredients in the alcohol (or oleaginous) portion and the water soluble ingredients in the water portion. Then add the aqueous solution to the alcohol solution, stirring constantly. This will keep the alcohol concentration as high as possible so that the final solution does not become turbid.

COMPOUNDING PRINCIPLES FOR DOSAGE FORMS (cont'd)

Suspensions

The term suspension refers to a two phase system consisting of a finely divided solid dispersed in a liquid. The smallest particle size that can be suspended is approximately 0.1 micrometer. The primary concern in formulating suspensions is that they tend to settle over time, so the dose is unevenly dispersed in the liquid. A well formulated suspension remains dispersed or settles very slowly, and can be redispersed easily with shaking. The settling properties of a suspension are controlled by (1) the addition of **flocculating agents** to enhance particle "dispersability" and (2) the addition of **thickening agents** to reduce the settling (sedimentation rate) of the suspension.

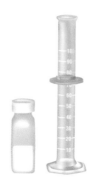

➡ Flocculating agents are electrolytes which carry an electrical charge. The flocculating agent imparts the electrical charge onto the suspended particle; since all of the particles will have the same charge, there is a slight repulsion between the particles as they settle. What results are clusters of particles or floccules which are loosely associated with each other and may be easily redispersed by shaking.

➡ Thickening agents are added to suspensions to thicken the suspending medium, thereby reducing the sedimentation rate of the floccules. Typical thickening agents include carboxymethylcellulose, methylcellulose, bentonite, and tragacanth.

To begin compounding a suspension, the solid drug to be suspended is levigated in a mortar with a pestle. This will reduce the drug's particle size. Common levigating agents are alcohol or glycerin. Then, a portion of the vehicle is added to the mortar, and mixed with the levigated drug until a uniform mixture results. This mixture is then put into the final container or a volumetric measuring device. The mortar and pestle are rinsed with portions of the remaining vehicle, and each rinsing is added to the final container or volumetric measuring device until the final volume is reached. Suspensions should be dispensed in containers that contain enough air space for adequate shaking. The bottle should contain the auxiliary label "Shake well."

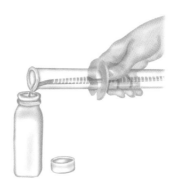

mixing

Some commercially available suspensions require reconstitution with water before they are dispensed. Water is added to the package container and shaken to form the suspension.

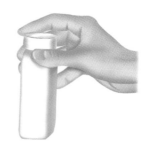

shaking

 flocculating agent electrolytes used in the preparation of suspensions to form particles that can easily be redispersed.
thickening agent an ingredient used in the preparation of suspensions to increase the viscosity of the liquid.

 Thickening agents are often referred to as viscosity enhancers or suspending agents.

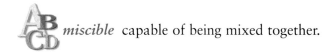

miscible capable of being mixed together.

Ointments and Creams

Ointments and creams are used for many different purposes, e.g., as protectants, antiseptics, emollients, antipruritics, kerotolytics, and astringents. Ointments are simple mixtures of a drug(s) in an ointment base. There are five types of ointment bases ranging from oleaginous to water **miscible**. A particular ointment base is chosen for its fundamental properties, or for its potential to serve as a drug delivery vehicle. Creams are emulsions that are used topically for their emollient properties. They are either thick liquids or soft semi-solids.

If the base is to be a drug delivery vehicle, the primary consideration will be its ability to release drug. Oleaginous (oil based) bases generally release substances slowly and unpredictably, since water cannot penetrate them well enough to dissolve the drug and allow for diffusion out of the ointment. Water miscible or aqueous bases tend to release drugs more rapidly.

Ointments are generally compounded on an ointment slab. In the simple case of combining two ointments or creams, each component is carefully weighed and placed on an ointment slab. The ointments are combined by geometric dilution using two spatulas to mix the ointments. One spatula will be used to continually remove ointment from the other spatula. Using the spatula, transfer the mixture into an ointment jar just big enough for the final volume. When filling the ointment jar, use the spatula to bleed out air pockets. Wipe any excess material from the outside of the jar, including the cap screw threads.

Drugs in powder or crystal form, such as salicylic acid, precipitated sulfur, or hydrocortisone, need to be triturated or levigated in a mortar with a pestle before incorporating them into an ointment base. This will prevent a gritty texture in the final product. Another technique to reduce particle size is to dissolve the drug (if soluble) in a very small amount of solvent, and then let the solvent evaporate.

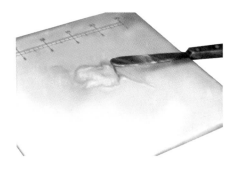

Ointments are generally compounded on an ointment slab.

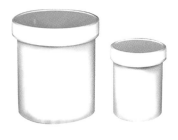

ointment jars

Properties of Ointment Bases

Property	Oleaginous Bases	Absorption Bases	Water/Oil Emulsion Bases	Oil/Water Emulsion Bases	Water Miscible Bases
Water Content	anhydrous	anhydrous	hydrous	hydrous	hydrous
Spreadability	difficult	difficult	moderate to easy	easy	moderate to easy
Washability	nonwashable	nonwashable	non- or poorly washable	washable	washable
Greasiness	greasy	greasy	greasy	nongreasy	nongreasy
Occlusiveness	yes	yes	sometimes	no	no
Examples	White Petrolatum, White Ointment	Hydrophillic Petrolatum, Aquaphor®	Hydrous Lanolin, Eucerin®, Nivea®	Hydrophillic Ointment	PEG Ointment

COMPOUNDING PRINCIPLES FOR DOSAGE FORMS (cont'd)

Emulsions

An emulsion is an unstable system consisting of at least two **immiscible** liquids, one of which is dispersed in the form of small droplets throughout the other, and a stabilizing agent. The dispersed liquid is known as the internal or discontinuous phase, whereas the liquid serving as the dispersion medium is known as the external or continuous phase.

emulsion before mixing

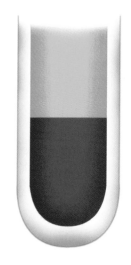

Oil-in-Water (o/w) Emulsions

When oils, petroleum hydrocarbons, and/or waxes are the dispersed phase, and water or an aqueous solution is the continuous phase, the system is called an oil-in-water (o/w) emulsion. An o/w emulsion is generally formed if the aqueous phase makes up greater than 45% of the total weight, and a **hydrophilic emulsifier** is used.

Water-in-Oil (w/o) Emulsions

When water or aqueous solutions are dispersed in an oleaginous (oil based) medium, the system is known as a water-in-oil (w/o) emulsion. W/O emulsions are generally formed if the aqueous phase constitutes less than 45% of the total weight and an **lipophilic emulsifier** is used.

Emulsifiers

Emulsions will separate into two distinct phases or layers over time. Some separation can be overcome with shaking. However, some separations results in emulsions that "break" and these cannot be redispersed. Emulsions are stabilized by adding an emulsifier or emulsifying agents. Emulsifiers provide a protective barrier around the dispersed droplets. Some commonly used emulsifying agents include tragacanth, sodium lauryl sulfate, sodium dioctyl sulfosuccinate, and polymers known as the Spans® and Tweens®.

a close-up after mixing

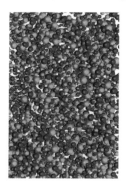

ABCD *immiscible* cannot be mixed.
emulsifier a stabilizing agent in emulsions.
water-in-oil emulsion an emulsion in which water is dispersed through an oil base.
oil-in-water emulsion an emulsion in which oil is dispersed through a water base.
hydrophilic emulsifier a stabilizing agent for water based dispersion mediums.
lipophilic emulsifier a stabilizing agent for oil based dispersion mediums.

 Stabilizing agents used in emulsions are called emulsifiers, surfactants, or surface active agents.

Methods for Preparing Emulsions

There are various methods used to make emulsions. Each requires that energy be put into the system in the form of either shaking, heat, or the action of a mortar and pestle.

The **Continental method** is one method for preparing emulsions. This is sometimes referred to as the **Dry Gum method**. In this method, the **initial or primary emulsion** is formed from oil, water, and a "gum" type emulsifier which is usually acacia. The primary emulsion is formed from 4 parts oil, 2 parts water, and 1 part emulsifier. The 4 parts oil and 1 part emulsifier represent their total amounts for the final product. In a dry wedgwood or porcelain mortar, the 1 part gum is triturated with the 4 parts oil until the powder is thoroughly levigated. Then the 2 parts water are added, and the mixture is vigorously and continually triturated until the primary emulsion is formed (usually 1 - 2 minutes). It appears as creamy white and produces a "cracking" sound as it is triturated. Additional ingredients are incorporated after the primary emulsion is formed, and the product is then brought to the final volume with the external phase vehicle.

In the **Wet Gum method,** the primary emulsion is formed by triturating the 1 part gum with 2 parts water to form a **mucilage,** and then slowly adding the 4 parts oil, in portions, with trituration after each addition. After all the oil is added, the mixture is triturated for several minutes to form the primary emulsion. Then other ingredients may be added as in the Continental method.

Some emulsions will have a consistency of a lotion or a cream (i.e., a semisolid). The method of choice in making these types of emulsions is the **beaker method.** The ingredients of the formulation are divided into water soluble and oil soluble components. All oil soluble components are dissolved in one beaker and all water soluble components are dissolved in a separate beaker. Both phases are then heated to approximately 70°C using a low temperature hotplate or steam bath. The two beakers are removed from the heat, and the internal phase is slowly added to the external phase with continual stirring. The product is allowed to cool to room temperature but is constantly stirred with a stirring rod, spatula, or magnetic stirring bar.

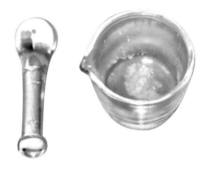

gum and water in preparation for the Wet Gum method

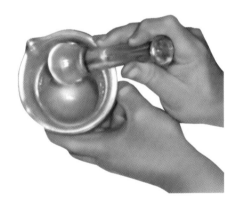

forming the mucilage

primary emulsion the initial emulsion to which ingredients are added to create the final product.

mucilage a wet, slimy liquid formed as an initial step in the wet gum method.

COMPOUNDING PRINCIPLES FOR DOSAGE FORMS (cont'd)

Suppositories

There are three classes of suppository bases defined by their composition and physical properties:

➡ Oleaginous bases

➡ Water soluble or miscible bases

➡ Hydrophilic bases

Oleaginous Bases

A well known oleaginous base is cocoa butter (Theobroma Oil) USP. At room temperature, cocoa butter is a solid, but at body temperature, it melts to a bland, nonirritating oil. Cocoa butter is no longer the base of choice because preparing suppositories with it is difficult, and the suppositories require refrigeration. Synthetic triglycerides can be used that do not have the formulation difficulties of cocoa butter, but they are more expensive. There are also newer bases composed of mixtures of fatty acids that do not have the formulation problems or the expense.

Water Soluble or Miscible Bases

Water soluble or miscible bases contain glycerinated gelatin or polyethylene glycol (PEG) polymers. Glycerinated gelatin is a useful suppository base, particularly for vaginal suppositories. Glycerinated gelatin suppositories are gelatinous solids that tend to dissolve slowly to provide prolonged release of active ingredients. **Polyethylene glycol (PEGs)** polymers are chemically stable, non irritating, miscible with water and mucous secretions, and can be formulated by molding or compression in a wide range of hardnesses and melting points. Like glycerinated gelatin, they do not melt at body temperature, but dissolve slowly to provide a prolonged release of drugs.

Polyethylene glycols are available in various molecular weight ranges. Those of 200, 400, or 600 molecular weight are liquids. Those with molecular weights over 1,000 are solids. Certain PEGs may be used individually as suppository bases but, more commonly, formulas call for combinations of two or more molecular weights mixed in various proportions to give a desired hardness or dissolution time. Since PEGs suppositories dissolve in body fluids and need not be formulated to melt at body temperature, they can be formulated with much higher melting points and can be safely stored at room temperature.

Hydrophilic Bases

Hydrophilic bases are mixtures of oleaginous and water miscible bases. They generally contain a small percentage of cholesterol or lanolin to assist in water absorption.

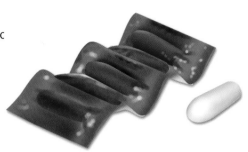

Some PEG Formulations

Molecular Weight	Percent
PEG 300	60%
PEG 8000	40%
PEG 300	48%
PEG 6000	52%
PEG 1000	95%
PEG 3350	5%
PEG 1000	75%
PEG 3350	25%
PEG 300	10%
PEG 1540	65%
PEG 3350	25%
PEG 8000	50%
PEG 1540	30%
PEG 400	20%
PEG 3350	60%
PEG 1000	30%
PEG 400	10%

compression molding a method of making suppositories in which the ingredients are compressed in a mold.

fusion molding a suppository preparation method in which the active ingredients are dispersed or dissolved in a melted suppository base.

Molding Methods

Suppositories are usually prepared by **compression molding** or **fusion molding.** Compression molding is a method of preparing suppositories by mixing the suppository base and the drug ingredients and forcing the mixture into a special compression mold.

Fusion molding is a method in which the drug is dispersed or dissolved in a melted suppository base. The fusion method can be used with all types of suppositories and must be used with most of them. In this method, the suppository base is melted on a low temperature hotplate, and the drug is dissolved or dispersed in the melted base. The mixture is then removed from the heat, and poured into a suppository mold, overfilling each cavity. The mixture is allowed to congeal (harden), and the excess material is removed from the top of the mold.

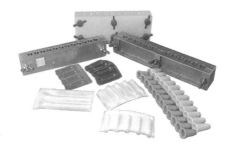

types of suppository molds

Suppository Molds

There are many types of suppository molds: metal (aluminum or steel) molds, plastic molds, or rubber molds. The metal molds come in a variety of cavity sizes, from six to one hundred. The two halves of the mold are held together with screws. When the suppository mixture has congealed, the excess mass on top of the suppository mold can be removed with a hot spatula or knife scraped flat across the surface of the mold. The screws on the mold are loosened, and the mold is separated. Never open a mold by prying it apart with a knife or spatula. This will damage the matching mold faces which have been accurately machined to give a tight seal. The suppositories are removed from the mold, generally wrapped in foil paper, and put in a suppository box.

Plastic suppository molds come in long strips and can be torn into any number of cavities. When the suppository has hardened in the cavity, the plastic mold is heat sealed, torn into individual suppository cavities, and put in a suppository box. Rubber molds come in long strips but cannot be separated into individual cavities. Suppositories are allowed to remain in the mold (i.e, unwrapped), and the entire mold is put in the dispensing box.

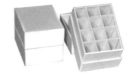

a suppository box

 Polyethylene glycol polyers (PEGs) are used in a wide variety of formulations. Low molecular weight PEGs (<1,000) are liquids and impart a softer texture to the formulation. High molecular weight PEGs (>1,000) are solids and add stiffness to the formulation.

COMPOUNDING PRINCIPLES FOR DOSAGE FORMS (cont'd)

Capsules

Hard gelatin capsules consist of a body and a cap which fits firmly over the body of the capsule. For human use, eight sizes of capsules are available. If the capsule is to be filled with a liquid then the volume of the capsule needs to be known. As a guide, the left-hand table below provides capsule sizes and their relative liquid fill capacities.

The total amount of a non-liquid formulation that can be placed in a capsule varies according to the bulk density of the formulation. Several methods have been devised to help select the appropriate size capsule for a particular powder formulation. One method is to compare the density of the formulation being compounded to the density of a known drug: Similar amounts of powder with similar densities will fit in the same size capsule. For example, if a formulation has a density similar to aspirin and 300 mg are needed for each dose, then a #1 capsule would be needed based on the information in the right-hand table below. In general, the smallest capsule that will contain the formulation is used since patients often have difficulty swallowing large capsules.

When filling a small number of capsules, the **"punch" method** is used. The ingredients are triturated to the same particle size and then mixed by geometric dilution. Since some powder will be lost in the punching process, calculate for the preparation of at least two extra capsules. The powder is placed on an ointment slab and smoothed with a spatula to a height approximately half the length of the capsule body. The body of the capsule is held vertically and the open end is repeatedly pushed or "punched" into the powder until the capsule is filled. The cap is then replaced to close the capsule. Each filled capsule is weighed using an empty capsule as a counterweight. Powder is added or removed until the correct weight has been placed in the capsule.

Capsule filling machines are available for filling 100 capsules at a time. The machines come with a capsule loader which correctly aligns all of the capsules in the machine base. The powder is poured onto the base plate and special spreaders and combs are used to fill the individual capsules. All of the caps are simultaneously returned to the capsule bodies, and the batch is complete. When using a capsule filling machine, it takes practice to ensure that each capsule has the same amount of drug. There is a tendency to overfill the capsules in the center, and underfill the capsules around the edges.

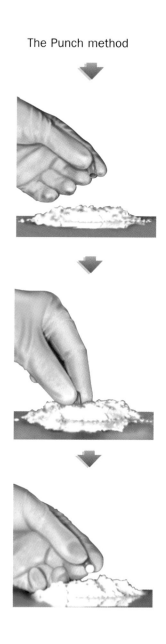

The Punch method

Capsule Size	Liquid Volume (ml)	Capsule Size	Liquid Volume (ml)
000	1.37	2	0.37
00	0.95	3	0.30
0	0.68	4	0.20
1	0.50	5	0.13

punch method a method for filling capsules by repeatedly pushing or "punching" the capsule into an amount of drug powder.
finger cots protective coverings for fingers.

Other Tips for Compounding Capsules:

➡ It is a good practice to remove the exact number of empty capsules needed from the capsule box before compounding begins. This will avoid preparing the wrong number of capsules and will prevent the contamination of other empty capsules with drug particles that cling to hands.

➡ The simplest method to keep a capsule free of moisture during compounding is to use the cap of one capsule as a holder for other capsule bodies during the filling operation. This avoids the capsules coming into contact with the fingers. Another way of protecting the capsules is to wear **finger cots** or rubber gloves.

➡ To remove traces of drug from the outside of the filled capsules, roll them between the folds of clean towel or shake in a towel that has been gathered into the form of a bag.

➡ Liquids that do not dissolve gelatin, e.g., alcohol and fixed oils, may be dispensed in capsules. By calibrated dropper or pipet, the correct volume of liquid is delivered into the empty capsule body. None of the liquid should touch the outside of the body and the size of the capsule should be chosen so that the liquid does not completely fill the body. The capsule is sealed by moistening the lower portion of the inside of the cap with warm water using a camel's hair brush. The moistened cap is placed on the body and given a half turn. The capsules should be placed on an absorbent paper and inspected for leakage.

➡ Capsules will absorb moisture and soften in high humidity. In a dry atmosphere, they become brittle and crack. To protect capsules from the extremes of humidity, dispense them in plastic or glass vials, and store in a cool, dry place. A piece of cotton may be added in the top of the vial to keep the capsules from rattling.

Capsule Size	Mg of Lactose	Mg of Aspirin
000	1250	975
00	850	650
0	600	490
1	460	335
2	350	260
3	280	195
4	210	130
5	140	65

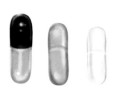

REVIEW

KEY CONCEPTS

COMPOUNDING

✔ Extemporaneous compounding is the on-demand preparation of a drug product according to a physician's prescription, formula, or recipe.

COMPOUNDING GUIDELINES

✔ Two professional organizations that have published guidelines for compounding are the National Association of Boards of Pharmacy and the American Society of Health-System Pharmacists.

EQUIPMENT

✔ Class A prescription balances can weigh as little as 120 mg of material with a 5% error.

✔ Aliquots can be used when weighing an amount of ingredient that is less than 120 mg.

USING A BALANCE

✔ Class A prescription balances need to be leveled from front-to-back and side-to-side before any ingredient is weighed.

✔ Weighing papers or weighing boats should always be placed on the balance pans before any weighing is done.

VOLUMETRIC EQUIPMENT

✔ Liquid drugs, solvents, or additives are measured in volumetric glassware or plasticware.

✔ Erlenmeyer flasks, beakers, and prescription bottles, regardless of markings, are not volumetric glassware.

LIQUID MEASUREMENT

✔ Always use the smallest device (graduated cylinder, pipet, syringe) that will accommodate the desired volume of liquid.

✔ When reading a volume of a liquid against a graduation mark, hold the graduated cylinder so the meniscus is at eye level and read the mark at the bottom of the meniscus.

MIXING SOLIDS AND SEMISOLIDS

✔ Trituration is the fine grinding of a powder. Levigation is the trituration of a powder drug with a solvent in which the drug is insoluble. Both techniques reduce the particle size of the drug.

COMPOUNDING PRINCIPLES FOR DOSAGE FORMS

✔ Aqueous solutions are clear liquids (but not necessarily colorless) made most commonly with purified water but which may also contain ethanol, glycerin, or propylene glycol.

✔ Nonaqueous solutions include elixirs, tinctures, spirits, collodions, liniments, and oleaginous solution.

✔ Suspensions are a two phase system consisting of a finely divided solid dispersed in a liquid.

✔ An emulsion is an unstable system consisting of at least two immiscible (unmixable) liquids, one that is dispersed as small droplets throughout the other, and a stabilizing agent.

✔ There are three classes of suppository bases defined by their composition and physical properties: oleaginous bases, water soluble or miscible bases, and hydrophilic bases.

✔ When preparing capsules, the smallest capsule capable of containing the final formulation is used since patients often have difficulty swallowing large capsules.

SELF TEST

MATCH THE TERMS.   *answers can be checked in the glossary*

arrest knob

flocculating agent

geometric dilution

hydrophilic emulsifier

levigation

lipophilic emulsifier

meniscus

punch method

stability

suspending agent

trituration

- the chemical and physical integrity of the dosage unit and its ability to withstand microbiological contamination.
- the knob on a balance that prevents any movement of the balance pans.
- the curved surface of a column of liquid.
- the fine grinding of a powder.
- triturating a powder drug with a solvent in which it is insoluble to reduce its particle size.
- a technique for mixing two powders of unequal quantity.
- electrolytes used in the preparation of suspensions.
- a thickening agent used in the preparation of suspensions.
- a stabilizing agent for water based dispersion mediums.
- a stabilizing agent for oil based dispersion mediums.
- a method for filling capsules.

CHOOSE THE BEST ANSWER   *the answer key begins on page 347*

1. _____ is the on-demand preparation of a drug product according to a physician's prescription.
   a. IVPB
   b. Extemporaneous compounding
   c. Trituration
   d. Spatulation

2. _____ is a term for the chemical and physical integrity of the dosage unit.
   a. Stability
   b. Suspensibility
   c. Solubility
   d. Miscibility

3. Which of the chemical grades listed below has the highest purity?
   a. USP/NF
   b. AR
   c. HPLC
   d. FCC

4. Which record will document how a compounded formula was actually prepared?
   a. formulation record
   b. compounding record
   c. standard operating procedure
   d. material safety data sheet

REVIEW

5. Aliquots can be used when a prescription calls for less than _____ of an ingredient.
   a. 120 gm
   b. 500 gm
   c. 500 mg
   d. 120 mg

6. When using a Class A prescription balance,
   a. the weight goes on the left pan and the powder goes on the right pan.
   b. the weight goes on the right pan and the powder goes on the left pan.
   c. no need to place weights, as the weight can be adjusted internally.
   d. Class A balances only have one pan to weigh powders.

7. The sensitivity requirement of a Class A prescription balance is
   a. 6 micrograms.
   b. 60 micrograms.
   c. 60 milligrams.
   d. 6 milligrams.

8. The maximum weighable amount for most Class A prescription balances is
   a. 60 micrograms.
   b. 60 grams.
   c. 6 milligrams.
   d. 6 grams.

9. _____ are used as mixing instruments for ointments and creams.
   a. Volumetric flasks
   b. Spatulas
   c. Erlenmeyer flasks
   d. Droppers

10. Which type of mortar and pestle is recommended for mixing liquids and semisolids?
    a. wedgwood
    b. porcelain
    c. glass
    d. earthenware

11. Which type of glassware is "TC" (i.e., "to contain"?
    a. Erlenmeyer flasks
    b. single volume pipet
    c. beaker
    d. volumetric flask

12. A 100 ml graduated cylinder cannot accurately measure volumes less than
    a. 20 ml.
    b. 50 ml.
    c. 30 ml.
    d. 40 ml.

13. _____ are volumetric vessels and can be used to accurately measure liquids for compounding.
    a. Volumetric flasks, graduated cylinders, pipets, and syringes
    b. Beakers
    c. Erlenmeyer flasks and beakers
    d. Erlenmeyer flasks

14. Medicine droppers
    a. cannot be used to deliver small doses of medication.
    b. can be used to deliver small doses of medication if they are calibrated.
    c. can be used to deliver small doses of medication without calibration.
    d. can only be used to deliver water.

15. Which type of syringe is used to administer a dose of liquid medication to a patient?
    a. hypodermic with Luer-Lok® tip
    b. oral syringe
    c. hypodermic with Slip-Tip®
    d. Adapt-a-Cap®

16. _____ is the technique used to mix two powders of unequal quantity.
    a. Volumetric dilution
    b. Volumetric emulsification
    c. Geometric emulsification
    d. Geometric dilution

17. The fine grinding of a powder is called
    a. extemporaneous compounding.
    b. suspension.
    c. emulsion.
    d. trituration.

18. Compounds that liquefy when they are brought together are called
    a. transitional.
    b. sublime.
    c. eutectic.
    d. valent.

19. Clear liquids in which the drug is completely dissolved are called
    a. sublimations.
    b. suspensions.
    c. solutions.
    d. emulsions.

20. Which of the following is not a method used to reduce particle size?
    a. melting
    b. trituration
    c. levigation
    d. suspension

21. Which is a required ingredient in a suspension?
    a. flocculating agent
    b. surface acting agent
    c. levigating agent
    d. emulsifying agent

22. A system containing two immiscible liquids with one dispersed in the other is called
    a. an emulsion.
    b. a suspension.
    c. a syrup.
    d. a solution.

23. Which of the following can have the consistency of an ointment?
    a. emulsion
    b. suspension
    c. syrup
    d. elixir

HOW DRUGS WORK

Drugs produce either desired or undesired effects on the body.

Once they are in the blood, drugs are circulated throughout the body. The properties of both the drug and the body influence where the drug will go, and what concentration it will have at each place. The place where a drug causes an effect to occur is called the **site of action**. Some of the effects caused by the drug are desired effects, and some are undesired. *The objective of drug therapy is to deliver the right drug, in the right concentration, to the right site of action, and at the right time to produce the desired effect.*

When a drug produces an effect, it is interacting at a molecular level with cellular material or structure.

The cellular material directly involved in the action of the drug is called its **receptor**. The receptor is often described as a lock into which the drug molecule fits as a key, and only those drugs able to bind chemically to the receptors in a particular site of action can produce effects at that site. This is why specific cells only respond to certain drugs, even though their receptors are exposed to any drug molecules that are present in the body. This is also why drugs are **selective** in their action, that is, they only act on specific targeted receptors and the tissues they affect.

Receptors are located on the surfaces of cell membranes and inside cells.

There are many different types of receptors, each type having a different influence on the body's processes. Most receptors can be found throughout the body, though some occur in only a few places.

---

 site of action the location where an administered drug produces an effect.

receptor the cellular material at the site of action that interacts with the drug.

selective (action) the characteristic of a drug that makes its action specific to certain receptors and the tissues they affect.

DRUG ACTION AT THE SITE OF ACTION

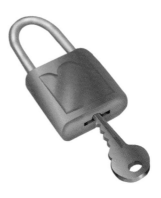

Like a lock and key, only certain drugs are able to interact with certain receptors.

Types of Action

When drugs interact with the site of action, they can:

➡ act through physical action, as with the protective effects of ointments upon topical application;

➡ react chemically, as with antacids that reduced excess gastric acidity;

➡ modify the metabolic activity of pathogens, as with antibiotics;

➡ change the osmolarity of blood and draw water out of tissues and into the blood;

➡ incorporate into cellular material to interfere with normal cell function;

➡ join with other chemicals to form a complex that is more easily excreted;

➡ modify the biochemical or metabolic process of the body's cells or enzyme systems.

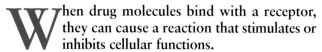

When drug molecules bind with a receptor, they can cause a reaction that stimulates or inhibits cellular functions.

The pharmacological effects of these interactions are termed **agonism** or **antagonism**. **Agonists** are drugs that activate receptors and produce a response that may either accelerate or slow normal cellular processes, depending on the type of receptor involved. For example, epinephrine-like drugs act on the heart to increase the heart rate, and acetylcholine-like drugs act on the heart to slow the heart rate. Both are agonists. **Antagonists** are drugs that bind to receptors but do not activate them. They block the receptors' action by preventing other drugs or substances from interacting with them.

The number of receptors available to interact with a drug will directly influence the effect.

A minimum number of receptors have to be occupied by drug molecules to produce an effect. If there are too few drug molecules to occupy the necessary number of receptors, there will be little or no effect. In this case, increasing the dosage will increase the effect. On the other hand, once all the receptors are occupied, increasing the dosage will not increase the effect.

Receptors can be changed by drug use.

For example, extended stimulation of cells with an agonist can reduce the number or sensitivity of the receptors, and the effect of the drug is reduced. Extended inhibition of cell functions with an antagonist can increase the number or sensitivity of receptors. If the antagonist is stopped abruptly, the cells can have an extreme reaction to an agonist. To avoid such withdrawal symptoms, some drugs must be gradually discontinued.

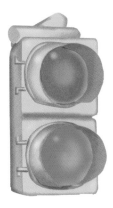

antagonists
block action

agonists activate
receptors

Other Drug Actions

➡ Some drugs work by changing the ability of ions to move into or out of cells. For example, sodium or calcium ion channels can open and allow movement of the ions into nerve cells, stimulating their function. With potassium channels, the opposite can happen. The channels can open and allow the movement of potassium ions out of nerve cells, obstructing their function.

➡ Some drugs modify the creation, release, or control of nerve cell hormones that regulate different physiological processes.

agonist drugs that activate receptors to accelerate or slow normal cellular function.

antagonist drugs that bind with receptors but do not activate them. They block receptor action by preventing other drugs or substances from activating them.

 The objective of drug therapy is to deliver the right drug, in the right concentration, to the right site of action, and at the right time to produce the desired effect.

CONCENTRATION & EFFECT

It is difficult to measure the amount of a drug at the site of action and therefore to predict an effect based upon that measurement.

One problem is that many factors influence a drug's movement from the site of administration to the site of action (metabolism, excretion, membrane permeability, etc.). It can also be physically impossible to measure the drug at the site of action either because of its unknown location or small size.

One way to monitor the amount of a drug in the body and its effect at the site of action is to use a dose-response curve.

Using a dose-response curve, you would expect a certain effect for any given dose. However, when a series of drug doses is given to a number of people, the results show that some people respond to low doses but others require larger doses for an equal response to be produced. This is due to human variability: different people have different characteristics that affect how a drug product behaves in them. Some differences are due to the product itself, but most come from how the drug is transported from the site of administration to the site of action, and how it interacts with the receptor. For these reasons, dose-response curves are not ideal for relating the amount of drug in the body to its effect.

A better way to relate the amount of a drug in the body to its effect is to determine drug concentrations in the body's fluids.

Of the body's fluids, blood is generally used because of its rapid equilibrium between the site of administration and the site of action. As a result, knowing a drug's concentration in the blood can be directly related to its effect and this is the most common way to analyze the potential effect of a drug.

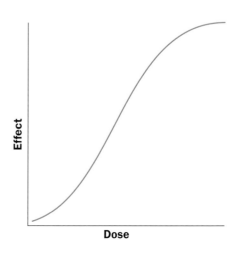

A typical dose-response curve shows that a response increases as the dose is increased.

Blood Concentration-Time Profiles

Blood concentration-time profiles have these applications:

➡ Manufacturers use the data to evaluate their drug products.

➡ Pharmacy professionals use them to visualize the consequences of incorrectly compounding a formulation or of using the wrong route of administration.

➡ Researchers and clinicians use them to measure human variability in drug product performance (e.g., influence of age, gender, nationality, or disease).

➡ Physicians and pharmacists use them to monitor the drug therapy of patients.

 biopharmaceutics the study of the factors associated with drug products and physiological processes, and the resulting systemic concentrations of the drugs.

minimum effective concentration (MEC) the blood concentration needed for a drug to produce a response.

onset of action the time MEC is reached and the response occurs.

therapeutic window a drug's blood concentration range between its MEC and MTC.

An advantage of using blood concentrations as a measure of the "drug amount in the body" is that blood can be repeatedly sampled.

When sampling covers several hours or more, a blood concentration-time profile can be developed. Plasma or serum concentrations can be used instead of blood concentrations, and the same type of profile will result.

For many drugs, changes in the blood concentration-time profile reflect changes in concentration at the site of action and therefore changes in effect.

There are exceptions to this. The concentration of some drugs in the site of action produces an action hours or days later. Other drugs show no relationship between blood concentrations and concentrations in the site of action. Still others don't depend on blood concentrations at all to produce an effect.

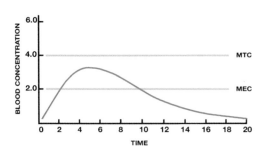

a blood concentration-time profile

A Sample Profile

The illustration above shows a typical blood concentration–time profile for a drug given orally. The blood concentration begins at zero at the time the drug is administered (before it has been absorbed into the blood). With time, the drug leaves the formulation and enters the blood, causing concentrations to rise. To produce an effect, the concentrations must achieve a **minimum effective concentration (MEC).** This is when there is enough drug at the site of action to produce a response. The time this occurs is called the **onset of action.** With most drugs, when blood concentrations increase, so does the intensity of the effect, since *blood concentrations reflect the concentrations at the site of action that produce the response.*

Some drugs have an upper blood concentration limit beyond which there are undesired or toxic effects. This limit is called the **minimum toxic concentration (MTC).** The range between the minimum effective concentration and the minimum toxic concentration is called the **therapeutic window.** *When concentrations are in this range, most patients receive the maximum benefit from their drug therapy with a minimum of risk.*

The last part of the curve shows the blood concentrations declining as absorption is complete and elimination is proceeding. The time between the onset of action and the time when the minimum effective concentration is reached by the declining blood concentrations is called the **duration of action.** The duration of action is the time the drug should produce the desired effect.

minimum toxic concentration (MTC) the upper limit of the therapeutic window. Drug concentrations above the MTC increase the risk of undesired effects.

duration of action the time drug concentration is above the MEC.

ADME PROCESSES & DIFFUSION

Blood concentrations are the result of four simultaneously occurring processes: absorption, distribution, metabolism, and excretion.

These four processes are referred to as the **ADME processes**, but may also be called **disposition**. Metabolism and excretion combined are called **elimination**.

The transfer of drug into the blood from an administered drug product is called absorption.

When a drug product is first administered, absorption is the primary process. Distribution, metabolism, and excretion will also occur, but the amount of drug available for them is much less than the amount of drug available for absorption. So these processes have little effect. As more of the drug is absorbed into the blood, it is available to undergo these other processes and their roles increase.

A drug's distribution will be affected by physiological functions and its own properties.

Though blood may deliver the drug to body tissue, if the drug cannot penetrate the tissue's membranes, it will not interact with the receptors inside. The opposite situation can also occur. A drug may be able to enter a tissue, but if there is not enough blood flow to the tissue, little of the drug will enter. Distribution is also influenced by drug binding to proteins in the blood or in tissues.

The ADME processes are all illustrated by blood concentration–time curves.

Concentrations rise during absorption, but as absorption nears completion, metabolism and elimination become the primary processes, and they cause the blood concentration to decline.

 Even though the ADME processes occur simultaneously, they are studied separately to understand the critical factors responsible for each process.

In the first part of a blood concentration–time curve, absorption is the primary process and concentrations rise. As absorption nears completion, metabolism and excretion become the primary processes, causing the concentration to decline. Distribution occurs throughout. The blue lines show the parts of the profile most influenced by the various ADME processes.

 disposition a term sometimes used to refer to all of the ADME processes together.

elimination the processes of metabolism and excretion.

passive diffusion the movement of drugs from an area of higher concentration to lower concentration.

active transport the movement of drugs from an area of lower concentration to an area of higher concentration. Cellular energy is required.

hydrophobic water repelling; cannot associate with water.

hydrophilic capable of associating with or absorbing water.

lipoidal fat like substance.

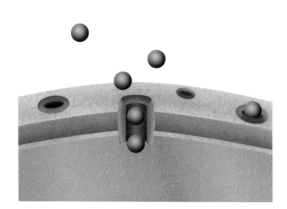

A diagram showing drug molecules penetrating a cell membrane.

Ionization and Unionization

Because they are weak organic acids and bases, most drugs will dissociate (come apart) and associate (attach to other chemicals) in solutions. When acids dissociate, they become ionized. When bases dissociate, they become unionized.

Unionized drugs penetrate biological membranes more easily than ionized drugs for these reasons:

- ➥ unionized drugs are more lipid soluble;
- ➥ charges on biological membranes bind or repel ionized drug;
- ➥ ionized drugs associate with water molecules, creating larger particles with reduced penetrating capability.

Besides the four ADME processes, a critical factor of drug concentration and effect is how drugs move through biological membranes.

Before an effective concentration of a drug can reach its site of action, it must overcome many barriers, most of which are biological membranes.

Biological membranes are complex structures composed of lipids (fats) and proteins.

They are generally classified in three types: those made up of *several layers of cells*, such as the skin; those made up of *a single layer of cells*, as in the intestinal lining; and those of *less than one cell* in thickness, as in the membrane of a single cell.

Most drugs penetrate biological membranes by passive diffusion.

Drugs in the body's fluids will generally move from an area of higher concentration to an area of lower concentration until the concentrations in each area are balanced, or in a state of equilibrium. This process is called **passive diffusion**. It is the most common way a drug penetrates biological membranes and is a primary factor in the distribution process. This movement from higher to lower concentration causes most orally administered drugs to move from the intestine to the blood and from the blood to the site of action.

Drug concentration is not the only factor influencing diffusion.

Membranes are **lipoidal** (fat-like), and drugs that are more lipid (fat) soluble will penetrate them better than those that are not. These drugs are called **hydrophobic drugs**. They hate or repel water and are attracted to fats. **Hydrophilic drugs** (drugs attracted to water) can also penetrate membranes. However, it is thought that they move through water-filled passages called **aqueous pores** which allow water (and any drug contained in it) to move into cells.

In addition to passive diffusion, some drugs may be carried across membranes by *specialized transport mechanisms*.

This type of **active transport** (as opposed to passive diffusion) is thought to explain how certain substances that do not penetrate membranes by passive diffusion nevertheless succeed in entering a cell.

ABSORPTION

Once a drug is released from its dosage formulation, the process that transfers it into the blood is called *absorption.*

Absorption occurs to some extent with any route of administration. For example, even a drug in an intravenous suspension or emulsion must first be released from the dosage form to be absorbed into the blood. However, since many drugs are given orally, this page will look at the ADME processes from the perspective of oral administration.

One of the primary factors affecting oral drug absorption is the *gastric emptying time.*

This is the time a drug will stay in the stomach before it is emptied into the small intestine. Since stomach acid can degrade many drugs and since most absorption occurs in the intestine, gastric emptying time can significantly affect a drug's action. If a drug remains in the stomach too long, it can be degraded or destroyed, and its effect decreased. Gastric emptying time can be affected by a various conditions, including the amount and type of food in the stomach, the presence of other drugs, the person's body position, and their emotional condition. Some factors increase the gastric emptying time, but most slow it.

Once a drug leaves the stomach, its rate of movement through the intestines affects its absorption.

Slower than normal intestinal movement can lead to increased drug absorption because the drug is in contact with the intestinal membrane longer. Faster than normal intestinal movement can produce the opposite result since the drug moves through the intestinal tract too rapidly to be fully absorbed.

Bile salts and enzymes from the intestinal tract also affect absorption.

Bile salts improve the absorption of certain hydrophobic drugs. Enzymes added to the intestinal tract's contents from pancreatic secretions destroy certain drugs and consequently decrease their absorption. Enzymes are also present in the intestinal wall and destroy drugs that pass from the gut into the blood, decreasing their absorption.

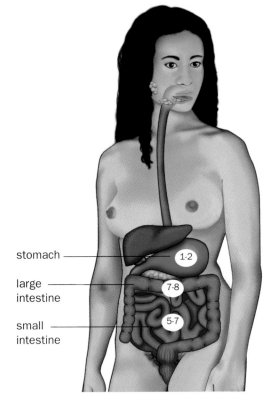

stomach

large intestine

small intestine

gastrointestinal organs and their pH

Most drugs are given orally and absorbed into the blood from the small intestine. The small intestine's large surface area benefits drug absorption. However, there are many conditions in the stomach that can affect absorption positively or negatively before the drug even reaches the small intestine. Once in the intestines, there are many additional factors that can affect a drug's absorption.

absorption the movement of the drug from the dosage formulation to the blood.

gastric emptying time the time a drug will stay in the stomach before it is emptied into the small intestine.

DISTRIBUTION

D istribution involves the movement of a drug within the body once the drug has reached the blood.

Blood carries the drug throughout the body and to its sites of action, as well as to the organs responsible for the metabolism and excretion of the drug.

The blood flow rates to certain organs have a significant effect on distribution.

Drugs are rapidly distributed to organs having high blood flow rates such as the heart, liver, and kidneys. Distribution to areas such as muscle, fat, and skin is usually slower because they have lower blood flow rates.

The permeability of tissue membranes to a drug is also important.

Most tissue membranes are easily penetrated by most drugs. Small drug molecules (those having a low molecular weight) and drugs that are hydrophobic will generally diffuse through tissue membranes with ease. Some tissue membranes have specialized transport mechanisms that assist penetration. A few tissue membranes are highly selective in allowing drug penetration. The blood-brain barrier, for example, limits drug access to the brain and the cerebral spinal fluid.

Protein binding can also affect distribution.

Many drugs will "bind" to proteins in blood plasma, forming a **complex**. The large size of such complexes prevents the bound drug from entering its sites of action, metabolism, and excretion — essentially making the drug inactive. Only free or "unbound" drug can move through tissue membranes and cellular openings. Another drug with a stronger binding capacity can displace a weaker bound drug from a protein, making the weakly bound drug pharmacologically active again or increasing its effect.

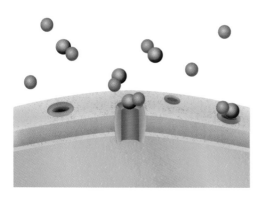

Protein Binding

Many drugs bind to proteins in blood plasma to form a complex that is too large to penetrate cellular openings. So the drug remains inactive.

Protein binding can be considered a type of drug storage within the body. Some drugs bind extensively to proteins in fat and muscle, and are gradually released as the blood concentration of the drug falls. These drugs remain in the body a long time, and therefore have a long duration of action.

Selective Action

Though drugs are widely distributed throughout the body once they reach the bloodstream, they can have action that is selective to certain tissues or organs. This is due both to the specific nature of receptor action as well as to various factors that can affect the distribution of the drug. This is why drugs can be targeted to specific therapeutic effects.

Since most receptors can be found in multiple areas throughout the body, most drugs have multiple effects. This is why a drug may be used for different therapies. It is also one reason they have side effects. For example, terbutaline is used for bronchodilation but it will also delay labor in pregnant women.

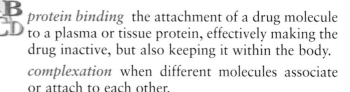

protein binding the attachment of a drug molecule to a plasma or tissue protein, effectively making the drug inactive, but also keeping it within the body.

complexation when different molecules associate or attach to each other.

METABOLISM

Drug metabolism refers to the body's process of transforming drugs.

The transformed drug is called a **metabolite.** Most metabolites are inactive molecules that are excreted. However, the metabolites of some drugs are active, and they will produce effects in the individual until they are further metabolized or excreted.

The primary site of drug metabolism in the body is the liver.

Enzymes are complex proteins that catalyze chemical reactions into other substances. The enzymes produced by the liver interact with drugs and transform them into metabolites.

In response to the chronic administration of certain drugs, the liver will increase its enzyme production.

This is called **enzyme induction,** and it results in greater metabolism of a drug. As a result, larger doses of the drug must be administered to produce the same therapeutic effects. Some drugs decrease or delay enzyme activity, a process called **enzyme inhibition.** In this case, smaller doses of the drug will be needed to avoid toxicity from drug accumulation.

The liver may secrete drugs or their metabolites into bile that is stored in the gall bladder.

The gall bladder empties the bile (and any drugs or metabolites in it) into the intestine in response to food entering the intestinal tract. Any drugs or metabolites contained in the bile may be reabsorbed or simply eliminated with the feces. If the drugs or metabolites are reabsorbed back into the blood circulation, this is called **enterohepatic cycling.**

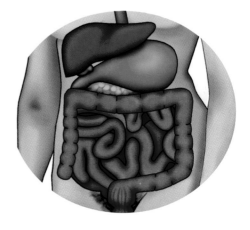

First-Pass Metabolism

With oral administration, once a drug is absorbed from the gastrointestinal tract, it is immediately delivered to the liver. It will then be transferred into the general systemic circulation.

However, before it reaches the circulatory system, the drug can be substantially degraded or destroyed by the liver's enzymes. This is called **"first-pass metabolism"** and is an important factor with orally administered drugs. Because of it, certain drugs must be administered by other routes. Any route of administration other than the oral route either partially or completely bypasses first-pass metabolism.

 metabolite the substance resulting from the body's transformation of an administered drug.

enzyme a complex protein that catalyzes chemical reactions into other substances.

enzyme induction the increase in enzyme activity that results in greater metabolism of drugs.

enzyme inhibition the decrease in enzyme activity that results in reduced metabolism of drugs.

enterohepatic cycling the transfer of drugs and their metabolites from the liver to the bile in the gall bladder, then into the intestine, and then back into circulation.

first pass metabolism the substantial degradation of a drug caused by enzyme metabolism in the liver before the drug reaches the systemic circulation.

EXCRETION

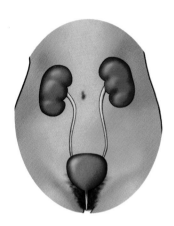

Factors Affecting Urinary Excretion

➡ If the kidney's process of filtration becomes impaired, excretion will be reduced and drugs will accumulate in the blood. In such cases, the dosage of drugs must be decreased or the dosing interval lengthened.

➡ Some drugs affect the excretion of others. In such cases, the affected drug will accumulate in the blood, and the dosage of the affected drug must be decreased or the dosing interval lengthened.

➡ The pH of the urine can affect the reabsorption of some drugs. A high pH can increase excretion of weak acids such as salicylates and phenobarbital. The opposite effect can occur with a low (acidic) pH.

Most drugs and their metabolites are excreted in the urine by the kidneys.

Some orally administered drugs are not easily absorbed from the gastrointestinal tract and as a result are significantly excreted in the feces. Excretion can also occur through the bile (if entero-hepatic cycling does not occur) and certain drugs are removed through the lungs in the expired breath.

The kidneys filter the blood and remove waste materials (including drugs and metabolites) from it.

As blood flows through a kidney, some of the plasma water is filtered from it into the kidney **nephron** (the functional unit of the kidney) in a process called **glomerular filtration**. As the water moves through the nephron, waste substances are secreted into the fluid, with urine as the end result. Some drugs can be filtered and reabsorbed back into the blood during this process, and some drugs are not filtered at all but are secreted into the urine by specialized processes.

The rate of urinary excretion is much faster than that of fecal excretion.

Drugs that will be excreted through the feces generally take a day to be excreted, whereas drugs may be excreted through the urine within hours of administration.

ABCD *nephron* the functional unit of the kidneys.
glomerular filtration the blood filtering process of the kidneys.

BIOEQUIVALENCE

The amount of a drug that is available to the site of action and the rate at which it becomes available is called the *bioavailability* of the drug.

By FDA definition, bioavailability is measured by determining *the relative amount of an administered dose of a drug that reaches the general systemic circulation and the rate at which this occurs.* As a result, it can be measured using a blood concentration-time profile.

Comparing the bioavailability of one dosage form to another determines their *bioequivalency*.

The FDA requires drug manufacturers to perform bioequivalency studies on their products before they are approved for marketing. In such studies, the bioavailability of the active ingredients in a test formulation is compared to that in a standard formulation. Bioequivalency studies are also used to compare bioavailability between different dosage forms (tablets, capsules, etc.), different manufacturers, and different production lots.

Bioequivalency can be graphically illustrated by placing the blood concentration-time profiles of the standard and test formulation on the same plot.

In the illustration below, the same dose is contained in both the standard and test formulations, but the two curves are not superimposed. The standard formulation has a faster rate of absorption than the test formulation but the test formulation has a longer duration of action.

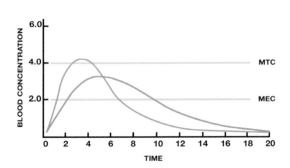

bioavailability the relative amount of an administered dose that reaches the general circulation and the rate at which this occurs.

bioequivalency the comparison of bioavailability between two dosage forms.

BIOEQUIVALENCE

Bioequivalent Drug Products

Bioequivalent drug products are pharmaceutical equivalents or alternatives which have *essentially* the same rate and extent of absorption when administered in the same dose of the active ingredient under similar conditions.

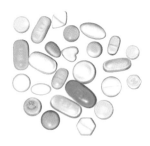

Differences Between Bioavailabilities

Exact bioequivalency between drug products (where blood concentration–time profiles for each product are identical) does not occur, and is not expected. There are simply too many variables that can contribute to differences between products. In tablets, for example, there can be different amounts or types of fillers, binders, lubricants, and other components. The particle size of the active drug itself may be slightly different. The manufacturing process may also produce different results in size, hardness, or other characteristics (especially for different manufacturers, but also for the same manufacturer at different times or different manufacturing facilities). Changes in these or various other factors can affect the bioavailability of a drug. Though there can be differences in the bioavailability different products, when the differences are not significant the products are bioequivalent.

The following terms are used by the FDA to define the type of equivalency between drug products:

Pharmaceutical Equivalents

Pharmaceutical equivalents are drug products that contain identical amounts of the same active ingredients in the same dosage form, and that meet the same applicable standards of identity, strength, quality, and purity, including potency and, where applicable, content uniformity, disintegration times, and/or dissolution rates. They do not have to contain the same inactive ingredients, or have the same shape, release mechanisms, packaging, or expiration time. Since pharmaceutical equivalents may have different inactive ingredients, different pharmaceutically equivalent products may not be equally suitable for a patient. Some patients may be unusually sensitive to an inactive ingredient in one product that another product does not contain.

➡ same active ingredients
➡ same amounts
➡ same dosage form
➡ inactive ingredients can be different

Pharmaceutical Alternatives

Pharmaceutical alternatives are drug products that contain the identical active ingredients, but not necessarily in the same amount or dosage form. Each such drug product must individually meet the applicable standards of its dosage form. They do not have to contain the same inactive ingredients, or have the same shape, release mechanisms, packaging, or expiration time.

➡ same active ingredients
➡ amounts can be different
➡ dosage form can be different

Therapeutic Equivalents

Therapeutic equivalents are pharmaceutical equivalents which produce the same therapeutic effect in patients.

Note: a related term is **therapeutic alternative**. This refers to drugs that have different active ingredients but produce similar therapeutic effect.

➡ pharmaceutical equivalents that produce the same effects in patients

 pharmaceutical equivalent drug products that contain identical amounts of the same active ingredients in the same dosage form.

pharmaceutical alternative drug products that contain the same active ingredients, but not necessarily in the same amount or dosage form.

therapeutic equivalent pharmaceutical equivalents that produce the same effects in patients.

REVIEW

KEY CONCEPTS

HOW DRUGS WORK

✔ The objective of drug therapy is to deliver the right drug, in the right concentration, to the right site of action, and at the right time to produce the desired effect.

✔ Only those drugs able to bind chemically to the receptors in a particular site of action can produce effects in that site. This is why specific cells only respond to certain drugs.

CONCENTRATION AND EFFECT

✔ To produce an effect, a drug must achieve a minimum effective concentration (MEC). This is when there is enough drug at the site of action to produce a response.

✔ The range between the minimum effective concentration and the minimum toxic concentration is called the therapeutic window. When concentrations are in this range, most patients receive the maximum benefit from their drug therapy with a minimum of risk.

ADME PROCESSES AND DIFFUSION

✔ Blood concentrations are the result of four simultaneously occurring processes: absorption, distribution, metabolism, and excretion (the ADME processes).

✔ Besides the four ADME processes, a critical factor of drug concentration and effect is how drugs move through biological membranes. Most drugs penetrate biological membranes by passive diffusion.

ABSORPTION

✔ One of the primary factors affecting oral drug absorption is the gastric emptying time.

DISTRIBUTION

✔ Many drugs bind to proteins in blood plasma to form a complex that is too large to penetrate cellular openings, essentially making the drug inactive.

METABOLISM

✔ Enzymes catalyze the transformation of drugs to metabolites. Most metabolites are inactive molecules that are excreted.

EXCRETION

✔ The kidneys filter blood and remove wastes (including drugs and metabolites) from it.

BIOEQUIVALENCE

✔ The amount of a drug that is available to the site of action and the rate at which it becomes available is called the bioavailability of the drug.

✔ Bioequivalent drug products are pharmaceutical equivalents or alternatives which have essentially the same rate and extent of absorption when administered in the same dose of the active ingredient under similar conditions.

✔ Pharmaceutical equivalents are drug products that contain identical amounts of the same active ingredients in the same dosage form, but may contain different inactive ingredients.

✔ Pharmaceutical alternatives are drug products that contain the identical active ingredients, but not necessarily in the same amount or dosage form.

SELF TEST

MATCH THE TERMS.

answers can be checked in the glossary

agonist

antagonist

bioavailability

bioequivalence

enzyme induction

first-pass metabolism

passive diffusion

protein binding

receptor

selective (action)

site of action

- the location where an administered drug produces an effect.
- the cellular material which interacts with the drug.
- the characteristic of a drug that makes its action specific to certain receptors.
- drugs that activate receptors to accelerate or slow normal cellular function.
- drugs that bind with receptors but do not activate them.
- the movement of drugs from an area of higher concentration to lower concentration.
- the attachment of a drug molecule to a protein, effectively making the drug inactive.
- the increase in enzyme activity that results in greater metabolism of drugs.
- the substantial degradation of a drug caused by enzyme metabolism in the liver before the drug reaches the systemic circulation.
- the relative amount of an administered dose that reaches the general circulation and the rate at which this occurs.
- the comparison of bioavailability between two dosage forms.

CHOOSE THE BEST ANSWER.

the answer key begins on page 347

1. The place where a drug causes an effect to occur is called the
   a. therapeutic window.
   b. site of administration.
   c. site of action.
   d. minimum toxic concentration (MTC).

2. When a drug produces an effect, it is acting at a/an _____ level.
   a. tissue
   b. atomic
   c. molecular
   d. organ

3. _____ is the study of the factors associated with drug products and physiological processes, and the resulting systemic concentration of the drugs.
   a. Disposition
   b. Therapeutics
   c. Equilibrium
   d. Biopharmaceutics

4. In a blood concentration-time curve, the range between the minimum toxic concentration (MTC) and the minimum effective concentration (MEC) is called the
   a. onset of action.
   b. concentration at site of action.
   c. duration of action.
   d. therapeutic window.

REVIEW

5. A typical dose-response curve shows that response increases as the dose
   a. increases.
   b. does not change.
   c. plateaus.
   d. decreases

6. In the blood concentration-time curve, the duration of action can be measured as the
   a. range between minimum effective concentration (MEC) and minimum toxic concentration (MTC).
   b. time from dose administration to when the blood concentrations first reach the MEC.
   c. time between dose administration and when declining blood concentrations reach the MEC.
   d. time from when blood concentrations first reach the MEC to when the declining blood concentrations reach the MEC.

7. The _____ is the blood concentration needed to produce a response.
   a. minimum toxic concentration (MTC)
   b. onset of action
   c. minimum effective concentration (MEC)
   d. therapeutic window

8. When studying concentration and effect, the _____ is the time MEC is reached and the response occurs.
   a. therapeutic window
   b. MTC
   c. onset of action
   d. duration of action

9. Blood concentrations are the result of _____ simultaneously occurring processes.
   a. two
   b. four
   c. three
   d. five

10. All of the ADME processes together are sometimes referred to as
    a. absorption.
    b. distribution.
    c. metabolism.
    d. disposition.

11. _____ involves the movement of drugs from an area of higher concentration to lower concentration.
    a. Active diffusion
    b. Active transport
    c. Absorption
    d. Passive diffusion

12. Most drugs penetrate biological membranes by
    a. disposition.
    b. active transport.
    c. active diffusion.
    d. passive diffusion.

13. Unionized drugs are more
    a. lipid soluble.
    b. charged.
    c. water soluble.
    d. hydrophilic.

14. Most drugs given orally are absorbed into the blood from the
    a. small intestine.
    b. kidneys.
    c. stomach.
    d. liver.

15. When drug molecules are bound to plasma or tissues proteins they are
    a. more potent.
    b. metabolized.
    c. inactive.
    d. excreted.

16. In metabolism, the breakdown of drugs into metabolites is caused by
    a. passive diffusion.
    b. glomerular filtration.
    c. enterohepatic cycling.
    d. enzymes.

17. An enzyme is a complex _____ that catalyzes chemical reactions into other substances.
    a. lipid
    b. mineral
    c. protein
    d. atom

18. First-pass metabolism refers to the substantial degradation of a drug caused by enzyme metabolism in the
    a. liver.
    b. blood.
    c. kidneys.
    d. small intestine.

19. Most drugs and their metabolites are excreted by the
    a. liver.
    b. kidneys.
    c. gall bladder.
    d. gastrointestinal tract.

20. Elimination is
    a. absorption and metabolism.
    b. metabolism and excretion.
    c. distribution and excretion.
    d. distribution and metabolism.

21. Glomerular filtration is the blood filter process of the
    a. liver.
    b. small intestine.
    c. gall bladder.
    d. kidneys.

22. The nephron is the function unit of the
    a. gall bladder.
    b. liver.
    c. small intestine.
    d. kidneys.

23. The percentage or fraction of the administered dose of a drug that actually reaches systemic circulation and the rate at which this occurs is the drug's
    a. bioequivalence.
    b. bioavailability.
    c. biotransformation.
    d. gastric emptying time.

HUMAN VARIABILITY

Human variability in biopharmaceutics and disposition is a significant factor in the outcome of drug blood concentration-time profiles and effect.

Differences in age, weight, genetics, and gender are among the significant factors that influence the differences in response to medication among people.

Age

Human life is a continuous process but it is usually characterized as having stages. The distinctions between the stages are open to individual interpretation, but they are based on physiological characteristics. The stages are generally considered as:

➡ Neonate, up to one month after birth

➡ Infant, between the ages of one month and two years

➡ Child, between the ages of two and twelve years

➡ Adolescent, between the ages of 13 and 19 years

➡ Adult, between 20 and 70 years

➡ Elder, older than 70 years

Neonates and Infants

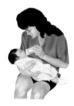

Drug distribution, metabolism, and excretion are quite different in the neonate and infant than in adults because their organ systems are not fully developed. They are not able to eliminate drugs as efficiently as adults. Older infants reach approximately adult levels of protein binding and kidney function, but liver function and the blood-brain barrier are still immature.

Children

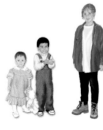

Children metabolize certain drugs more rapidly than adults. Their rate of metabolism increases between 1 year and 12 years of age depending on the child and the drug. Afterwards, metabolism rates decline with age to normal adult levels. Some of the drugs eliminated faster in children include clindamycin, valproic acid, ethosuximide, and theophylline.

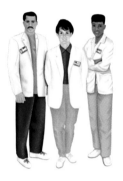

Adults

Adults experience a decrease in many physiological functions between 30 to 70 years of age, but these decreases and their affects on drug activity are gradual.

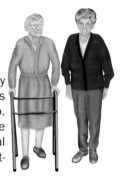

The Elderly

The elderly typically consume more drugs than other age group. They also experience more physiological changes that significantly affect drug action.

➡ Changes in gastric pH, gastric emptying time, intestinal motility, and gastrointestinal blood flow all tend to *slow the rate of absorption.*

➡ Changes in the cardiovascular system (including lower cardiac output) tend to *slow distribution* of drug molecules to their sites of action, metabolism, and excretion.

➡ Though there is probably a decrease in the liver's production of metabolizing enzymes, the metabolism of most drugs does not appear to decrease.

➡ A decline in kidney function (including glomerular filtration and secretion) occurs which tends to *slow urinary excretion* of drugs.

pharmacogenetics a new field of study which defines the hereditary basis of individual differences in absorption, distribution, metabolism, and excretion (the ADME processes).

Gender

Most research has involved men, with findings applied to women. One particular reason has been to avoid exposing a fetus or potential fetus to unknown risks. But now, many studies have been completed in both genders and show differences depending on the drug. For example, males and females have similar elimination for antipyrine, cimetidine, and lorazepam, but women eliminate propranolol, isosorbide dinitrate, diazepam, and temazepam more slowly than men. Acetaminophen and clofibric acid are eliminated more rapidly in women than men.

However, some gender based differences in drug response appear to be related to hormonal fluctuations in women during the menstrual cycle. For women with clinical depression, for example, higher dosages of antidepressant medication may be necessary when menstrual symptoms are worse.

Distribution may also be somewhat different between men and women simply as a result of differences in body composition (males have more muscle, women more fat).

Pregnancy

A number of physiological changes (including delayed gastric emptying and decreased motility in the gastrointestinal tract) occur in women in the latter stages of pregnancy. These changes tend to *reduce the rate of absorption.*

Drug plasma protein binding may be reduced and metabolism increased in pregnant women for a number of drugs. The rate of urinary excretion for a number of drugs is much greater in pregnant women than in non-pregnant women.

Genetics

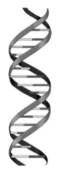 Genes determine the types and amounts of proteins produced in the body, with each person being somewhat different. Since drugs interact with proteins in plasma, tissues, receptor sites, and elsewhere, genetic differences can result in differences in drug action.

A new field of study, **pharmacogenetics**, has arisen to define the hereditary basis of individual differences in absorption, distribution, metabolism and excretion (the ADME processes.) The largest contributing factor to inherited variability is metabolism. For example, people with certain genetic characteristics will not metabolize a drug that most people metabolize, or will metabolize it at an abnormal rate. In such cases, the individual may experience no therapeutic effect at all, or perhaps even an adverse or toxic effect instead.

Body Weight

Dosage adjustments based on weight are generally not made for adults who are slightly overweight. However, weight is often considered in infants, children, or unusually small, emaciated, or obese patients. Adults who are obese (i.e., body fat content greater than 30% of total body weight) will have significant changes in the distribution and renal excretion of a number of drugs.

Psychological Factors

Though the specific reasons are unknown, it is clear that psychological factors can influence individual responses to drug administration. For example, in clinical trials in which placebos are used, patients receiving them often report both therapeutic and adverse effects. This may account for some variability in patient responses to an administered (non-placebo) drug. At a fundamental level, it is a factor in patient willingness to follow prescribed dosage regimens.

ADVERSE DRUG REACTIONS

Drugs generally produce a mixture of *therapeutic* (desired) and *adverse* effects (undesired effects).

An adverse drug reaction can be any symptom in any disease process and involve any organ. They may be common or rare, localized or widespread, mild or severe depending on the drug and the patient. Some adverse drug reactions occur with usual doses of drugs (often called side effects). Others are more likely to occur only at higher than normal dosages.

COMMON ADVERSE DRUG REACTIONS

Central Nervous System Effects

CNS effects may result from CNS stimulation (e.g., agitation, confusion, delirium, disorientation, hallucinations) or CNS depression (e.g., dizziness, drowsiness, sedation, coma, impaired respiration and circulation).

Hepatotoxicity

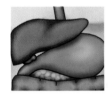

"Hepato" means "of the liver." Hepatotoxicities include hepatitis, hepatic necrosis, and biliary tract inflammation or obstruction. These are relatively rare but potentially life-threatening. Commonly used hepatotoxic drugs include acetaminophen, halothane, isoniazid, chlorpromazine, methotrexate, nitrofurantoin, phenytoin, and aspirin.

Hypersensitivity or Allergy

Almost any drug, in almost any dose, can produce an **allergic** or **hypersensitive reaction** in a patient. This generally happens because a patient developed antibodies while previously taking the drug or a drug with a similar chemical structure. The drug will interact with the antibodies, releasing histamines and other substances that produce reactions that can range from mild rashes to potentially fatal **anaphylactic shock.**

Allergic reactions can occur within minutes or weeks of drug administration. Anaphylactic shock occurs within minutes. It is a hypersensitivity reaction that can lead to cardiovascular collapse and death if untreated. Its symptoms include severe respiratory distress and convulsions. Immediate emergency treatment with epinephrine, antihistamines, or bronchodilator drugs is required.

Gastrointestinal Effects

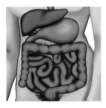

Anorexia, nausea, vomiting, constipation, and diarrhea are among the most common adverse reactions to drugs. More serious effects include ulcerations and colitis (e.g., irritable bowel disease).

hepato a prefix meaning "of the liver."

hypersensitivity an abnormal sensitivity generally resulting in an allergic reaction.

anaphylactic shock a potentially fatal hypersensitivity reaction producing severe respiratory distress and cardiovascular collapse.

Nephrotoxicity

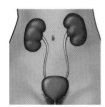

Kidney failure can occur with gentamicin and other aminoglycosides, and with ibuprofen and other nonsteroidal anti-inflammatory drugs.

Idiosyncrasy

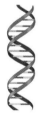

Idiosyncrasy is the unexpected reaction to a drug the first time it is given to a patient. Such reactions are thought to be caused by genetic characteristics that alter the patient's drug metabolizing enzymes.

Hematological Effects

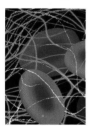

Blood coagulation, bleeding, and bone marrow disorders are potentially life threatening and can be caused by various drugs. Anticoagulants can cause excessive bleeding. Antineoplastic drugs may cause bone marrow depression.

Drug Dependence

Chronic usage of narcotic analgesics, sedative-hypnotic agents, antianxiety agents, and amphetamines often results in physiological or psychological dependence. Physiological dependence is accompanied by unpleasant physical withdrawal symptoms when the dose is discontinued or reduced. Psychological dependence involves an emotional or mental fixation on drug usage.

Teratogenicity

This is the ability of a substance to cause abnormal fetal development when given to pregnant women. Drug groups considered teratogenic include analgesics, diuretics, antihistamines, antibiotics, and antiemetics.

Carcinogenicity

This is the ability of a substance to cause cancer. Several drugs are carcinogens, including some hormones and anticancer drugs.

idiosyncrasy an unexpected reaction the first time a drug is taken, generally due to genetic causes.

nephrotoxicity the ability of a substance to harm the kidneys.

carcinogenicity the ability of a substance to cause cancer.

DRUG-DRUG INTERACTIONS

The administration of more than one drug at a time to a patient can cause *drug-drug interactions.* The probability of a drug-drug interaction increases with the number of drugs a patient takes and in certain disease states. Such interactions can affect the disposition of one or more drugs and *result in either increases or decreases in therapeutic effects or side effects.* Some drug-drug interactions may not alter drug disposition but will still change the therapeutic effect.

An understanding of the ways drug-drug interactions occur is important. Examples of some common types are on these pages.

➡ **Additive effects** occur when two drugs with similar pharmacological actions result in an effect equal to the sum of the individual effects.

> **Example:** trimethoprim + sulfamethoxazole for antibiotic effect

> **Example:** amiodarone + disopyramide for prolongation of heart's QT interval

➡ **Synergism** occurs when two drugs with similar pharmacological actions produce greater effects than the sum of individual effects.

> **Example:** acetaminophen + codeine = increased analgesia

> **Example:** penicillin + gentamicin = increased anti-bacterial effects

➡ **Potentiation** occurs when one drug with no inherent activity of its own increases the activity of another drug that produces an effect.

> **Example:** carbidopa + dopa = prolonged half-life of dopa and increased duration of anti-Parkinsonian effect

➡ An **antidote** to a particular drug is given to block or reduce its toxic effects.

> **Example:** naloxone + morphine = relief of morphine induced respiratory depression. Naloxone displaces morphine from their receptor sites, preventing morphine from causing further depressive effects.

> **Example:** vitamin K + warfarin = opposition of the anticoagulant effect of warfarin and a return to normal blood clotting time.

➡ Decreased intestinal absorption of oral drugs occurs when drugs **complex** to produce nonabsorbable compounds.

> **Example:** aluminum or magnesium hydroxide + tetracycline = binding of tetracycline to aluminum or magnesium ions. This causes decreased tetracycline absorption and antibiotic effect.

> **Example:** cholestyramine + thyroxine = binding of thyroxine to cholestyramine reduces the absorption of the thyroid hormone.

---

additive effects the summation in effect when two drugs with similar pharmacological actions are taken.

synergism when two drugs with similar pharmacological action produce greater effects than the sum of individual effects.

antidote a drug that antagonizes the toxic effect of another drug.

potentiation when one drug with no inherent activity of its own increases the activity of another drug that produces an effect.

complexation when two different molecules associate or attach to each other.

displacement a drug bound to a plasma protein is removed when another drug of greater binding potential binds to the same protein.

inhibition a drug blocks the activity of metabolic enzymes in the liver.

induction a drug causes more metabolic enzymes to be produced, thus increasing the metabolic activity.

➥ **Displacement** of one drug from protein binding sites by a second drug increases the effects of the displaced drug. This occurs because the blood concentration of the now free displaced drug is increased. For some drugs this increased effect may be transitory.

  Example: aspirin + warfarin = increased anticoagulant effect

  Example: chloral hydrate + warfarin = increased anticoagulant effect

➥ **Inhibition** by one drug with the elimination of a second drug may intensify the effects of the second drug.

  Example: Cimetidine inhibits drug metabolizing enzymes in the liver and therefore interferes with the metabolism of many drugs. When these drugs are given at the same time as cimetidine, their blood concentration increases and they are more likely to cause adverse reactions or toxic effects.

  Example: Alcohol is metabolized first to acetaldehyde and then subsequently to carbon dioxide and water. Disulfiram blocks the subsequent metabolic steps so acetaldehyde accumulates in the body. This Disulfiram Reaction (flushing, nausea, breathlessness, and tachycardia) is used to deter alcoholic patients from drinking.

➥ **induction** increases the concentration of metabolizing enzymes in the liver, and increases the metabolism of other drugs affected by the same enzymes. Enzyme inducing drugs include some anticonvulsants, barbiturates, and antihistamines.

  Example: phenobarbital + warfarin = decreased effects of warfarin

  Example: phenytoin + oral contraceptives = decreased contraception effect

➥ **Urinary excretion** of some drugs can be altered by raising urinary pH and decreasing renal reabsorption.

  Example: sodium bicarbonate + phenobarbital = increased excretion of phenobarbital. The sodium bicarbonate raises urine pH and increases the ionization of phenobarbital, increasing its excretion.

Time Course of Drug Interactions

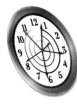 The time it takes for drug-drug interactions to occur can vary substantially. Some interactions occur almost immediately while others may take weeks. Knowing the time course of an interaction allows quick identification and treatment of potential interactions. It also allows clinicians to evaluate the relative importance of an interaction from two drugs compared to their therapeutic effects. For example, if an interaction requires one to two weeks to occur, short term administration over a few days will not cause a significant adverse effect.

DRUG-DRUG INTERACTIONS (cont'd)

ABSORPTION

There are several means by which one drug may affect the gastrointestinal absorption of another:

Binding in GI Tract

Some drugs can form nonabsorbable complexes by binding to other drugs, resulting in decreased absorption. For example, iron salts can affect the absorption of several tetracyclines, methlydopa, and levodopa in this way. Antacids and sucralfate appear to reduce the absorption of norfloxacin and ciprofloxacin by this mechanism.

Gastric Emptying

Certain drugs will affect gastric emptying and therefore the absorption of other drugs. For example, use of propantheline will delay acetaminophen absorption. On the other hand, use of metoclopramide will increase acetaminophen absorption, since metoclopramide increases the rate of gastric emptying. Another problem with reducing gastric emptying time is that drugs that are degraded by gastric acid have a longer time to degrade, resulting in a decreased amount of drug available for absorption from the intestine.

Gastric pH

Drugs that alter the gastrointestinal pH can have varied effects on other administered drugs. Some of the factors affected by pH are:

➡ the amount of unionized drug available for absorption;

➡ the rate of dissolution;

➡ intestinal motility;

➡ degradation.

Intestinal Metabolism

Alterations in metabolism are involved in the interaction between oral contraceptives and oral antibiotic therapy. The antibiotic kills the normal bacterial flora in the GI tract, which disrupts the enterohepatic recycling of the oral contraceptive's estrogens.

DISTRIBUTION

Displacement

One drug can displace another from a plasma protein binding site and so increase the amount of the free drug available for distribution. This will increase its pharmacological effect and its elimination, since more of the drug is available for metabolism and excretion.

Such displacement interactions generally occur within the first week or two of administration. When they do occur, many turn out to be self-correcting after a few days, at which point the concentration of displaced drug often returns to pre-interaction levels, even if the patient continues to take both drugs.

The biggest consequence of displacement interactions is the *change in pharmacological effect*. If drugs are highly protein bound, displacement tends to have a greater effect than with drugs that are not highly bound. For example, warfarin is 98% plasma protein bound, with only 2% free or unbound. If a drug interaction displaces only 2% of the bound warfarin, then 96% will be bound, but 4% will now be free. That is a 100% increase in the free concentration of warfarin, and it might double its pharmacological effect. By comparison, for a drug that is only 60% bound, displacing 2% will cause only a 5% increase in the concentration.

METABOLISM

Enzyme Induction

Some drugs are capable of increasing the concentration of metabolizing enzymes in the liver. This process is called **enzyme induction**. It increases the metabolism of drugs that use the same enzyme system and usually results in a *reduction in pharmacological effect.* Examples of enzyme inducers include phenobarbital, carbamazepine, phenytoin, and rifampin. Cigarette smoking and chronic alcohol use may also induce metabolism.

The time course of drug interactions from enzyme induction is slower than for many other types of interactions. Though enzyme induction may be dose related, it can also be caused by age, genetics, or liver disease. As a result, it is a difficult type of interaction to predict.

Enzyme Inhibition

Another alteration in metabolism is called **enzyme inhibition,** which usually occurs when two drugs compete for binding sites on the same metabolizing enzyme. This generally *increases the plasma concentration (and consequently the pharmacological effect) of at least one of the drugs.* Enzyme inhibition is one of the most common drug interactions. In fact, if a drug is known to be metabolized by the liver, manufacturers often study its potential for enzyme inhibition early in the drug development process. Examples of enzyme inhibitors include allopurinol, cimetidine, erythromycin, disulfiram, isoniazid, ketoconazole, and verapamil.

Unlike enzyme induction, which has a much slower time course, enzyme inhibition has a rapid onset, generally within 24 hours, and tends to disappear quickly once the inhibitor is discontinued. Enzyme inhibition is also easier to predict since it appears to be dose related. It is also true that drugs that share a similar chemical structure often share the potential for enzyme inhibition.

EXCRETION

Glomerular Filtration

Drug interactions that actually change the filtration rate itself are rare. Changes in the filtration rate are more likely to occur in response to specific drugs, such as those that change the systemic blood pressure, for example. Whatever the cause, changes in the filtration rate will also change the rate of drug excretion.

Renal Secretion

There are different secretory systems in the kidneys for basic drugs and acidic drugs. Basic drugs do not seem to compete for the acidic drug transport system, or visa versa. However, two basic drugs or two acidic drugs may compete for the same transport system and this can cause one or both of the drugs to accumulate in the blood. For example, probenecid competes with penicillin and reduces penicillin's secretion. Probenecid also inhibits the secretion of cephalosporins. The interaction between NSAIDS and methotrexate is another example. Some of these interactions can increase methotrexate concentrations two- to three-fold. An example of such a competition involving basic drugs is quinidine and digoxin. Quinidine reduces digoxin excretion by 30% to 50%.

Urinary Reabsorption

Urinary reabsorption, a passive transport process, is influenced by the pH of the urine and the extent of ionization of the drug. In acidic urine, acidic drugs tend to be reabsorbed while basic drugs are not. As a result, basic drugs are excreted in the urine. In alkaline urine, acidic drugs will not be reabsorbed but will instead be excreted in the urine, while basic drugs will be reabsorbed. An example of these interactions is quinidine, which is a base. The excretion of quinidine is reduced nearly 90% when the urine pH is increased from less than 6.0 to over 7.5.

DRUG-DIET INTERACTIONS

Dietary intakes and patterns vary widely among individuals and can contribute to variability in the disposition of drugs. Differences may be attributed to various factors including food preferences and availability, diets designed for weight gain or loss, and variations for seasonal, religious, and therapeutic reasons.

ABSORPTION

The physical presence of food in the gastrointestinal tract can alter absorption in several ways:

➥ interacting chemically (e.g., tetracycline and iron);

➥ improving the solubility of some drugs by increasing bile secretion;

➥ affecting the performance of the dosage form (e.g., altering the release characteristics of polymer coated tablets);

➥ altering gastric emptying;

➥ altering intestinal motility;

➥ altering liver blood flow.

As a result, some drugs have increased bioavailability and some have decreased bioavailability in the presence of food. For example, the bioavailability of propranolol, metoprolol, hydralazine, erythromycin, and phenytoin is enhanced by the presence of food.

The bioavailability of a drug is generally decreased when the presence of food slows absorption. For example, when tablets or capsules are taken with food, they dissolve more slowly, slowing absorption as a result.

Food may also combine with a drug to form an insoluble drug-food complex. This is how tetracycline interacts with dairy products, such as milk and cheese. It combines with the calcium in milk products to form an insoluble, nonabsorbable compound that is excreted in the feces. In general, dietary fiber decreases the absorption of drugs.

DISTRIBUTION

The presence of food can also influence drug distribution. For example, high fat meals can increase fatty acid levels in the blood. The fatty acids bind to the same plasma protein binding sites as many drugs. This displaces previously bound drug and increases the free concentration of that drug, leading to an increased effect.

There are also differences in the plasma protein binding of certain drugs between well nourished and undernourished people.

ADMINISTRATION TIMES

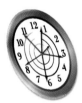

Interactions that alter drug absorption can be minimized by separating the administration of drugs and food intake about 2 hours.

drug-diet interactions when elements of ingested nutrients interact with a drug and this affects the disposition of the drug.

METABOLISM

Most foods are complex mixtures of carbohydrate, fat, and protein. Research studies designed to determine the influence of diet on drug metabolism use diets in which one of these nutrients is increased, another decreased, and the third nutrient and total caloric intake are kept constant. In general, high protein (low carbohydrate) diets are associated with accelerated metabolism while high carbohydrate (low protein) diets appear to decrease metabolism. The substitution of fat calories for carbohydrate seems not to affect drug metabolism rates.

In general, mildly or moderately undernourished adults have normal or enhanced metabolism of drugs and severely malnourished adults have decreased drug metabolism. As with any diet, however, there are many variables in malnourishment that can produce an affect on metabolism.

EXCRETION

Increasing protein in the diet appears to increase glomerular filtration, decrease reabsorption, and decrease secretion in the kidney. The total effect of restricted protein intake will depend on the urinary excretion characteristics of the specific drug.

Effect of Dietary Factors on Metabolism

Change in Food Composition	Effect on Metabolism
increased protein	increased metabolism
increased carbohydrate	decreased metabolism
increased fat	no effect
decreased calories	decreased metabolism

SPECIFIC FOODS

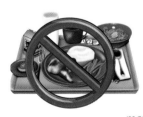 Some foods contain substances that react with certain drugs. For example, eating foods containing tyramine while using monoamine oxidase (MAO) inhibitors may produce severe hypertension or intracranial hemorrhage. MAO inhibitors include isocarboxazid, phenelzine, and procarbazine. Foods containing tyramine include beer, red wine, aged cheeses, yeast products, chicken livers, and pickled herring.

Certain cruciferous vegetables (i.e., brussels sprouts, cabbage) stimulate the metabolism of a few drugs. Other foods that might also have the similar effect are alfalfa, turnips, broccoli, cauliflower, or spinach. Some of the same foods are also involved with an interaction with oral anticoagulants such as warfarin. Spinach and other greens contain vitamin K, and vitamin K inhibits the action of oral anticoagulants. A patient ingesting foods containing vitamin K while taking an anticoagulant would not receive the full therapeutic effect from the drug.

DISEASE STATES

The disposition and effect of some drugs can be influenced by the presence of diseases other than the one for which a drug is used. Hepatic, cardiovascular, renal, and endocrine disease all increase the variability in drug response.

HEPATIC

There are a variety of liver diseases that affect hepatic function differently. Some, but not all, hepatic diseases require that the patient be monitored when receiving certain drugs.

Cirrhosis and **obstructive jaundice** appear to decrease hepatic metabolism and thereby diminish drug elimination. With **acute viral hepatitis** changes in drug disposition vary, generally are of little significance, and return to normal as the condition clears.

The effect of hepatic disease on drug absorption is not well understood. However, to the extent that liver activity is decreased, it appears that the first-pass effect is also reduced. This results in increased bioavailability for drugs that are usually severely degraded by first-pass metabolism. Another factor that increases bioavailability is that patients with cirrhosis can develop a condition in which a significant amount of the blood coming from the intestine bypasses liver cells and enters the circulatory system directly. When this happens, the bioavailability of drugs that would otherwise be degraded by first-pass metabolism rises substantially.

Selected Drugs with Decreased Elimination in Cirrhosis

➡ Encainide	➡ Caffeine
➡ Lidocaine	➡ Diazepam
➡ Meperidine	➡ Metronidazole
➡ Metropolol	➡ Theophylline
➡ Verapamil	➡ Erythromycin

CIRCULATORY

Circulatory disorders are generally characterized by diminished blood flow to one or more organs of the body. Since blood flow influences drug absorption, distribution, and elimination, this may also affect the action of drugs.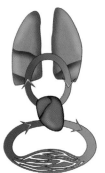

Decreased blood flow from cardiovascular disorders can delay or cause erratic drug absorption. As a result, intravenous administration may be needed to obtain a desired effect.

Decreased blood flow can also affect the metabolizing action of the liver. For example, when blood flow to the liver is decreased, the metabolism of lidocaine also decreases.

 cirrhosis a chronic and potentially fatal liver disease which occurs after long term alcohol abuse; it causes loss of function and increase resistance to blood flow through the liver.

acute viral hepatitis an inflammatory condition of the liver caused by viruses; the effects are less than in cirrhosis but long term exposure can progress into chronic disease with the same characteristics as cirrhosis.

obstructive jaundice an obstruction of the bile duct that causes hepatic waste products and bile to accumulate in the liver.

RENAL

Reduced renal function, especially end-stage renal disease, can affect the elimination of many drugs and affect the plasma protein binding of drugs.

Effects on drug elimination: As renal function decreases, the dosage of a drug that is eliminated by the kidney should be reduced to avoid accumulation of the drug in the body.

Effects on plasma protein binding: While the plasma protein binding of *acidic* drugs is markedly reduced in patients with severe renal insufficiency, the plasma protein binding of *basic* drugs is expected to be increased.

Decreases in renal function can be measured by monitoring the amount of creatinine excreted in the urine. Creatinine is produced by muscles in the body, and is excreted at a constant rate primarily by glomerular filtration. In diseased kidneys, the rate of creatinine excretion decreases.

THYROID

Changes in thyroid function can affect many of the aspects of absorption, excretion, and metabolism.

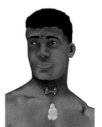

In **hypothyroidism** (a condition in which the thyroid is underactive), the bioavailability of a few drugs (e.g., riboflavin, digoxin) is increased. In **hyperthyroidism** (an overactive thyroid condition) their bioavailability is decreased because of changes in gastrointestinal motility.

Some other changes affected by thyroid conditions are:

➡ Renal blood flow is decreased in hypothyroidism and increased in hyperthyroidism.

➡ The activity of metabolizing enzymes in the liver is reduced in hypothyroidism and increased in hyperthyroidism.

➡ The metabolism of theophylline, propranolol, propylthiouracil, and methimazole is increased by hyperthyroidism.

Bioavailabilty of Selected Drugs in Patients with Renal Disease

➡ Decreased	Furosemide
➡ Increased	Propranolol
➡ Unchanged	Cimetidine, ciprofloxacin, digoxin, labetalol, sulfamethoxazole, trimethoprim

A
B
C
D *hypothyroidism* a condition in which thyroid hormone secretions are below normal, often referred to as an underactive thyroid.

hyperthyroidism a condition in which thyroid hormone secretions are above normal, often referred to as an overactive thyroid.

REVIEW

KEY CONCEPTS

HUMAN VARIABILITY

✔ Differences in age, weight, genetics, and gender are among the significant factors that influence the differences in medication responses among people.

✔ Drug distribution, metabolism, and excretion are quite different in the neonate and infant than in adults because their organ systems are not fully developed.

✔ Children metabolize certain drugs more rapidly than adults.

✔ The elderly typically consume more drugs than other age groups. They also experience more physiological changes that significantly affect drug action.

✔ Genetic differences can cause differences in the types and amounts of proteins produced in the body, which can result in differences in drug action.

ADVERSE DRUG REACTIONS

✔ Almost any drug, in almost any dose, can produce an allergic or hypersensitive reaction in a patient. Anaphylactic shock is a potentially fatal hypersensitivity reaction.

✔ Anorexia, nausea, vomiting, constipation, and diarrhea are among the most common adverse reactions to drugs in the GI tract.

✔ Teratogenicity is the ability of a substance to cause abnormal fetal development when given to pregnant women.

DRUG-DRUG INTERACTIONS

✔ Drug-drug interactions can result in either increases or decreases in therapeutic effects or side effects.

✔ Additive effects occur when two drugs with similar pharmacological actions result in an effect equal to the sum of the individual effects.

✔ Synergism occurs when two drugs with similar pharmacological actions produce greater effects than the sum of the individual effects.

✔ Displacement of one drug from protein binding sites by a second drug increases the effects of the displaced drug.

✔ Decreased intestinal absorption of oral drugs occurs when drugs complex to produce nonabsorbable compounds.

✔ When drugs induce metabolizing enzymes in the liver, it increases the metabolism of other drugs affected by the same enzymes.

✔ Some drugs increase excretion by raising urinary pH and lessening renal reabsorption.

DRUG-DIET INTERACTIONS

✔ Some foods contain substances that react with certain drugs, e.g., foods containing tyramine can react with monoamine oxidase (MAO) inhibitors.

DISEASE STATES

✔ The disposition and effect of some drugs can be influenced by the presence of diseases other than the one for which a drug is used. For example, renal disease has been correlated with decreased renal excretion of many drugs.

SELF TEST

MATCH THE TERMS.   *answers can be checked in the glossary*

additive effects

anaphylactic shock

antidote

carcinogenicity

cirrhosis

hepato

hypersensitivity

idiosyncrasy

nephrotoxicity

synergism

teratogenicity

- a prefix meaning "of the liver."
- the ability of a substance to cause abnormal fetal development when given to pregnant women.
- an abnormal sensitivity generally resulting in an allergic reaction.
- a potentially fatal hypersensitivity reaction producing severe respiratory distress and cardiovascular collapse.
- an unexpected reaction the first time a drug is taken, generally due to genetic causes.
- the ability of a substance to harm the kidneys.
- the ability of a substance to cause cancer.
- when two drugs with similar pharmacological actions result in an effect equal to the sum of the individual effects.
- when two drugs with similar pharmacological actions produce greater effects than the sum of the individual effects.
- a drug that antagonizes the toxic effect of another drug.
- a chronic and potentially fatal liver disease causing loss of function and increased resistance to blood flow through the liver.

CHOOSE THE BEST ANSWER.   *the answer key begins on page 347*

1. Drug distribution, metabolism, and excretion are quite different in _____ than in adults because their organ systems are not fully developed.
   a. children and adolescents
   b. elders
   c. infants and adolescents
   d. neonates and infants

2. Children between the ages of _____ metabolize certain drugs more rapidly than adults.
   a. 0 and 6 months
   b. 6 and 18 months
   c. 1 and 2 years
   d. 1 and 12 years

3. Distribution of drugs may be different between men and women due to
   a. hormonal fluctuations.
   b. age.
   c. differences in body composition.
   d. activity.

4. The placebo effect is a
   a. psychological variable.
   b. gender variable.
   c. hypersensitive reaction.
   d. drug dependence variable.

REVIEW

5. Examples of CNS depression include
   a. agitation, confusion, coma.
   b. disorientation, hallucinations, confusion.
   c. delirium, dizziness, hallucinations.
   d. dizziness, drowsiness, sedation, impaired respiration.

6. Drugs that cause hepatotoxicity cause damage to the
   a. liver.
   b. gall bladder.
   c. pancreas.
   d. kidneys.

7. An unexpected adverse effect to a drug the first time it is given to a patient is considered what type of reaction?
   a. hypersensitivity
   b. anaphylaxis
   c. idiosyncrasy
   d. autoimmune

8. Anaphylactic shock usually occurs within
   a. micro-seconds.
   b. minutes.
   c. hours.
   d. days.

9. What organ is associated with the adverse effect of nephrotoxicity?
   a. liver
   b. kidney
   c. gall bladder
   d. gastrointestinal tract

10. Pharmacogenetics is the study of
    a. genetic effects on the ADME processes.
    b. patient variability to placebos.
    c. teratogenicity.
    d. gender differences in the ADME processes.

11. _____ is accompanied by unpleasant physical withdrawal symptoms.
    a. Psychological dependence
    b. Teratogenicity
    c. Physiological dependence
    d. Nephrotoxicity

12. The ability of a drug to cause cancer is called
    a. carcinogenicity.
    b. hepatotoxicity.
    c. nephrotoxicity.
    d. teratogenicity.

13. _____ occur(s) when two drugs with similar pharmacological actions result in an effect equal to the sum of their individual effects.
    a. Additive effects
    b. Displacement
    c. Inhibition
    d. Synergism

14. When two drugs with similar pharmacological actions produce greater effects than the sum of the individual effects the interaction is called
    a. an additive effect.
    b. a synergistic effect.
    c. an induction effect.
    d. a displacement effect.

15. The increased sedation seen when alcohol and a sedative are taken together is a/an
    a. distributional drug-diet interaction.
    b. idiosyncrasy.
    c. enzyme inhibition reaction.
    d. additive drug-drug interaction.

16. A/an _____ is a drug that antagonizes the toxic effects of another drug.
    a. agonist
    b. synergist
    c. antidote
    d. inducer

17. Displacement drug interactions occur at
    a. hepatocytes.
    b. nephrons.
    c. protein binding sites.
    d. glomerulus.

18. Enzyme induction and inhibition would effect which ADME process?
    a. absorption
    b. distribution
    c. metabolism
    d. excretion

19. Glomerular filtration is a part of
    a. excretion.
    b. absorption.
    c. adsorption.
    d. metabolism.

20. Interactions that alter drug absorption can be minimized by separating the administration of the drug and food intake by
    a. 15 minutes.
    b. 30 minutes.
    c. 2 hours.
    d. 4 hours.

21. Cruciferous vegetables like cabbage and brussel sprouts may _____ metabolism of a few drugs.
    a. decrease
    b. increase

22. Spinach and other green vegetables contain vitamin _____ that inhibits the action of oral anticoagulants.
    a. A
    b. E
    c. B-complex
    d. K

23. A patient who has cirrhosis from long term alcohol abuse may experience a/an _____ in metabolism of many drugs.
    a. decrease
    b. increase

24. Acute hepatitis is an inflammatory condition caused by
    a. chronic alcohol abuse.
    b. glomerular filtration.
    c. decreased renal blood flow.
    d. viruses.

25. Which endogenous compound is used to monitor renal function?
    a. ciprofloxacin
    b. creatinine
    c. cimetidine
    d. caffeine

INFORMATION

The tremendous amount of drug research being done results each year in the appearance of many new drugs on pharmacy shelves. As a pharmacy technician, you may find it difficult to absorb all this pharmaceutical information. Even if you do not, however, your knowledge and skills will become outdated in a very short time. Therefore, becoming familiar with the various pharmaceutical information sources will allow you to keep current with information necessary to perform your job on an on-going basis.

Pharmacy literature can be thought of as a pyramid divided into three sections.

Primary literature sits at the base. It provides the foundation for the development of **secondary** and **tertiary** sources of professional literature.

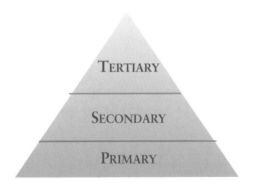

Primary Literature

Primary literature provides direct access to the most current information resulting from contemporary research. It is the largest and most current source of information. This type of literature includes original reports of scientific, clinical, technological, and administrative research projects and studies, and is found in professional and scientific journals such as The Journal of Pharmacy Technology. The need for large storage spaces and the varying quality of journal articles constitute the greatest disadvantage of this type of literature.

primary literature original reports of clinical and other types of research projects and studies.

secondary literature general reference works based upon primary literature sources.

tertiary literature condensed works based on primary literature, such as textbooks, monographs, etc.

PHARMACY LITERATURE

Secondary Literature

Secondary literature consists of general reference works based upon primary literature sources. This type of literature includes **abstracting services**, indexing or bibliographic services, and specialized microfiche systems.

Abstracting services (e.g., *Drugdex*) summarize information contained in a finite number of professional and scientific journals. Indexing or bibliographic services (e.g., *Index Medicus*) contain a comprehensive listing of current articles that have appeared in professional and scientific international journals. You can usually find these indexing services in hospital or university libraries as well as on-line. It's important to remember that a lag time (the time between a discovery or idea and the time of publication), varying from one week to twelve months, exists for secondary literature references.

Tertiary Literature

Tertiary literature sources contain condensed and compact information based on primary literature. This type of literature reference includes: textbooks, monographs, standard reference books, and review articles.

Of the three types of literature reference materials, the pharmacist and pharmacy technicians find the tertiary, which are now also available on CD-ROM and on-line, the easiest and most convenient to use. However, no single tertiary reference source contains all the information needed by the pharmacy department. View tertiary references carefully, since authors of the information may misinterpret or misquote the original literature. In addition, these references may be published one or more years after the original literature and may no longer be current.

abstracting services services that summarize information from various primary sources for quick reference.

LEGAL ASPECTS

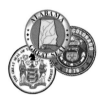

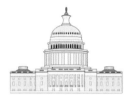

Federal

At present, no federal law exists that mandates the professional literature to be maintained in a pharmacy. The Occupational, Safety, Health Administration (OSHA) does require pharmacies to have Material Safety Data Sheets (MSDS) for each hazardous chemical they use. A pharmacy can obtain these MSDS's from the manufacturer of the hazardous chemical or the local OSHA area office. The MSDS provides information you need to ensure the implementation of proper protective measures for exposure to hazardous chemicals.

The Health Insurance Portability and Accessibility Act (HIPAA) of 1996 affects many of the daily activities that take place in the pharmacy. The act's privacy regulation, *HIPAA Privacy Standards: A Compliance Manual for Pharmacies*, was created to protect the privacy of patient health records and requires pharmacies to set boundaries on the use and disclosure of patients' protected health information (PHI).

State

Most states have Pharmacy Statutes and State Board of Pharmacy Rules and Regulations that require pharmacies to maintain specific professional literature references. For example, the Colorado State Board of Pharmacy requires a professional reference library located in the pharmacy area to contain the *Drug and Druggist Act*; the *Colorado Licensing of Controlled Substances Act*; the *Pharmacy Peer Health Assistance Diversion Program*; the *Uniform Controlled Substances Act of 1992*; the current *Rules and Regulations of the Board of Pharmacies*; the current edition of *21 Code of Federal Regulations (CFR)*; the *Guide to Parenteral Admixtures* or *Handbook of Injectable Drugs;* and *Technical Manual Section IV: Chapter 2, Controlling Occupational Exposure to Hazardous Drugs* or *ASHP Technical Assistance Bulletin on Handling Cytotoxic and Hazardous Drugs* if cytotoxic drugs are compounded.

Legal References

An awareness of the legal aspects of pharmacy protects both the pharmacy technician and the patients. The pharmacy law references described below provide information of laws concerning controlled substances, drug control, and those critical to the practice of pharmacy.

➡ *United States Pharmacopoeia Drug Information (USP DI) Volume III: Approved Drug Products and Legal Requirements* contains the USP and NF drug standards and dispensing requirements, as well as relevant state and federal legal requirements.

➡ *Handbook of Federal Drug Law* by James Robert Nielson provides an understanding of federal drug law as it affects the practice of pharmacy.

➡ *Pharmacy Law Digest of Facts and Comparisons* provides information on controlled substance, pharmacy inspection, drug control, civil liability and business laws. It also contains the addresses of the boards of pharmacy and a survey of the state pharmacy laws compiled and published by the National Association of Boards of Pharmacy (NABP).

COMMON REFERENCES

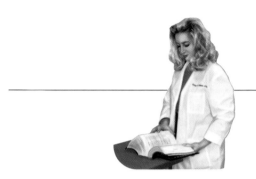

Pharmacists and pharmacy technicians routinely use pharmaceutical reference information in the course of their work.

The ten tertiary literature sources described on these pages are the pharmacy references most commonly available in drug information centers and pharmacies in the United States. Many of these common references are available in a CD-ROM format.

Drug Facts and Comparisons (DFC) (www.factsandcomparisons.com)

The DFC is a preferred reference for comprehensive and timely drug information, containing information about prescription and OTC products. DFC divides drugs into therapeutic groups. Similar drugs are grouped together with easy-to-use comparative tables. The loose-leaf edition provides the most up-to-date drug reference, with new or revised information sent each month.

Martindale, *The Complete Drug Reference*

Formerly known as Martindale, *The Extra Pharmacopoeia,* this reference provides the best source of information on drugs in clinical use internationally. It contains drug monographs that provide information of the properties, actions and uses of drugs. Martindale lists proprietary drug names and their country of origin.

AHFS Drug Information (www.ashp.org/products-services)

The AHFS is accepted as the authority for drug information questions. It groups drug monographs by therapeutic use. Various organizations and programs recognize it as a leading source of drug information for determining reimbursement of prescriptions and as a resource for Drug Utilization Reviews (DUR). The AHFS master volume appears in January. Updates on newly approved uses, new drugs, and other timely information are released periodically. Online updates are available at www.ashp.org/ahfs.

Handbook on Injectable Drugs

This is a collection of monographs on commercially available parenteral drugs that include concentration, stability, dosage and compatibility information.

Physicians' Desk Reference (PDR) (www.pdr.net)

The PDR is an annual publication intended for physicians that provides prescription information on major pharmaceutical products. You will find that PDR information is similar to the pharmaceutical manufacturer's drug package inserts since manufacturers prepare the essential drug information found in the PDR. The PDR contains five color-coded sections: an alphabetical brand name drug index, a drug classification index by company, a generic and chemical name index, a product identification section, and a product information section of drug monographs. New and revised information is published periodically in supplements. Be aware that the PDR is not a comprehensive source of drug information.

The Merck Index (www.merck.com)

This is an encyclopedic source of chemical substance data, contains monographs referenced by trade, code, chemical, investigational and abbreviated drug names. The index also provides the pharmacy technician with two additional features: an extensive section of tables, and a formulary index.

American Drug Index

This index provides the most exhaustive list of drugs and drug products. It contains trade and generic drug names, phonetic pronunciations, indications, manufacturers and schedule information in a dictionary format. The index cross-references drugs by generic, brand, and chemical names.

Drug Topics Red Book

The *Red Book* is the pharmacist's guide to accurate product information and prices on prescription drugs, OTC items, and reimbursable medical supplies., provide annual price lists of drug products including manufacturer, package size, strength and wholesale and retail prices. It contains nationally-recognized AWP's, NDC numbers for all FDA-approved drugs, complete package information, common lab values, buying groups and billing standards, drug interaction information and directories for manufacturers, wholesalers and third party administrators.

United States Pharmacopoeia Drug Information (USP DI) (www.usp.org)

The *USP DI* provides comprehensive and clinically relevant information on drugs in current use. Divided into three volumes: *Volume I* is *Drug Information for the Health Care Professional*, *Volume II* is *Advice for the Patient*, and *Volume III* is *Approved Drug Products and Legal Requirements*. This volume includes the "Orange Book", which is the common name for the FDA's *Approved Drug Products* publication.

Stedman's Medical Dictionary (www.stedmans.com)

This dictionary provides the medical word reference needed in the pharmacy.

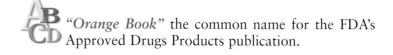 *"Orange Book"* the common name for the FDA's Approved Drugs Products publication.

OTHER REFERENCES

Professional Practice Journals

These journals are official publications of pharmacy organizations and can reflect the political views or policies of these groups. They also reflect changes in standards of practice and indicate trends in the profession. They may publish some original research studies. Examples are *Today's Technician (NPTA)*, *America's Pharmacist* (NCPA), *American Journal of Health-System Pharmacists* (ASHP) and *Journal of the American Pharmacists' Association* (APhA).

Trade Journals

Trade journals are published commercially for pharmacist but are not produced by the profession. They tend to contain large amounts of advertising material. Examples are: *American Druggist*, *Pharmacy Times* (www.pharmacytimes.com), *US Pharmacist* (www.uspharmacist.com), and *Community Pharmacist* (www.communityrph.com).

Primary Literature

Primary literature can be accessed by printed indexes and abstracts or by CD-ROM and online database searching. The continuing development of online and CD-ROM databases has increased the efficiency of the access, retrieval, and storage of information. *Micromedex* (www.micromedex.com) and MEDLINE (www.nlm.nih.gov) are two databases of importance to the pharmaceutical researcher. *Micromedex* provides a compilation of full-text databases covering drug information, toxicology and critical care. It includes *Drugdex*, *Poisondex*, and *Identidex* as well as *Index Nominum*, *Martindale*, *The Physician's Desk Reference* (PDR), *Red Book*, and *USP DI Volume I* and *Volume III*. *Index Medicus*, online as MEDLINE, contributes the most comprehensive index of international medical literature. Citations are arranged alphabetically by first author and by subject headings.

Newsletters

Newsletters are published rapidly and frequently and provide a useful source of current information. *The Medical Letter* and *The Pink Sheet* are a few examples of the many newsletters available to pharmacy personnel.

➡ *The Medical Letter on Drugs and Therapeutics* (www.medicalletter.org) contains short abstracts from journal articles. It also provides information on clinical trials and profiles on products recently granted New Drug Application (NDA) status.

➡ *The Pink Sheet* (www.thepinksheet.com) reports on important regulatory issues, company marketing business and new products.

 Except generally for textbooks, many of these resources (including a considerable amount of primary literature) are available (at least in part) over the Internet. For more information on using the Internet, turn the next page.

Textbooks

Textbooks can provide basic information on a particular topic or a range of topics. As with any publications, there is a wide range in the quality, level, and usefulness of textbooks. It is important to not accept the information in them as the last word on a subject. However, textbooks are very useful for explaining basic concepts and in refreshing your understanding of a topic. The texts below are noted for their authoritativeness and reliability in providing pharmaceutical information and in including the citations of primary material.

➥ *Handbook of Nonprescription Drugs*

The *Handbook* provides the most comprehensive source available for OTC products. It serves both as a textbook for the pharmacy student and an information source for the practicing pharmacist. It is also a useful source for patient education. Infrequent revision is the main drawback of this reference.

➥ Remington, *The Science and Practice of Pharmacy*

Published every 5 years since 1885, Remington's is the most comprehensive work in the pharmaceutical sciences. Remington's covers all aspects of pharmacy for students, practitioners and researchers, including evolution of pharmacy, ethics, pharmaceutics, pharmaceutical testing and manufacturing, pharmacodynamics, and pharmacy practice.

➥ *Goodman and Gilman's The Pharmacological Basis of Therapeutics* (www.goodmanandgilman.com)

This is a principal pharmacy text on pharmacology and therapeutics, emphasizing clinical pharmacy practice. It guides the reader to citations in the primary literature.

Personal Digital Assistants (PDA's)

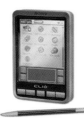

A PDA is a fully functioning computer the size of a paperback book. In 1996, the original Palm Pilot was introduced. It ran for weeks on AAA batteries, was easy to use and could store thousands of contacts, appointments and notes. PDA's have evolved into machines for downloading information from the Internet. They fall into two major categories, hand-held and palm-sized. Hand-held computers are larger, have larger liquid crystal displays (LCD's) and use a miniature keyboard. Palm-sized computers are smaller, have smaller LCD's and rely on stylus/touch-screen technology for data entry. All PDA's come with personal information management (PIM) software. Pharmacists use these devices to provide drug information to patients and health care professionals. Pharmacy software is available on the Internet from a variety of sources including www.epocrates.com, www.micromedex.com, www.lexi.com, and www.ashp.org.

THE INTERNET

A computer network is a series of computers connected by a communication line that allows the computers to exchange information. The Internet is a "supernetwork," with many networks from around the world all connected to each other by telephone lines, and all using a common "language" (software and rules for communication) that enable them to communicate with each other.

The Internet is the world's largest network.

It has grown from a skeletal experimental network used by scientists to a gigantic commercial "information superhighway" used daily by over fifty million people in 1998. It also contains the world's largest source of information, the **World Wide Web**.

The World Wide Web is a "virtual" library in which electronic information existing on hundreds of thousands of Web sites is accessible to Internet users.

Among this information is a growing amount of pharmacy literature and reference. In addition, patients are increasingly using the World Wide Web to find pharmaceutical and health information.

What It Costs

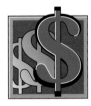

There's a monthly fee for the ISP. Most heavy Internet users set up both their ISP and local phone service on an "unlimited" basis. That is, they pay a flat rate for unlimited local calls and unlimited time on the Internet. In addition to phone lines we now have DSL, cable and Satellite High-Speed Internet Access.

World Wide Web a collection of electronic documents at addresses called Web sites.

modem a piece of hardware that enables a computer to communicate through telephone lines.

browser a software program that allows users to view Web sites on the World Wide Web.

Internet Service Provider (ISP) a company that provides access to the Internet.

URL(uniform resource locator) a web address.

search engine software that searches the web for information related to criteria entered by the user.

GETTING CONNECTED

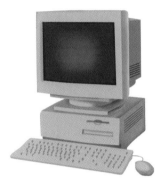

A computer user can connect to the Internet and explore the World Wide Web if they have the following:

➡ **An Internet ready computer:** this is a computer with a **modem**, a small hardware item that can connect the computer to a telephone line.

➡ **A connection:** the modem needs to be connected to a telephone line, the same kind of connection a standard telephone uses.

➡ **Internet software:** Typically, this has been called a **browser**, the most popular of which are Netscape Navigator and Microsoft Explorer. Browsers have many functions that allow you to move around the Web, view Web sites, print their contents, save information, and so on. They generally include an Email function that allows you to send messages to anyone on the Internet with an email address.

➡ **An Internet Service Provider (ISP):** America Online, Earthlink, and Microsoft Network are just some of the popular providers. Generally, people use providers with local area code "access numbers" so their Internet "calls" cost no more than a local phone call.

Web addresses can and do change. If one of the addresses on this page doesn't work, try looking up the address in a search engine.

FINDING WHAT YOU WANT

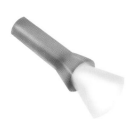

Connecting to the Internet is only a starting point. To find information, you must have the specific addresses of Web sites you want to visit. (Web addresses are also referred to as **URLs** – uniform resource locators). For example, to go to the USP site, you enter **www.usp.org** in the address line of your browser.

If you don't know the address you want, you can use a **search engine** to look for it. This is software that will search the Web for specific information you enter. Different search engines have different rules for entering search criteria, but they are very easy to use, and most Internet users rely on them heavily. Here are addresses for a few:

➨ **AltaVista**: www.altavista.digital.com

➨ **Infoseek**: www.infoseek.com

➨ **HotBot**: www.hotbot.com

➨ **Google**: www.google.com

➨ **Dogpile**: www.dogpile.com

PLACES TO VISIT

Pharmacy Education and Related Information

➨ www.altimed.com
Ratiopharm – The pharmacist's guide to the internet

➨ www.rxlist.com
RxList: Internet Drug Index – The top 200 drugs

➨ www.pharmacylaw.buffalo.edu/
Covers New York state pharmacy practice laws

➨ www.pharmacy.org
The virtual library in pharmacy

➨ www.micromedex.com
Provides the most trusted information for health-care safety and the environment

➨ www.lexi.com
 Provides unique knowledge and tools to improve the quality of patient care.

➨ www.ismp.org
The Institute for Safe Medication Practices: provides medication safety alerts, error reporting and self-assessment guidelines

Pharmacy Organizations

➨ www.nacds.org
National Association of Chain Drug Stores

➨ www.ncpanet.org
National Community Pharmacists Association

➨ www.aphanet.org
American Pharmacists Association

➨ www.ashp.org
American Society of Health-System Pharmacists

➨ www.jcaho.org
Joint Commission on Accreditation of Healthcare Organizations

➨ www.nabp.net
National Association of Boards of Pharmacy

Government

➨ www.usdoj.gov/dea
U.S. Drug Enforcement Administration

➨ www.fda.gov/cder
U.S. Food and Drug Administration

➨ www.access.gpo.gov
U.S. Government Printing Office: provides access to government information products

➨ www.osha.gov
Occupational Safety & Health Administration

➨ www.hipaa.org
Information on how to handle HIPAA

➨ www.os.dhhs.gov
US Department of Health and Human Services

TECHNICIAN REFERENCES

There are many references that provide valuable information on the pharmacy technician profession.

They are useful for those interested in entering the field, technicians wishing to improve their skills and professionalism, and instructors.

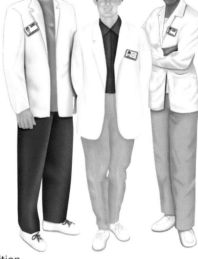

Occupational Information

These references present an overview of the profession for those interested in becoming pharmacy technicians.

➡ Rudman, Jack. *Pharmacy Technician* . Career Examination Serv.; Vol. C-3822. This is available at www.amazon.com.

➡ *The Pharmacy Technician Companion: Your Road Map to Technician Training and Careers.* Washington, DC: American Pharmacist Association, 1998. This is available at the www.pharmacist.com store.

➡ *Occupational Outlook Handbook.* Washington, D.C.: Bureau of Labor Statistics. This is annual edition.

Occupational Information on the Internet

A considerable amount of information is available on the Internet regarding the responsibilities of a pharmacy technician, the training required, salary, and job opportunities. A good first stop for this information is the Educational Testing Service's SIGI PLUS® site: www.ets.org/sigi/pharmtec.html.

You can also visit the Bureau of Labor Statistics' Occupational Outlook Handbook site (http://www.bls.gov/oco and use the Index to look up pharmacy technicians and pharmacy assistants.

Another good way to look up job descriptions, training programs, opportunities, and other information is to use a search engine. Just enter "pharmacy technician" and start exploring!

Training Programs

Many pharmacy technicians receive informal, on-the-job training but formal training programs are becoming more widespread. These programs differ in many respects, from credentials to program length. A directory of ASHP-accredited training programs can be found at www.ashp.org/directories/technicians. The Pharmacy Technician Educators' Council (PTEC) recommendations for pharmacy technology program content can be found at www.rxptec.org under links.

Pharmacy Technician Organizations and Publications

➡ American Association of Pharmacy Technicians (www. pharmacytechnician.com)

➡ National Pharmacy Technician Association (www.pharmacytechnician.org)

➡ *The Journal of Pharmacy Technology* (www.jpharmtechnol.com): provides information covering the entire body of pharmacy practice and includes CE articles.

➡ *Today's Technician* (www.pharmacytechnician.org/magazine): a bimonthly journal specifically for pharmacy technicians including news briefs, technician spotlight, new products, compounding corner and technician specific CE programs.

➡ *CPhT Connection* (www.ptcb.org): the newsletter of the Pharmacy Technician Certification Board (PTCB).

Certification Examination Preparation

In 1995 the Pharmacy Technician Certification Board (PTCB) began administering the National Pharmacy Technician Certification Examination (PTCE). These texts, and the Pharmacy Technician Certification Board website at www.ptcb.org, offer information to help individuals prepare for the PTCE.

➡ *Pharmacy Technician Certification Review and Practice Exam.* Bethesda, MD: American Society of Health-System Pharmacists, 1998. This is the APHA's complete review for the pharmacy technician.

➡ *Pharmacy Certified Technician Training Manual.* Washington, DC: American Pharmacist Association.

➡ *APHA's Complete Math Review for the Pharmacy Technician.* Washington DC: American Pharmacist Association.

➡ *Pharmacy Technician Workbook and Certification Review, 2nd edition.* Englewood, CO: Morton Publishing, 2004.

➡ *Certification Review for Pharmacy Technicians.* Evergreen, CO: Ark Pharmaceutical Consultants.

➡ Math Master *Pharmaceutical Calculations.* Evergreen, CO: Ark Pharmaceutical Consultants

Continuing Education and Information

Once certified, the PTCB requires you to obtain 20 hours of continuing education credit every two years to maintain your certification. At least one contact hour in pharmacy law is required. This publication offers the certified pharmacy technician ten contact hours of continuing education.

➡ *C.E. for Pharmacy Technicians.* Washington, DC: American Pharmaceutical Association., 1997

➡ www.techlectures.com: continuing education for technicians

➡ www.rxtrek.net: information for technicians

Professional Liability

Since the pharmacy technician is a recognized professional, Pharmacist Mutual (www.phmic.com) offers a pharmacy technician liability policy that meets the needs of today's pharmacy technician.

Whether you are considering becoming a pharmacy technician, receiving certification or recertification, or simply maintaining your competency and skills, it's always a good idea to research and read about your job. There's a lot you learn on your own, if you make the effort.

REVIEW

KEY CONCEPTS

INFORMATION

✔ Primary literature provides direct access to the most current contemporary research. Secondary literature primarily consists of general reference works based upon primary literature sources. Tertiary literature sources contain condensed information based on primary literature.

✔ OSHA requires pharmacies to have Material Safety Data Sheets (MSDS) for all their hazardous chemicals.

✔ States have laws and State Board of Pharmacy rules and regulations that require pharmacies to maintain specific professional literature references.

COMMON REFERENCES

✔ *Drug Facts and Comparisons* (DFC) is a preferred reference for comprehensive and timely drug information, containing information about prescription and OTC products.

✔ Martindale, *The Complete Drug Reference* provides the best source of information on drugs in clinical use internationally.

✔ *AHFS* is accepted as the authority for drug information questions. It groups drug monographs by therapeutic use.

✔ The *USP DI* Volume I-III provides comprehensive and clinically relevant information on drugs and drug standards as well as state and federal law requirements. Volume III contains the FDA's Approved Drug Products publication, commonly known as "The Orange Book."

✔ The *Handbook on Injectable Drugs* is a collection of monographs on commercially available parenteral drugs that include concentration, stability, dosage and compatibility information.

✔ The *Drug Topics Red Book* is the pharmacist's guide to products and prices and provides annual price lists of drug products including manufacturer, package size, strength and whole sale and retail prices.

OTHER REFERENCES

✔ *Index Medicus*, online as MEDLINE, contributes the most comprehensive index of international medical literature.

✔ A personal digital assistant (PDA) is a fully functioning computer the size of a paperback book. Pharmacists use it to provide drug information. Pharmacy software for PDA's can be downloaded from the internet.

THE INTERNET

✔ The Internet is a supernetwork, with many networks from around the world all connected to each other by telephone lines, cable or satellite and all using a common "language."

✔ A search engine will search the Web for specific information you enter.

TECHNICIAN REFERENCES

✔ The Pharmacy Technician Certification Board (PTCB) administers the National Pharmacy Technician Certification Exam (PTCE). The PTCB website at www.ptcb.org provides information regarding exam application and preparation.

✔ Once certified as a Pharmacy Technician, the PTCB requires you to obtain 20 hours of continuing education credit every two years to maintain your certification.

SELF TEST

MATCH THE TERMS.   *answers can be checked in the glossary*

abstracting services

HIPAA

Internet Service Provider (ISP)

PDA

professional practice journals

primary literature

search engine

secondary literature

tertiary literature

World Wide Web

- original reports of clinical and other types of research projects and studies.
- general reference works based upon primary literature sources.
- condensed works based on primary literature, such as textbooks, monographs, etc.
- services that summarize information from various primary sources for quick reference.
- regulation created to protect the privacy of patient health records.
- a fully functioning computer the size of a paperback book.
- a collection of electronic documents at internet addresses.
- a company that provides access to the Internet.
- software that searches the web for information related to criteria entered by the user.
- official publications of pharmacy organizations

CHOOSE THE BEST ANSWER.   *the answer key begins on page 347*

1. _____ literature contains original reports of clinical and other types of research projects and studies.
   a. Secondary
   b. Abstract
   c. Primary
   d. Tertiary

2. _____ literature contains general reference works based upon primary literature sources.
   a. Orange
   b. Tertiary
   c. Secondary
   d. Abstract

3. The Occupational, Safety and Health Administration (OSHA) requires pharmacies to have this literature on hand:
   a. Material Safety Data Sheets
   b. *The Merck Index*
   c. policy and procedure manuals
   d. Remington, *The Science and Practice of Pharmacy*

4. HIPAA has established boundaries for use and disclosure of _____ (PHI).
   a. patient health information
   b. private health information
   c. protected health information
   d. portable health information

REVIEW

5. The *USP DI* has _____ volumes.
   a. one
   b. two
   c. three
   d. four

6. This common reference provides comprehensive and timely drug information about prescriptions and OTC products.
   a. *American Hospital Formulary Service*
   b. *Drug Facts and Comparisons*
   c. *Physicians' Desk Reference*
   d. *USP DI*

7. Which common reference would you use to find information on a drug from England?
   a. *Drug Facts and Comparisons*
   b. Martindale, *The Complete Drug Reference*
   c. *The Merck Index*
   d. *USP DI*

8. _____ loose leaf with updates provides the up-to-date drug information with new or revised information sent each month.
   a. *The Merck Index*
   b. *Drug Facts and Comparisons*
   c. *Physicians' Desk Reference*
   d. *USP DI Volume II*

9. _____ is an encyclopedic source of chemical substance data.
   a. *Drug Facts and Comparisons*
   b. *Physicians' Desk Reference*
   c. *American Drug Index*
   d. *The Merck Index*

10. _____ provides nationally recognized AWPs and NDCs for FDA approved drugs.
    a. *USP DI Volume I*
    b. Orange Book
    c. *USP DI Volume II*
    d. *Red Book*

11. *Today's Technician* is an example of a
    a. pink sheet.
    b. trade journal.
    c. professional practice journal.
    d. newsletter.

12. *Pharmacy Times* is an example of a
    a. textbook.
    b. primary literature.
    c. pharmacopoeia.
    d. trade journal.

13. _____ is an example of a newsletter.
    a. *Drug Facts and Comparisons*
    b. *The Merck Index*
    c. *The Medical Letter*
    d. *Physicians' Desk Reference*

14. The most comprehensive text covering pharmaceutical sciences is
    a. Remington, *The Science and Practice of Pharmacy.*
    b. *Goodman and Gilman's The Pharmacological Basis of Therapeutics.*
    c. the Orange Book.
    d. the *American Drug Index.*

15. A _____ is a piece of computer hardware that enables a computer to communicate through telephone lines.
    a. mother board
    b. modem
    c. monitor
    d. keyboard

16. A company that provides access to the Internet is a/an
    a. browser.
    b. isp.
    c. search engine.
    d. url.

17. Internet Explorer and Netscape Navigator are examples of
    a. modems.
    b. browsers.
    c. search engines.
    d. uniform resource locators.

18. DSL provides internet connections that are _____ than telephone modem connections.
    a. slower
    b. faster

19. The Bureau of Labor Statistics provides information about careers on the internet in the
    a. *Occupational Outlook Handbook.*
    b. "Orange Book."
    c. *Red Book.*
    d. *Pink Sheet.*

20. The directory of accredited technician training programs can be found at the website for
    a. BLS.
    b. ASHP.
    c. APhA.
    d. PTEC.

21. How many hours of continuing education does PTCB require you to obtain every two years to maintain your certification?
    a. 10
    b. 15
    c. 20
    d. 30

22. What bimonthly journal provides information and continuing education specifically for pharmacy technicians?
    a. *The Journal of Pharmacy Technology*
    b. *Today's Technician*
    c. *Pharmacy Times*
    d. *The Pink Sheet*

23. How many contact hours of continuing education in pharmacy law is required every two years to maintain your certification?
    a. one
    b. two
    c. three
    d. four

INVENTORY MANAGEMENT

An *inventory* is a listing of the goods or items that a business will use in its normal operation.

Pharmacies generally develop an inventory of medications based upon what they expect to need. Rarely used medications might not be kept in inventory but instead ordered as needed.

The goal of inventory management is to ensure that drugs are available when they are needed.

Because medication needs are often urgent, pharmacies must maintain good control of their stock or inventory. This means that all drugs which are likely to be needed are both on hand and usable—that is, they have not expired or been damaged, contaminated, or otherwise made unfit for use. The technician plays a critical role in inventory management, but there are many participants in the process—the pharmacy, the institution, the wholesaler, the manufacturer, the government, insurers and other third parties.

Inventory management is an integral part of the technician's job responsibility.

Each technician is required to master the specific inventory system in use at their workplace. In some cases, inventory management may be the technician's primary responsibility, and the technician has the opportunity to become a "pharmaceutical buyer." At hospitals and other institutions, for example, a **purchasing/inventory technician** is often responsible for obtaining and maintaining the institution's medication and device supply.

Why Use Wholesalers?

The thousands of medications that a pharmacy stocks represent many manufacturers. Obtaining them from individual manufacturers would be a difficult and costly process. Besides the paperwork involved (individual purchase orders, invoices, payments, etc.), there would be many different procedures to learn: how orders could be placed, how they would be shipped, returns policies, and so on.

Wholesalers stock inventories of the most used medications, obtain less-used medications as they are needed, and make frequent deliveries, often on a daily basis. They also provide added-value services such as emergency delivery, automated inventory systems, automated purchasing systems, generic substitution options, private label products, and many others. Obtaining most medications from a single wholesaler greatly simplifies the purchasing process and reduces the staff needed for it.

THE INVENTORY ENVIRONMENT

There are many participants in the inventory process—the pharmacy, the institution, the wholesaler, the manufacturer, the government, insurers and other third parties.

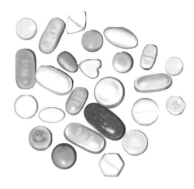

The Formulary

Many hospitals, HMOs, insurers, and other health-care systems maintain a list of medications called a **formulary.** These are the medications that are approved for use in the system.

➡ An **open formulary** is one that allows purchase of any medication that is prescribed.

➡ A **closed formulary** is a limited list of approved medications. A physician must receive permission to use a medication that is not on the list. Closed formularies are generally used as a cost savings tool, in which less expensive substitutes are stocked. Though these substitutes are mainly generic equivalents, in some hospitals a drug on the formulary that is **therapeutically equivalent** (chemically different but with similar actions and effects) may be substituted for a drug not on the formulary.

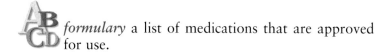 *formulary* a list of medications that are approved for use.

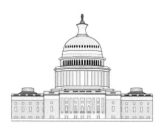

The Government

In the United States, the Drug Enforcement Administration (DEA) regulates the distribution of controlled substances and has various distribution, inventory, record keeping, and ordering requirements. Schedule II substances must be stocked separately in a secure place and require a special order form for reordering. Their stock also must be continually monitored and documented.

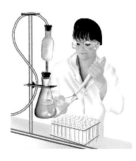

Drug manufacturers

Drugs are not always available from wholesalers due to expense, storage requirements, or other reasons. When this is the case, they can be obtained directly from the manufacturer. When ordering from a manufacturer, a **purchasing account** for the pharmacy must be set up with the manufacturer.

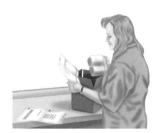

The Pharmacy

Individual pharmacies (whether in community or institutional environments) may use their own inventory system or one provided by another party such as a wholesaler or a corporate parent if they are part of a chain. When drugs need to be purchased, pharmacies buy them directly from wholesalers and sometimes manufacturers, or participate in a large purchasing group which buys the drugs in bulk for its members. Because of the savings that bulk purchasing provides, independent pharmacies often join buying groups that negotiate bulk contracts.

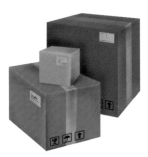

Wholesalers

More than three-quarters of pharmaceutical manufacturers' sales are directly to drug wholesalers*, who in turn resell their inventory to hospitals, pharmacies, and other pharmaceutical dispensers. Wholesalers stock tens of thousands of items from hundreds of manufacturers, everything from disposable razors to Activase, a life saving emergency use drug. They are government-licensed and regulated and offer their customers dependable one-stop-shopping for most of their medication needs. Using wholesalers simplifies the drug purchasing process and saves time, effort, and expense.

source: National Wholesale Drug Association

INVENTORY SYSTEMS

A pharmaceutical inventory system is able to track inventory, forecast needs, and generate reorders to maintain adequate inventory.

This means that neither too many nor too few drugs are on hand at all times. Too many drugs on hand involves unnecessary cost and maintenance and may result in spoilage. Too few drugs means that medications won't be available when needed. The goal of a good inventory system is to have the right amount of stock available at all times.

In order to maintain an adequate supply of medications, pharmacies use a perpetual inventory system.

A perpetual inventory system maintains a continuous record of every item in inventory so that it always shows the stock on hand. This is a requirement for Schedule II substances, but it is also important for many medications since their availability has health consequences.

Spoilage

Time or storage conditions may cause the chemical compounds in medications to break down, resulting in either lost potency or changed function. This is called inventory spoilage. Use of such medications may be dangerous. As a result, medications carry expiration dates and storage requirements that must be honored. It is an important task of the pharmacy technician to constantly check all stock for drugs going out of date.

✔ **Note:** As an expiration date approaches, it may already be too late to dispense the medication, since it must be used before the date passes. If an expiration date for a medication has passed, or the medication cannot be completely used before that date, the medication must be appropriately disposed of or returned to the supplier for credit. In some cases, wholesalers will not accept expired drugs, but the drug manufacturer will. When returned, packages must generally be unopened.

turnover the rate at which inventory is used, generally expressed in number of days.

point of sale system (POS) an inventory system in which the item is deducted from inventory as it is sold or dispensed.

reorder points minimum and maximum stock levels which determine when a reorder is placed and for how much.

INVENTORY CONCEPTS

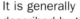

Turnover

Turnover is the rate at which inventory is used. It is generally described by the number of days it takes for the complete stock of an item to be used.

Besides quality and spoilage issues, there's a financial consideration to rapid stock turnover. If a supplier's payment terms are "thirty days net" and stock turnover averages less than thirty days, the stock will be sold before the supplier must be paid for it. The more this is true of the turnover, the lower the cost is of the stock.

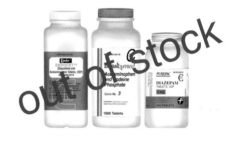

Availability

Besides monitoring stock on hand, it is important to monitor the market availability of medications. At any time, a particular drug may be unavailable due to manufacturing difficulties, raw material unavailability, recalls, etc. This can increase market demand for substitutes for the unavailable drug, sometimes causing shortages in the substitutes as well.

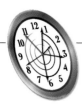

TOOLS FOR PERPETUAL INVENTORY

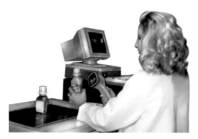

Point of sale (POS)

Pharmacy operations generally use a point of sale system in which the item is deducted from inventory as it is sold or dispensed. The transaction is often triggered by the scanning of a bar code on the medication packaging, though it can also be keyed into the system.

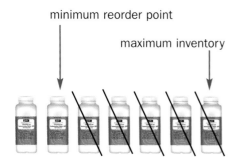

Reorder Points

In order to maintain adequate inventory for their needs, community and institutional pharmacies maintain computer databases of their inventory using drug reorder points. These are **maximum** and **minimum** inventory levels for each drug. As the minimum reorder point of a medication is reached, most computer systems will generate an automatic purchase order for more of it. What medications should be ordered (and how much) is automatically identified on a daily basis. The order amount will be calculated to reach the maximum reorder point. Reorder points for any item can generally be set according to the needs of the facility.

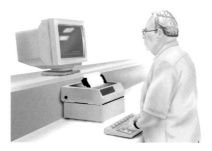

Automated Reports

Computerized inventory systems provide a continuous picture of the inventory situation through automated reports that allow users to analyze and monitor their inventory a variety of ways. They automatically update stock amounts, track turnover, produce purchase orders based on reorder points, and forecast future needs.

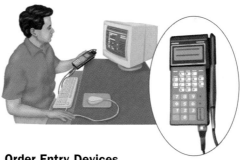

Order Entry Devices

Portable hand held devices are widely used to enter ordering data. When inspection of stock shows that a drug is approaching the minimum inventory level, the reorder can be made using one of these devices. The drug's ID number is entered by hand or scanned into the device using a bar coded shelf tag and the wand attached to the device. A desired quantity, generally enough to reach the maximum inventory level, is then entered to complete the order. The data is sent over a phone line to the institution's ordering computer, which processes the data and sends an order based on it via modem to the supplier's computer.

COMPUTERS & INVENTORY

Computerized inventory systems automatically adjust inventory and generate orders based on maintaining set inventory levels.

The inventory system is often just a component of a comprehensive pharmacy management system that includes elements like patient profiling, management reporting, and so on. In many cases, the drug wholesaler provides the system to its customers as part of the wholesaler service. The customer's system interacts with the wholesaler's so that various types of information (pricing, order information, etc.) can be exchanged automatically between the two systems.

Entering correct information is essential to any computer system.

Computerized systems may automatically create and maintain records based on each inventory transaction. However, many of these transactions are manually entered into the system. So there is always a possibility of error. For this reason, each system produces reports that cover virtually every aspect of the inventory process from stock to turnover to reorders. These reports can be read on screen or in printed form so that errors can be detected.

To protect against possible abuses, users are given passwords to access different features of the system.

This not only protects the employer, but the employee as well. It prevents unauthorized activities and also documents who did what and when.

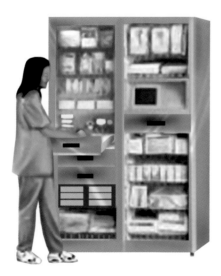

Supply Station, courtesy of Pyxis

AUTOMATED DISPENSING SYSTEMS

Baker Cells® is an example of an **automated counting/filling device** which is sometimes used by pharmacies that process a high volume of prescriptions. These devices have cells, each of which is filled with a particular drug. When a drug is ordered, the device quickly counts the appropriate amount of capsules or tablets into the a prescription vial. Some devices also produce the prescription label. Technicians keep the cells stocked and must record all lot numbers of drugs used.

Pyxis Supply Station® is an example of an **automated point-of-use storage system** for making floor stock items available to nurses in the hospital setting. A network of storage stations are located throughout a facility and are connected to a Pyxis server which in turn links to the hospital's ADT, billing, and materials management information systems. The system not only tracks inventory per se but keeps a record of which drugs/supplies were taken by which nurse for which patient.

Homerus® is an example of a centralized **robotic unit-dose dispensing device.** It can individually package and store large amounts of medications from bulk supplies, deliver bar-coded medications to 24-hour patient-specific medication bins, and return medications to storage after a patient is discharged.

Some hospitals have **mobile robots** that travel throughout a facility delivering drugs to various nursing units and departments.

database a collection of information structured so that specific information within it can easily be retrieved and used.

KEY COMPUTER CONSIDERATIONS

Manual Checking

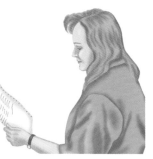

Checking reports manually is an important step in ensuring that records are correct. Simple data entry errors can result in serious mistakes affecting orders, stock availability, prices, and other issues. For example: If a box containing 150 u/d tablets of Tylenol (R) is set up in the system as one unit, but is incorrectly keyed into the system as 150 units, the system's information will be grossly incorrect.

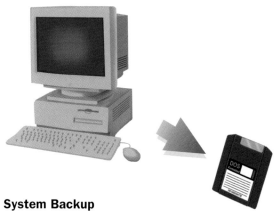

System Backup

Each system's **database** of information is a critical component of the pharmacy or institution in which it functions. These files must be regularly **backed-up** or copied to an appropriate storage media. There are many types of such media but whatever the media, it is important to know its reliability. Depending on the operation, back up may need to be performed daily.

System Care and Maintenance

Computer systems have become very durable, but they need care and maintenance. It is important to know and follow the operating instructions for any system. Some factors that can cause damage to computers are:

- ✔ temperature;
- ✔ dust;
- ✔ moisture;
- ✔ movement;
- ✔ vibrations;
- ✔ power surges.

PC Based Systems

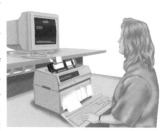

Personal computer-based systems require periodic maintenance, such as **defragmentation** of the files on the system. This is essentially a reorganization of files that have been automatically stored in pieces or fragments on the system. Up to a point, this is not a problem. However, too many fragmented files on a system will slow it down and may cause other problems. Each system contains software that defragments its files. Some work automatically. Some require a user to start the program.

The Operation Manual

Computer systems have operation manuals that explain how to use and maintain the system. It is of course necessary that users of the system follow the manual's instructions. It is also important that they store the manual in a safe and accessible location so they can refer to it when they need to.

 It is important to know the system care, maintenance, backup, and hard copy requirements that apply to the system you use at your workplace.

ORDERING

Ordering systems involve automated and manual activities.

Much of the work is done by computer systems, both the orderer's and the supplier's. However, manual checking, editing, and confirmation are essential to making such systems work as required.

AUTOMATED ORDERING

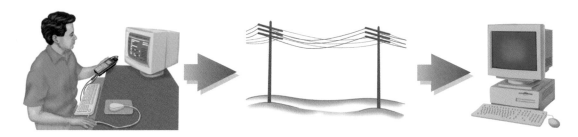

Orders can be generated using an order entry device or automatically generated by the system based on stock levels and reorder points. These reports must then be checked and confirmed. If changes are needed, they can be made manually. The system then produces a revised order, which should again be checked and edited until it is ready for sending to the supplier.

When an order is ready, the ordering system and the supplier's system are connected over phone lines so the order can be "downloaded" from one system to the other.

The supplier's computer system analyzes the order line by line to determine if it can be filled as requested. It checks to see if there is enough of each item in the supplier's inventory to fill the order. If there is more than one warehouse in the system, it may check multiple locations to see if the items are available.

➡ If the order can be filled as ordered, a message will automatically confirm the order to the ordering system. This confirmation can be read onscreen by the orderer but should also be printed for their records.

➡ If the order cannot be filled exactly as ordered, a message containing the **exceptions** will be sent. This report should be printed and appropriate action taken to fill the order. It may be necessary to create a second purchase order, talk with the supplier personally, or find an alternative supplier. Some common reasons for omissions are: temporarily out-of-stocks, back-ordered drugs, or the item may no longer be carried.

ORDER DETAILS

Shipping

When a purchase order is sent to a supplier, the type of shipping is indicated by the orderer. This will determine both the time and cost of shipping.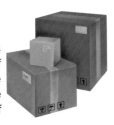

When the order is shipped, it may be a single shipment or multiple shipments. For example, if a single distribution center of a supplier does not have all the items ordered, a partial shipment at a later time or from another distribution center may be needed to fill the order.

Material Safety Data Sheets (MSDS) for hazardous substances such as chemotherapeutic agents indicate when special handling and shipping is required. The Postal Service, Federal Express, United Parcel Service, and others all have specific policies for shipping hazardous substances that must be followed. Some substances are not allowed to be shipped by plane, because the Federal Aviation Administration (FAA) will not allow them onboard. Often these drugs are shipped via a courier.

Credits/Returns

Each supplier has a policy and procedure for returns and credit that must be followed in order to receive the credit. As with orders, the documentation must be carefully checked item by item to make sure it is accurate. A printed copy must be kept on file in addition to any electronic version.

There are companies that specialize in returns to the manufacturer of expired drugs and drugs removed from a formulary. These companies complete each manufacturer's return form, follow their procedures, as well as package, mail and track the drugs. They also return and fill out the paper work for **C-II drugs** and other controlled substances. Their fee is generally a percentage of the return credit, and is deducted automatically from the refund so there is not a separate bill.

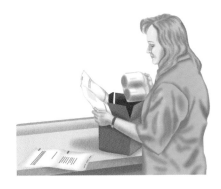

Receiving

Accuracy is essential in checking in the medications received from suppliers. It is important to be alert for drugs that have been incorrectly picked, received damaged, are outdated or missing entirely from the supplier. In many settings, items are stickered with bar codes that can be scanned to do an automatic count.

✔ Shipments, invoices and purchase orders must be reconciled item by item.

✔ The strength and amount of each item must be checked to make sure they are correct. A common mistake is an item sent in bulk instead of unit dose (or the reverse).

✔ Shipment prices on the supplier invoice should match the purchase order exactly. Individual price changes must be identified and may have to be entered into the system manually to make sure the system has the correct information.

✔ If there are any discrepancies, the supplier should generally be notified immediately.

✔ Controlled substances are shipped separately and should be checked in by a pharmacist.

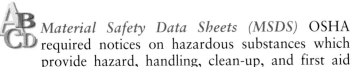

Material Safety Data Sheets (MSDS) OSHA required notices on hazardous substances which provide hazard, handling, clean-up, and first aid information.

FORMS

The Online Ordering Screen

Online ordering systems generally contain abbreviated descriptions of drug products in the formulary. The technician uses an "Select" (or similar) function to choose products and may then "Add" it to an order. Quantities may be manually entered or edited—if they have been automatically recorded by the system.

The system automatically assigns to each order a **purchase order number** for identification. Once the order is finished, checked, and ready, it is sent to the supplier's system.

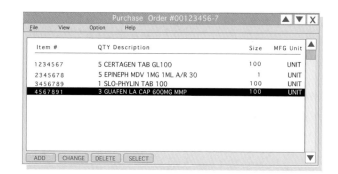

The Confirmation Printout

When an online purchase order is received by the supplier, the supplier's system checks the order to see what items it will be able to ship to the orderer. Once it completes this process, a confirmation of the order is sent back to the orderer's system. This confirmation indicates which items will be shipped, which will not (due to unavailability), and what the cost of the items and any related costs may be. The confirmation comes in the form of a file that is saved on the system, but is also printed out so a hard copy of the confirmation is available for checking.

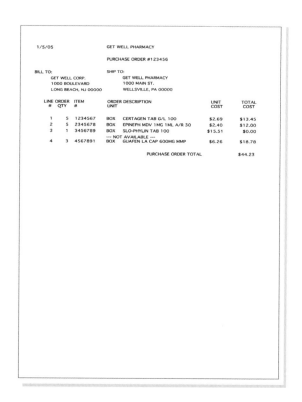

The Shipping Invoice

When the items are shipped, the supplier includes an **invoice** listing the items in the shipment, items that may be shipped separately, items that are unavailable, and the cost of the shipment. The invoice must be checked item by item against the items in the shipment to make certain nothing is missing.

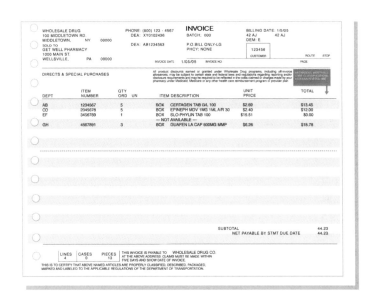

The Returns Form

Preprinted multipart forms are often used for returns, though some computer inventory systems generate their own form. When returning items, the following information is usually required:

➡ original p.o. number
➡ item number
➡ quantity
➡ reason for return

Reasons for returning products can include overshipments, damaged or expired products, or changed needs.

STOCKING & STORING

Most medications are received from the supplier in bulk "stock bottles" that carry FDA required information on the label. This information includes the brand name, generic name, prescription legend, storage requirements, dosage form, quantity, controlled substance mark, manufacturer's name, lot number, expiration date, and NDC number (National Drug Code). These bottles often contain bulk quantities from which individual prescriptions will be filled.

Some medications, particularly in hospitals, are packaged in individual doses called "unit/dose" packaging.

Unit dose packaging allows the dispensing of individual doses to patients in hospitals and other settings. Because the dose information is on each dose, it is easily checked before leaving the pharmacy to the nursing unit. In many settings, technicians prepare unit-dose packaging under the supervision of a pharmacist as part of their job.

Drugs must be stored according to manufacturer's specifications.

Most drugs are kept in a fairly constant room temperature of 59°-86°F (and not below, unless stated by the manufacturer to do so). The storage room must have adequate ventilation or proper air distribution. Drug shelves should be sturdy and allow proper air flow around the medications and room.

ABCD *unit-dose packaging* a package containing a single dose of a medication.

Unit-Dose Packaging

Unit-dose packaging can take many forms: plastic packs, vials, tubes, ampules, etc. Some unit-dose drugs are packaged in individual bubbles on cards containing ten doses. A box of one hundred unit doses would contain ten such cards. Each unit dose package contains the name of the drug, its strength, and the expiration date. In some settings, technicians are hired specifically to create unit-dose packaging from bulk supplies.

PACKAGING

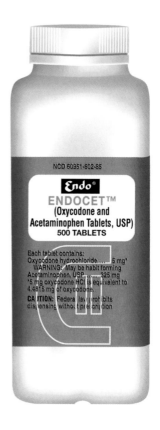

bulk container with 500 tablets of Endocet

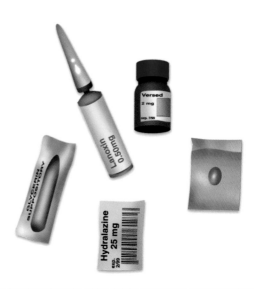

STORAGE

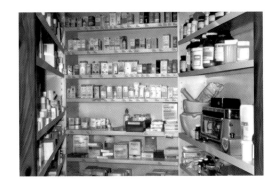

Physical Organization

Drugs may be organized by various methods. Storing by manufacturer would locate the drug using its brand name and is often done in a retail pharmacy. Storing **alpha-generically** organizes drugs alphabetically by their generic names. For example, if the generic name "cimetidine" is on the shelf, Tagamet may be placed there along with the generic.

Whatever the overall organization, the following basic guidelines should be met:

✔ Each medication should be organized in a way that will dispense the oldest items first so that the medications will remain fresh.

✔ The location of each drug should be quickly identifiable through a locator system in which each drug is assigned a location number that is stored in the computer system. This allows quick retrieval of any drug.

✔ Enough space should be provided for each medication to minimize breakage and to make it difficult to accidentally select the wrong medication.

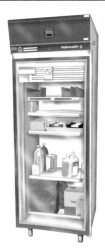

Refrigeration

Some drugs must be stored at a constant temperature in a controlled commercial refrigerator designed for medications. If refrigerated or frozen medications are left out for a period of time longer than stated in the literature, they may begin to break down chemically or lose potency. Commercial refrigerators and freezers have gauges on the outside that indicate the internal temperature and allow it to be monitored. The temperature of refrigeration should generally be 40-42°.

The refrigerator or freezer should be plugged into a wall receptacle that is marked for emergency use and will switch to emergency power generators if there is a power failure. If any medication is left out of refrigeration beyond the recommendations of the manufacturer, it should be discarded.

Point of Use Stations

In hospitals and other settings, medications are stocked in dispensing units throughout the facility that may be called supply stations or med-stations. Since they are at the **point of use**, they greatly simplify the dispensing of medications to patients.

Items stocked in these stations differ based upon the needs of the patients. For example, a station in an operating room would contain many anesthetics.

All withdrawals and restocks of stations are recorded just as they would be from a central dispensary. As discussed earlier in this chapter, some stations may be linked into the facility computing system so the information can be automatically communicated to it.

 Stock that has expired, been damaged, recalled, or has otherwise been targeted for return or disposal must be segregated and clearly marked to avoid contamination and/or mix-up with the good stock.

REVIEW

KEY CONCEPTS

INVENTORY MANAGEMENT'

✔ Good inventory management ensures that drugs which are likely to be needed are both on hand and usable—that is, not expired, damaged, contaminated, or otherwise unfit for use.

✔ An open formulary is one that allows purchase of any medication that is prescribed. A closed formulary is a limited list of approved medications.

✔ Schedule II substances must be stocked separately in a secure place and require a special order form for reordering. Their stock must be continually monitored and documented.

✔ More than three-quarters of pharmaceutical manufacturers' sales are directly to drug wholesalers, who in turn resell their inventory to hospitals, pharmacies, and other pharmaceutical dispensers.

INVENTORY SYSTEMS

✔ A perpetual inventory system maintains a continuous record of every item in inventory so that it always shows the stock on hand.

✔ Turnover is the rate at which inventory is used.

✔ Pharmacy operations generally use a point of sale system in which the item is deducted from inventory as it is sold or dispensed.

✔ Drug reorder points are maximum and minimum inventory levels for each drug.

✔ Important reports (especially purchase orders) should be regularly printed out and filed as hard copy both for convenience and as a backup record-keeping system.

COMPUTERS AND INVENTORY

✔ Pharmacy computer files must be regularly backed-up or copied to an appropriate storage media.

✔ In a computerized inventory system, orders can be generated using an order entry device or automatically generated by the system based on stock levels and reorder points.

ORDERING

✔ In an online ordering system, if an order can be filled as ordered, a message from the supplier will automatically confirm the order to the ordering system. The system automatically assigns to each order a purchase order number for identification.

✔ Material Safety Data Sheets (MSDS) for hazardous substances such as chemotherapeutic agents indicate when special handling and shipping is required.

✔ Controlled substances are shipped separately and should be checked in by a pharmacist.

STOCKING AND STORING

✔ Most medications are received from the supplier in bulk "stock bottles."

✔ Drugs must be stored according to manufacturer's specifications.

✔ Most drugs are kept in a fairly constant room temperature of 59°-86°F. The temperature of refrigeration should generally be 40-42°.

✔ Medications should be organized in a way that will dispense the oldest items first.

✔ In hospitals and other settings, medications are stocked in dispensing units throughout the facility that may be called supply stations or med-stations.

SELF TEST

MATCH THE TERMS.   *answers can be checked in the glossary*

closed formulary

database

Material Safety Data Sheets

open formulary

perpetual inventory

point of sale system (POS)

purchase order number

reorder points

turnover

unit-dose packaging

- a system that allows purchase of any medication that is prescribed.
- a limited list of approved medications.
- the rate at which inventory is used, generally expressed in number of days.
- an inventory system in which the item is deducted from inventory as it is sold or dispensed.
- minimum and maximum stock levels which determine when a reorder is placed and for how much.
- a collection of information structured so that specific information within it can easily be retrieved and used.
- OSHA required notices on hazardous substances which provide hazard, handling, clean-up, and first aid information.
- the number system assigned to each order for identification.
- a package containing a single dose of a medication.
- a system that maintains a continuous record of every item in inventory so that it always shows the stock on hand.

CHOOSE THE BEST ANSWER.   *the answer key begins on page 347*

1. A listing of the goods or items that a business will use in its normal operation is called a(an)
   a. purchasing.
   b. inventory.
   c. open formulary.
   d. closed formulary.

2. The goal of inventory management is
   a. to ensure that drugs are available when they are needed
   b. to maintain MSDS sheets
   c. to develop closed formularies
   d. to increase use of wholesalers

3. In an open formulary, when a medication is ordered that is not on the formulary
   a. the medication may be ordered without obtaining additional permission.
   b. the patient must obtain the medication at another pharmacy.
   c. the physician must first receive permission to use the medication.
   d. the pharmacist is required to choose a therapeutic equivalent.

4. In a closed formulary, when a medication is ordered that is not on the formulary
   a. the physician must receive permission to use that medication.
   b. the medication may be ordered without obtaining additional permission.
   c. the formulary is changed to an open formulary.

REVIEW

5. Wholesalers who provide medications to hospitals, pharmacies, and other medication dispensers account for about _____ of pharmaceutical manufacturers' sales.
   a. half
   b. one-quarter
   c. three-quarters
   d. one-third

6. As an expiration date approaches, the pharmacy technician should be aware that it must be _____ before the expiration date passes.
   a. returned to the manufacturer for credit
   b. dispensed
   c. used
   d. returned to the wholesaler for credit

7. If a supplier's terms are thirty days net,
   a. it would be best to have a turnover less than thirty days
   b. it would be best to have a turnover equal to thirty days
   c. it would be best to have a turnover greater than thirty days
   d. none of the above

8. _____ is an inventory system in which the item is deducted from inventory as it is sold or dispensed.
   a. Point of sale system
   b. Turnover
   c. Automated reports
   d. Reorder point system

9. Minimum and maximum stock levels used to determine when a reorder is placed and for how much are
   a. reorder points.
   b. automatic ordering.
   c. POS.
   d. turnovers.

10. Checking of order reports to ensure the order contains no gross errors is done
    a. by computer.
    b. manually.
    c. by the corporate office.
    d. by the wholesaler.

11. Hard copies of order reports
    a. are only needed if there is a computer failure.e
    b. are not needed since everything is on the computer
    c. are kept for an established amount of time for business and legal reasons
    d. are only needed if there is a power failure

12. A(an) _____ is a collection of information structured so that specific information can be easily retrieved and used.
    a. database
    b. turnover
    c. POS
    d. system backup

13. Items that cannot be filled by the wholesaler exactly as ordered are included on a list of
    a. MSDSs.
    b. exceptions.
    c. OSHA.
    d. returns.

14. Material Safety Data Sheets (MSDS) provide
    a. protocols for fire hazards in the pharmacy setting
    b. safety codes by OSHA in the storage of inventory
    c. information concerning hazardous substances
    d. none of the above

15. In receiving an order, it is important to be alert for drugs that have been incorrectly picked, received damaged, are outdated, or missing, so orders are reconciled
    a. once per month.
    b. item by item.
    c. every two years
    d. once per year.

16. When reconciling an order, if a technician detects a discrepancy, the supplier should be notified
    a. immediately.
    b. before the end of the current reporting period.
    c. before the end of the month.
    d. before the end of the week.

17. A purchase order number is
    a. a number that is used to identify the pharmacy.
    b. is the same on all orders from a given pharmacy.
    c. is assigned by the FDA.
    d. a number used to identify an order.

18. The shipping invoice is provided by the
    a. supplier or wholesaler.
    b. pharmacy.
    c. pharmacy technician.
    d. pharmacist.

19. Most drugs are kept at room temperature between
    a. 59 - 86 degrees C.
    b. 33 - 45 degrees C.
    c. 59 - 86 degrees F.
    d. 33 - 45 degrees F.

20. A package that contains a single dose of a medication is called a(an)
    a. MSDS package.
    b. single use package.
    c. POS package.
    d. unit dose package.

21. The temperature of a refrigerator in a pharmacy should generally be
    a. 40 - 42 degrees F.
    b. 28 - 32 degrees C.
    c. 40 - 42 degrees C.
    d. 28 - 32 degrees F.

22. Supply stations or med-stations that are stocked dispensing units located throughout the facility are called
    a. Unit-Doses.
    b. POS.
    c. MSDS.
    d. Point of Use Stations.

FINANCIAL ISSUES

Financial issues have a substantial influence on health care and pharmacy practice.

In 1985, the average prescription price was approximately $10. By 2002 the average prescription price approached $60. The increase is due to a number of reasons, including inflation and the aging of the population. It is also due to the use of new medications that enhance the quality of health care, but which are often costly.

The use of third party programs to pay for prescriptions has also increased dramatically.

Third party programs are simply another party besides the patient or the pharmacy that pays for some or all of the cost of medication: essentially, an insurer. Although many individuals are uninsured, most people have some form of private or public health insurance. These include both public programs such as Medicaid and Medicare and private programs such as HMOs and basic health insurance. Many but not all such programs include prescription drug coverage. While the growth of these programs is largely a response to the rising costs of health care, in many cases third party programs allow patients to benefit from new and often more expensive drug therapies than they would otherwise be able to afford.

Because of the pharmacy technician's role in the prescription filling process, he or she must understand the different types of health insurance and how drug benefits differ among the programs.

A patient's prescription drug program determines important considerations for filling their prescription. Generic substitution may be required. There may be limits on the quantity dispensed (tablets, capsules, etc.) per fill, or on the frequency and number of refills, and so on.

PHARMACY BENEFITS MANAGERS

Regardless of how the claims are submitted and processed, participating pharmacies must sign contracts with insurers or pharmacy benefit managers before patients can get their prescriptions filled at that pharmacy and billed to their insurer or pharmacy benefit manager. A pharmacy benefit manager (PBM) is a company that administers drug benefit programs. Many insurance companies, HMOs, and self-insured employers use the services of more than 75 PBMs to manage drug benefit coverage for employees and health plan members. The following are the names of some pharmacy benefit managers (PBMs).

➥ AdvancePCS
➥ Argus
➥ Caremark
➥ Express Scripts
➥ Medco Health
➥ MedImpact
➥ RESTAT

pharmacy benefits managers companies that administer drug benefit programs

online adjudication the resolution of prescription coverage through the communication of the pharmacy computer with the third party computer.

co-insurance an agreement for cost-sharing between the insurer and the insured.

co-pay the portion of the price of medication that the patient is required to pay.

dual co-pay co-pays that have two prices: one for generic and one for brand medications.

maximum allowable cost (MAC) the maximum price per tablet (or other dispensing unit) an insurer or PBM will pay for a given product.

U&C or UCR the maximum amount of payment for a given prescription, determined by the insurer to be a usual and customary (and reasonable) price.

COMPUTERS AND THIRD PARTY BILLING

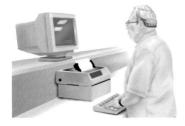

Procedures used by pharmacies to submit third party claims vary. Most insurers or pharmacy benefit managers mail checks to pharmacies (or their accounts receivable departments) at regular intervals along with listings of the prescriptions covered and those not covered (i.e., rejected).

Before the computer age, prescriptions were billed to third parties using paper claims. Although paper claims are still used, most claims are now filed electronically by online claim submission and **online adjudication** of claims. This electronic submission and adjudication process benefits both third party programs as well as pharmacies. The online communication between the prescription-filling computer in the pharmacy and the claim-processing computer of the insurer or pharmacy benefit manager results in improved accuracy and control. It is also much faster and more direct than processing paper claims. The benefits of computerizing the claims process have also been a factor in the rise of third party programs.

CO-PAYS

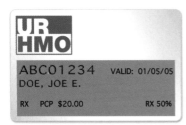

One of the common aspects of many third party programs is **co-insurance**, which is essentially an agreement between the insurer and the insured to share costs. One aspect of this is the requirement for the patient to **co-pay** for the filled prescription. That is, the patient must pay a portion of the price of the medication and the insurance company is billed for the remainder.

The amount paid by the insurer is not equal to the retail price normally charged, but is determined by a formula described in a contract between the insurer and the pharmacy. There is a **maximum allowable cost (MAC)** per tablet or other dispensing unit that an insurer or PBM will pay for a given product. This is often determined by survey of the **usual and customary (U&C)** prices for a prescription within a given geographic area. This is also referred to as the **UCR (usual, customary, and reasonable)** price for the prescription.

Many third party plans have **dual co-pays**, which means that a lower co-pay applies to prescriptions filled with generic drugs and a higher co-pay applies to prescriptions filled with brand name drugs that have no generic equivalent. Some plans have three different co-pays: the lowest co-pay applies to prescriptions filled with generic drugs, a higher co-pay applies to prescriptions filled with brand name drugs which have no generic equivalent, and a third higher co-pay applies to prescriptions filled with brand name drugs which have a generic equivalent.

THIRD PARTY PROGRAMS

PRIVATE HEALTH INSURANCE

Basic private health insurance policies may pay for prescribed expenses (such as prescriptions) when the patient is covered by a supplementary **comprehensive major medical policy** or when the patient's coverage includes an additional prescription drug benefit. Patients covered by comprehensive major medical policies pay out-of-pocket for their prescriptions. Once a **deductible** is met, the insurer may pay a portion of the cost of prescriptions filled the rest of the year. In other words, once a patient has paid a certain dollar amount for prescribed medical expenses (usually including prescriptions), the insurance company will reimburse a portion of the cost of filled prescriptions for the rest of the year. Whether or not a patient is required to get generic drugs when they are available is determined by individual plans and may not be obvious before filling the prescription. Major medical claims frequently involve paper claims. However, the use of electronic claim processing for major medical claims is growing.

Prescription Drug Coverage

Some traditional health insurance policies have the added benefit of prescription drug coverage. Patients with prescription drug coverage through a private insurance company are issued **prescription drug benefit cards** to carry in their wallets. These cards contain necessary billing information for pharmacies, including the patient's identification number, group number, and co-pay amount.

As with other prescription plans, there may be various types of co-pays and patients may be required to get generic drugs (when available). However, basic private health insurance policies often do not require generic substitution because the patient or their employer pays a higher premium for coverage.

Most prescription claims are processed through online adjudication: the pharmacy computer communicates with the insurer's or PBM's computer to determine the prescription drug benefit. When the claim is adjudicated or processed by the insurer or pharmacy benefit manager it becomes obvious if generic substitution is mandatory.

ABCD *deductible* a set amount that must be paid by the patient for each benefit period before the insurer will cover additional expenses.

prescription drug benefit cards cards that contain third party billing information for prescription drug purchases.

MANAGED CARE PROGRAMS

Managed care programs include health maintenance organizations (HMOs), point-of-service programs (POS), and preferred provider organizations (PPOs). Managed care programs provide all necessary medical services (usually including prescription coverage) in return for a monthly premium and co-pays. Most managed care prescription drug plans require generic substitution when a generic is available. Some managed care plans have single co-pays, some have dual co-pays, and some have three types of co-pays.

HMOs

HMOs are made of a network of providers who are either employed by the HMO or have signed contracts to abide by the policies of the HMO. HMOs usually will not cover expenses incurred outside their participating network. *HMOs often require generic substitution.*

POSs

POS programs are made of a network of providers contracted by the insurer. Patients enrolled in a POS choose a primary care physician (PCP) who is a provider in the insurer's network. Patients may receive care outside of the POS network, but the primary care physician is required to make referrals for such care. POSs often partially reimburse expenses incurred outside of their network. *POSs usually require generic substitution.*

PPOs

PPOs are also a network of providers contracted by the insurer. Of the managed care options, PPOs offer the most flexibility for their members. PPOs often partially reimburse expenses incurred outside of their participating network and do not require a primary care physician within their network to make referrals. *PPOs usually require generic substitution.*

Patients with prescription drug coverage through managed care organizations are issued prescription drug benefit cards with billing and co-pay information. Most claims for these programs are processed through online adjudication. Many HMOs, POSs, and PPOs use pharmacy benefit managers (PBMs) to manage drug benefit coverage.

 HMOs a network of providers for which costs are covered inside but not outside of the network.

POSs a network of providers where the patient's primary care physician must be a member and costs outside the network may be partially reimbursed.

PPOs a network of providers where costs outside the network may be partially reimbursed and the patient's primary care physician need not be a member.

THIRD PARTY PROGRAMS (cont'd)

PUBLIC HEALTH INSURANCE

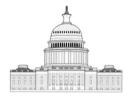

The largest public health insurance plans in the United States are Medicare and Medicaid.

Medicare

Medicare is a federal program that covers people over the age of 65, as well as disabled people under the age of 65, and people with kidney failure. Medicare Part A basically covers inpatient hospital expenses for patients who meet certain conditions, and it may also cover some hospice expenses. Medicare Part B basically covers doctors' services as well as some other medical services that are not covered by Part A. Medicare beneficiaries who pay a monthly premium for this medical coverage are covered by Medicare Part B.

Until 2006, some Medicare beneficiaries may pay a fee to obtain prescription drug discount cards that are approved by Medicare. After 2006, some Medicare beneficiaries may choose to enroll in the Medicare Prescription Drug Plan. The Medicare Prescription Drug Plan requires participants to pay a monthly premium and also meet certain deductibles and co-payments. Medicare beneficiaries that do not participate in the Medicare Prescription Drug Plan may have prescription drug coverage through a current or former employer. Some Medicare beneficiaries may not have any prescription drug coverage if they do not participate in either the Medicare Drug Plan or a prescription drug plan from a current or previous employer. Furthermore, some Medicare beneficiaries may qualify for medication management services provided by pharmacists.

Medicaid

Medicaid is a federal-state program. **ADC (Aid to Dependent Children)** is one type of Medicaid program. State welfare departments usually operate Medicaid. Each state decides who is eligible for Medicaid benefits and what services will be covered. A prescription drug formulary is a listing of the drugs that are covered by Medicaid. Prescription drug formularies for Medicaid recipients are determined by each state. *Medicaid programs do not automatically cover drugs that are not on the state formulary.* Completion of a prior authorization form is sometimes required to justify the need for a medication that is not on the state Medicaid formulary. Completion of the form does not imply the drug will be covered. Medicaid recipients can also qualify for HMO programs.

OTHER PROGRAMS

Workers' Compensation

In the United States, the federal government and every state have enacted workers' compensation laws. Under workers' compensation legislation, procedures for *compensation for employees accidentally injured on-the-job* are established. Administrative guidelines require that accidents be reported to a public board that grants compensation awards to injured workers.

In recent years, state workers' compensation programs have been broadened to provide for coverage of occupational diseases. Prescriptions related to the occupational injury or disease can be billed to the state's bureau of workers' compensation or to the employer (if the employer is self-insured). Many workers' compensation claims can be processed through online adjudication. However, some claims require paper claims. It is important to realize the billing procedure can be slightly different for self-insured claims. Pharmacy benefit managers (PBMs) may administer workers' compensation prescription drug benefits.

Patient Assistance Programs

Patient assistance programs are programs offered by some pharmaceutical manufacturers to help needy patients who require medication they cannot afford and do not have insurance coverage. Patient assistance programs require patients and their physicians to complete applications and submit them to the pharmaceutical manufacturer offering the program. Patients who qualify for patient assistance programs are often given cards issued by pharmacy benefit managers.

Medicare a federal program providing health care to people with certain disabilities over age 65; it includes basic hospital insurance and voluntary medical insurance.

Medicaid a federal-state program, administered by the states, providing health care for the needy.

workers' compensation an employer compensation program for employees accidentally injured on the job.

patient assistance programs manufacturer sponsored prescription drug programs for the needy.

ONLINE ADJUDICATION

In online adjudication, the technician uses the computer to determine the exact coverage for each prescription with the appropriate third party. The pharmacy computer communicates with the insurer's or pharmacy benefit manager's computer to determine this. Most community pharmacy computer programs are designed so the prescription label does not print until confirmation of payment is received from the insurer or PBM.

THE ONLINE PROCESS

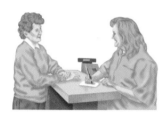

While non-patient information (NABP number, prices, co-pay, etc.) is provided by the computer system, it is generally the pharmacy technician's responsibility to obtain the patient, prescription, and billing information. In a typical community pharmacy, a patient presents a prescription (and often a prescription drug card) to a technician who must then obtain all of the patient and billing information required to enter the prescription and claim. If the patient has had prescriptions filled previously at the pharmacy, much of this information will be in the system already (though it is important for the technician to verify that this information is still correct).

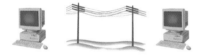

Once the necessary information is obtained, the pharmacy technician enters it into the pharmacy computer. Billing information for the prescription is then transmitted to a processing computer for the insurer or PBM. If all information has been entered correctly and is in agreement with data on-file with the insurer, the prescription claim is processed using online adjudication and an online response is received in less than one minute in the pharmacy. The claim-processing computer instantly determines the dollar amount of the drug benefit and the appropriate co-pay.

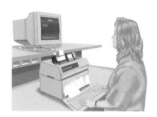

The pharmacy technician usually has an opportunity to review the data provided by the claim-processing computer before giving the OK for the prescription label and receipt to print in the pharmacy. The receipt indicates how much of the price of the prescription the patient must pay as determined by the insurer. The prescription can then be filled. The pharmacy technician should carefully review this adjudication information before proceeding to make sure the claim was processed properly. The pharmacy may be underpaid if the drug dispensed has a generic equivalent. The pharmacy technician should also look for claim processing messages such as drug or disease interaction alerts.

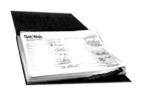

When prescriptions are billed online, pharmacies must keep records to verify prescriptions that prescriptions were actually dispensed. Insurers or PBMs require pharmacies to maintain hard copies of each prescription that must be readily retrievable upon request. Insurers or PBMs also require pharmacies to maintain signature logs for all claims submitted electronically that must be readily retrievable upon request.

ONLINE CLAIM INFORMATION

Although there are many different types of health care insurance, the information required for online processing of claims is remarkably similar. The following information is usually required for online claim processing:

- cardholder identification number (usually the social security number of the employee or a variation of this number)
- group number (a number assigned by the insurer to the employer of the cardholder)
- name of patient
- birthdate
- sex (M or F)
- relationship to cardholder (cardholder (C), spouse (S), dependent (D), other (O))
- date RX written
- date RX dispensed
- is this a new or refill prescription
- national drug code (NDC) of drug
- DAW indicator
- amount or quantity dispensed
- days supply
- identification number of prescribing physician
- identification of the pharmacy (pharmacies are often identified by the NABP Number which has been assigned by the National Association of Boards of Pharmacy or NABP)
- ingredient cost
- dispensing fee
- total price
- deductible or co-pay amount
- balance due

Dispense As Written (DAW)

When entering patient and prescription information, it is important to verify whether the patient's plan covers the brand name of a particular drug or if the patient is required to get generic drugs. When brand name drugs are dispensed, numbers corresponding to the reason for submitting the claim with brand name drugs are entered in a DAW (Dispense as Written) indicator field. Most health plan members have a choice between brand and generic drugs.

In some programs, if a patient receives a brand name drug when a generic is available, the patient must pay the difference between the cost of the brand and the cost of the generic. The following lists DAW indicators.

0 No DAW (No Dispense As Written)

1 DAW handwritten on the prescription by the prescriber

2 Patient requested brand

3 Pharmacist selected brand

4 Generic not in stock

5 Brand name dispensed but priced as generic

6 N/A

7 Substitution not allowed; brand mandated by law

8 Generic not available

 Billing special medications such as compounded prescriptions requires somewhat different procedures. These procedures are different for each insurer or PBM. When billing compounded medications or special medications the pharmacy technician should refer to informational booklets provided to the pharmacy by the insurer or PBM or call the pharmacy help desk as listed on the prescription drug card.

REJECTED CLAIMS

In the online adjudication process, the insurer sometimes rejects the claim as submitted.

This occurs before the prescription is dispensed and provides an opportunity to resolve the problem before it becomes larger. There are various reasons for rejections, and most problems can be resolved by telephoning a representative of the insurer or discussing the rejection with the patient. Rejections are best resolved during normal business hours.

REJECTIONS

At right are common reasons for rejection of pharmacy third party claims and suggestions on how to correct such rejections.

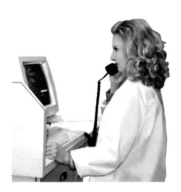

Resolving Rejections

When there is a question on coverage, the pharmacy technician can telephone the insurance plan's **pharmacy help desk** to determine if the patient is eligible for coverage. Pharmacy help desk personnel are often very helpful in resolving problems. If an employer has changed insurers, sometimes pharmacy help desk personnel can advise the pharmacy technician who the new insurer is. Many pharmacies maintain a list of phone numbers for insurers and their processors. If the prescription drug card is not available, the pharmacy technician can obtain the phone number of the insurer from this list.

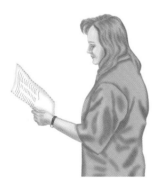

Handling Paper Claim Rejects

When paper claims are rejected by third parties, rejections often do not appear for several weeks after the claim was submitted. Rejections of paper claims are almost always accompanied by an explanation of the rejection and give details on what the technician can do to obtain successful payment of the claim. In many cases, the paper claim form was not completed correctly, information is missing, and the technician needs to only complete the missing information and resubmit the claim. Sometimes a telephone call must be made to the patient and/or the insurer to resolve the problem.

Dependent exceeds age limit as specified by plan

Many prescription drug plans have age limitations for children or dependents of the cardholder. Often, full-time college students are eligible for coverage as long as appropriate paperwork is on file with the insurer.

Invalid birthdate

The birthdate submitted by the pharmacy sometimes does not match the birthdate in the insurer's computer. To solve this problem, first double-check that you have the correct birthdate for the patient.

Invalid person code

The person code (e.g. 00,01,02,03) does not match the person code for the patient with the same sex and birthdate information in the insurer's computer.

Invalid sex

The sex (M or F) submitted by the pharmacy does not match the sex in the insurer's computer for the patient. To solve this problem, change the sex code (if M change to F) and resubmit the claim.

Prescriber is not a network provider

This type of reject is common to Medicaid programs and is sometimes seen with HMO programs. Simply stated, only prescriptions issued by network prescribers are covered by the insurer.

Unable to connect with insurer's computer

Sometimes, due to computer problems, an insurer's computer may be unavailable for claim processing. Under these circumstances, the technician must follow the guidelines of their employer.

Patient not covered (coverage terminated)

This can occur when a patient has a new insurance card, whether the new card is issued by the same insurer or a new one. If the insurer has not changed, perhaps billing numbers have changed (new cardholder identification number, group number, etc.).

Refill too soon

Most third party plans require that most of the medication has been taken before the plan will cover another dispensing of the same medication. Early refills should always be brought to the attention of the pharmacist. If the pharmacist thinks it is appropriate to dispense a refill early (for example, if a patient is going on vacation), the next step is to contact the insurer to determine if it will pay for an early refill.

Refills not covered

Many managed care health programs require mail order pharmacies to fill prescriptions for maintenance medications. Patients often are not aware of mail order requirements of their prescription drug coverage. Ideally the employer is responsible to explain mail order requirements if their employees are required to use mail order for maintenance medications. Sometimes, patients do not realize this restriction until prescription claims are rejected at their community pharmacy. In such cases, the pharmacy technician will have to contact the insurer to determine if emergency refills are covered at the community pharmacy.

NDC not covered

This type of rejection is common with state Medicaid programs and managed care programs with closed formularies. Ideally, the patient is aware that the insurer has a limited formulary for prescription drug coverage. However, often patients are not aware of how this works. The pharmacy technician can determine by calling the pharmacy help desk of the insurer the requirements of the patient's plan. Sometimes, the insurer will consider prior authorization to cover medications that are not on the formulary. Sometimes, the insurer will not cover the prescribed medication and a pharmacist may determine what should be done next.

OTHER ISSUES

PAPER CLAIMS

Processing paper claims usually involves the pharmacy and the patient completing a form that has been issued by the insurer. Most insurers require completion of a form that they provide. A **universal claim form** (UCF) is a standardized form accepted by many insurers. Before online claim submission, most pharmacy third party claims were submitted on universal claim forms. Instructions for completing paper claims (insurer provided forms as well as universal claim forms) are printed on the claim forms so that anyone can complete the forms as long as they have access to the required information. Usually there is a requirement for signature by the patient and the pharmacist or health care provider. Incomplete forms or forms that have not been completed following directions printed on the forms are returned to the pharmacy for correction before the insurer will consider paying the claim. Generally, the same type of information required for online claims is also required for paper claim processing.

IN-HOUSE BILLING PROCEDURES

Pharmacy billing is not limited to billing insurers. Some pharmacies have in-house billing procedures. For example, the finances of an elderly or disabled patient may be handled by a family member or legal representative who does not live with the patient. In these cases, a monthly bill is mailed to the family member or legal representative, who then pays the pharmacy. Most pharmacies do not have in-house billing. When a pharmacy does do in-house billing, the pharmacy technician must carefully follow the policies and procedures of the employer.

DISEASE STATE MANAGEMENT SERVICES

Disease state management services are evolving as a component of pharmaceutical care. PBMs are selling disease management services to employers and health plans. Conditions most often targeted for disease state management include diabetes, hypertension,asthma, smoking cessation, and cholesterol management.

Both electronic and paper billing systems can be used for billing disease state management services; however, currently, paper billing systems are more common. Pharmacy technicians must properly document services as well as submit and follow-up on paper claims. Note that the paper claims for these services are submitted to a department within an insurance company or PBM that is different from the department that processes claims for prescription drugs. The claims should include a cover letter, a copy of the order for the service from the physician (also known as the statement of medical necessity), an appropriate billing form (usually the standard **CMS-1500 form**, formerly named the HCFA1500 form, shown at right), and accurate documentation of the services provided by the pharmacy.

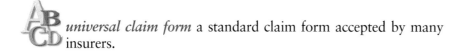

universal claim form a standard claim form accepted by many insurers.

CMS-1500 (formerly HCFA 1500) form the standard form used by health care providers, such as physicians, to bill for services. It can be used to bill for disease state management services and is available at http://cms.hhs.gov/providers/edi/cms1500.pdf.

PLEASE
DO NOT
STAPLE
IN THIS
AREA

CARRIER

HEALTH INSURANCE CLAIM FORM

| PICA | | | | | | | | PICA |

1. MEDICARE (Medicare #)   MEDICAID (Medicaid #)   CHAMPUS (Sponsor's SSN)   CHAMPVA (VA File #)   GROUP HEALTH PLAN (SSN or ID)   FECA BLK LUNG (SSN)   OTHER (ID)

1a. INSURED'S I.D. NUMBER   (FOR PROGRAM IN ITEM 1)

2. PATIENT'S NAME (Last Name, First Name, Middle Initial)

3. PATIENT'S BIRTH DATE MM DD YY   SEX M F

4. INSURED'S NAME (Last Name, First Name, Middle Initial)

5. PATIENT'S ADDRESS (No., Street)

6. PATIENT RELATIONSHIP TO INSURED   Self Spouse Child Other

7. INSURED'S ADDRESS (No., Street)

CITY   STATE

8. PATIENT STATUS   Single Married Other   Employed Full-Time Student Part-Time Student

CITY   STATE

ZIP CODE   TELEPHONE (Include Area Code) ( )

ZIP CODE   TELEPHONE (INCLUDE AREA CODE) ( )

9. OTHER INSURED'S NAME (Last Name, First Name, Middle Initial)

10. IS PATIENT'S CONDITION RELATED TO:

11. INSURED'S POLICY GROUP OR FECA NUMBER

a. OTHER INSURED'S POLICY OR GROUP NUMBER

a. EMPLOYMENT? (CURRENT OR PREVIOUS) YES NO

a. INSURED'S DATE OF BIRTH MM DD YY   SEX M F

b. OTHER INSURED'S DATE OF BIRTH MM DD YY   SEX M F

b. AUTO ACCIDENT?   PLACE (State) YES NO

b. EMPLOYER'S NAME OR SCHOOL NAME

c. EMPLOYER'S NAME OR SCHOOL NAME

c. OTHER ACCIDENT? YES NO

c. INSURANCE PLAN NAME OR PROGRAM NAME

d. INSURANCE PLAN NAME OR PROGRAM NAME

10d. RESERVED FOR LOCAL USE

d. IS THERE ANOTHER HEALTH BENEFIT PLAN? YES NO *If yes*, return to and complete item 9 a-d.

READ BACK OF FORM BEFORE COMPLETING & SIGNING THIS FORM.

12. PATIENT'S OR AUTHORIZED PERSON'S SIGNATURE I authorize the release of any medical or other information necessary to process this claim. I also request payment of government benefits either to myself or to the party who accepts assignment below.

SIGNED _____ DATE _____

13. INSURED'S OR AUTHORIZED PERSON'S SIGNATURE I authorize payment of medical benefits to the undersigned physician or supplier for services described below.

SIGNED _____

PATIENT AND INSURED INFORMATION

14. DATE OF CURRENT: MM DD YY ILLNESS (First symptom) OR INJURY (Accident) OR PREGNANCY(LMP)

15. IF PATIENT HAS HAD SAME OR SIMILAR ILLNESS. GIVE FIRST DATE MM DD YY

16. DATES PATIENT UNABLE TO WORK IN CURRENT OCCUPATION FROM MM DD YY TO MM DD YY

17. NAME OF REFERRING PHYSICIAN OR OTHER SOURCE

17a. I.D. NUMBER OF REFERRING PHYSICIAN

18. HOSPITALIZATION DATES RELATED TO CURRENT SERVICES FROM MM DD YY TO MM DD YY

19. RESERVED FOR LOCAL USE

20. OUTSIDE LAB? YES NO $ CHARGES

21. DIAGNOSIS OR NATURE OF ILLNESS OR INJURY. (RELATE ITEMS 1,2,3 OR 4 TO ITEM 24E BY LINE)

1. |___.__| 3. |___.__|
2. |___.__| 4. |___.__|

22. MEDICAID RESUBMISSION CODE   ORIGINAL REF. NO.

23. PRIOR AUTHORIZATION NUMBER

24. A DATE(S) OF SERVICE						B Place of Service	C Type of Service	D PROCEDURES, SERVICES, OR SUPPLIES (Explain Unusual Circumstances) CPT/HCPCS | MODIFIER	E DIAGNOSIS CODE	F $ CHARGES	G DAYS OR UNITS	H EPSDT Family Plan	I EMG	J COB	K RESERVED FOR LOCAL USE
From MM	DD	YY	To MM	DD	YY										
1															
2															
3															
4															
5															
6															

25. FEDERAL TAX I.D. NUMBER   SSN EIN

26. PATIENT'S ACCOUNT NO.

27. ACCEPT ASSIGNMENT? (For govt. claims, see back) YES NO

28. TOTAL CHARGE $

29. AMOUNT PAID $

30. BALANCE DUE $

31. SIGNATURE OF PHYSICIAN OR SUPPLIER INCLUDING DEGREES OR CREDENTIALS (I certify that the statements on the reverse apply to this bill and are made a part thereof.)

SIGNED _____ DATE _____

32. NAME AND ADDRESS OF FACILITY WHERE SERVICES WERE RENDERED (If other than home or office)

33. PHYSICIAN'S, SUPPLIER'S BILLING NAME, ADDRESS, ZIP CODE & PHONE #

PIN# _____ GRP# _____

PHYSICIAN OR SUPPLIER INFORMATION

(APPROVED BY AMA COUNCIL ON MEDICAL SERVICE 8/88)   *PLEASE PRINT OR TYPE*   APPROVED OMB-0938-0008 FORM CMS-1500 (12-90), FORM RRB-1500, APPROVED OMB-1215-0055 FORM OWCP-1500, APPROVED OMB-0720-0001 (CHAMPUS)

REVIEW

KEY CONCEPTS

FINANCIAL ISSUES

✔ Third party programs are simply another party besides the patient or the pharmacy that pays for some or all of the cost of medication: essentially, an insurer.

✔ A pharmacy benefit manager (PBM) is a company that administers drug benefit programs for insurance companies, HMOs, and self-insured employers.

✔ Co-insurance is essentially an agreement between the insurer and the insured to share costs. One aspect of it is the requirement for patients to co-pay a potion of the cost of prescriptions.

✔ The amount paid by insurers for prescriptions is not equal to the retail price normally charged, but is determined by a formula described in a contract between the insurer and the pharmacy.

THIRD PARTY PROGRAMS

✔ Prescription drug benefit cards contain necessary billing information for pharmacies, including the patient's identification number, group number, and co-pay amount.

✔ HMOs usually will not cover expenses incurred outside their participating network and often require generic substitution.

✔ POSs often partially reimburse expenses incurred outside of their network and usually require generic substitution.

✔ PPOs usually require generic substitution.

✔ Workers' compensation is compensation for employees accidentally injured on-the-job.

✔ Medicare covers people over the age of 65, disabled people under the age of 65 and people with kidney failure.

✔ Medicaid is a federal-state program for the needy.

ON-LINE ADJUDICATION

✔ In online adjudication, the technician uses the computer to determine the exact coverage for each prescription with the appropriate third party.

✔ When brand name drugs are dispensed, numbers corresponding to the reason for submitting the claim with brand name drugs are entered in a DAW (Dispense as Written) indicator field in the prescription system.

REJECTED CLAIMS

✔ Many prescription drug plans have age limitations for children or dependents of the cardholder.

✔ Most third party plans require that most of the medication has been taken before the plan will cover a refill of the same medication.

✔ Many managed care health programs require mail order pharmacies to fill prescriptions for maintenance medications.

OTHER ISSUES

✔ When a claim is rejected, the pharmacy technician can telephone the insurance plan's pharmacy help desk to determine if the patient is eligible for coverage.

✔ Claims for disease management services are submitted using a paper system and often require follow-up.

SELF TEST

MATCH THE TERMS.   *answers can be checked in the glossary*

co-insurance

co-pay

maximum allowable cost (MAC)

Medicaid

Medicare

online adjudication

pharmacy benefits

U&C or UCR

universal claim form

- companies that administer drug benefit programs
- the resolution of prescription coverage through the communication of the pharmacy computer with the third party computer.
- a standard paper claim form accepted by many insurers.
- the portion of the price of medication that the patient is required to pay.
- the maximum price per tablet (or other dispensing unit) an insurer or PBM will pay for a given product.
- the maximum amount of payment for a given prescription, determined by the insurer to be a usual and customary (and reasonable) price.
- a federal program providing health care to people with certain disabilities over age 65.
- a federal-state program, administered by the states, providing health care for the needy.
- a cost-sharing agreement between the insurer and the insured.

CHOOSE THE BEST ANSWER.   *the answer key begins on page 347*

1. Companies that administer drug benefit programs are called
   a. pharmacy benefit managers.
   b. MACs.
   c. HMOs.
   d. employers.

2. Another party, beside the patient or the pharmacy, that pays some or all of the cost of the medication is a(an)
   a. third party.
   b. co-insurance.
   c. MAC.
   d. UCR.

3. An agreement for cost-sharing between the insurer and the insured is called
   a. MAC.
   b. dual co-pay.
   c. co-insurance.
   d. co-pay.

4. The portion of the price of the medication that the patient is required to pay is called the
   a. co-insurance.
   b. co-pay.
   c. maximum allowable cost.
   d. Usual and customary price.

REVIEW

5. Pharmacies receive payment from third parties equal to
   a. the retail price of the drug.
   b. the manufacturer's cost.
   c. a wholesaler's price.
   d. none of the above.

6. Plans in which the patient pays a different amount depending on whether a generic or brand name medication is dispensed have
   a. dual co-pays.
   b. MAC.
   c. duplicate pricing.
   d. UCR.

7. If a third party plan has a dual co-pay, the patient usually pays _____ for generic drugs compared to brand name drugs.
   a. the same amount
   b. less
   c. more

8. HMOs, POS, and PPOs are examples of
   a. co-insurance.
   b. managed care programs.
   c. MAC.
   d. co-pays.

9. A(an) _____ is a network of providers for which costs are covered inside, but not outside of the network.
   a. POS
   b. HMO
   c. MAC
   d. PPO

10. A(an) _____ is a network of providers where costs outside the network may be partially reimbursed and the patient's primary care physician need not be a member.
    a. PPO
    b. HMO
    c. POS
    d. MAC

11. Which type of managed care program is least likely to require generic substitution?
    a. POS
    b. PPO
    c. Medicaid
    d. HMO

12. Medicaid
    a. is a federal/state program for the needy.
    b. is a federal program for people over 65.
    c. offers a completely open formulary.
    d. none of the above.

13. _____ is a federal-state program, administered by states, providing health care for the needy.
    a. Medicaid
    b. HMO
    c. Medicare
    d. PPO

14. Closed formulary programs, such as Medicaid, may cover drugs that are not on the formulary through a process called
    a. dual co-pay.
    b. co-insurance.
    c. POS.
    d. prior authorization.

15. Patient assistance programs are offered by
    a. HMOs.
    b. pharmacies.
    c. physicians.
    d. pharmaceutical manufacturers.

16. Which of the following information is generally not required in online claim processing?
    a. birth date
    b. weight
    c. sex
    d. group number

17. The DAW indicator that is appropriate for online adjudication if a physician has handwritten DAW on the prescription is
    a. 4.
    b. 2.
    c. 1.
    d. 3.

18. When there is a question on insurance coverage for an online claim, the pharmacy technician can
    a. telephone the insurance plan's pharmacy help desk.
    b. immediately refer the problem to the pharmacist.

19. When a technician receives a rejected claim "NDC Not Covered", this probably means
    a. the insurance plan has a closed formulary.
    b. the insurance plan has an open formulary.
    c. the birthdate submitted does not match the birthdate in the insurer's computer.
    d. the patient has mail order.

20. When a technician receives a rejected claim "Invalid Person Code", this probably means
    a. the patient is on Medicare.
    b. the patient has a mail order program.
    c. the person code entered does not match the birthdate &/or sex in the insurer's computer.
    d. the patient is on Medicaid.

21. When a technician receives a rejected claim "Unable to Connect", this probably means
    a. the insurer has an incorrect birthday for the patient.
    b. the patient's coverage has expired.
    c. the connection with the insurer's computer is temporarily unavailable due to computer problems.
    d. the insurer has a closed formulary.

22. A standard form that is often used to submit paper claims for prescriptions to a pharmacy benefit manager is called a
    a. MAC.
    b. DSM.
    c. NDC.
    d. universal claim form (UCF).

23. Pharmacists can provide services that are billed to third parties for conditions such as diabetes, hypertension, and asthma and these services are called
    a. POS.
    b. MAC.
    c. PPO.
    d. Disease State Management Services

COMMUNITY PHARMACY

Community or retail pharmacy practice is the practice of providing prescription services to the public.

In addition to prescription drugs, community pharmacies sell over-the-counter medications as well as other health and beauty products. A pharmacy may be owned independently or by a chain. Chains may specialize in pharmacy or be part of a broader mass merchandise or food store business.

One of the key characteristics of community pharmacy is the close interaction with patients.

The patient is a customer with alternatives as to where they can bring their business. So good customer service is a requirement, and for this, good interpersonal skills are needed.

Almost two thirds of all prescription drugs in the U.S. are dispensed by community pharmacies.

As a result, more pharmacists and technicians are employed in community pharmacy than any other area. An additional factor in employment is that the role of the community pharmacist in counseling and educating patients has been steadily increasing. This in turn has increased the role of the pharmacy technician in assisting pharmacists to dispense prescriptions. As a result, community pharmacy practice provides great opportunity for pharmacy technicians to find employment and serve the community.

Types of Community Pharmacies

There are about 60,000 community pharmacies in the United States which provide convenient access to medications and medication information. They can be found in a variety of business settings:

➡ **Independent Pharmacies**
  Individually owned local pharmacies.

➡ **Chain Pharmacies**
  Regional or national pharmacy chains such as Walgreens, CVS and Eckerd.

➡ **Mass Merchandiser Pharmacies**
  Regional or national mass merchandise chains such as Walmart, KMart, and Costco that sell various mass merchandise and have in-store pharmacies.

➡ **Food Store Pharmacies**
  Regional or national food store chains such as A&P, Giant Eagle, and Kroger's that have in-store pharmacies.

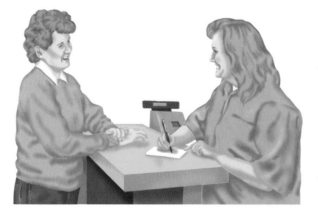

Customer Service

In contrast to institutional and other environments, technicians in the community pharmacy constantly interact with patients as customers. As a result, customer service is a major area of importance in the community pharmacy and technicians employed there must have strong interpersonal skills.

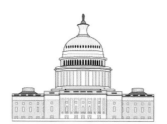

ABCD *interpersonal skills* skills involving relationships between people.

United States Government Regulations

The *1990 Omnibus Budget and Reconciliation Act (OBRA)* required community pharmacists to offer counseling to Medicaid patients regarding medications. Specifically, it required pharmacists to offer counseling and instruction regarding prescription drugs including such information as the name and description of the medication; generic name; the dosage form, dosage, route of administration, and duration of administration; special directions and precautions for preparation, administration and use by the patient; common severe side affects or interactions and therapeutic contraindications, how to avoid them, and what to do if they occur; techniques for patients to monitor their drug therapy; proper storage of the medication; what to do if a dose is missed; and refill information.

In 1996, the United States federal government passed the *Health Insurance Portability and Accountability Act (HIPAA)*. The regulations in this act, which went into effect in April, 2003, require that all healthcare professionals protect the privacy of patients. Any information related to a patient or their medical condition is considered "protected health information" and must be kept confidential. This information includes but is not limited to the patient's name and address, date of birth, diagnosis, medical history, and medications.

Some practical ways of protecting patients' privacy include:

➡ Never discussing patients outside of the pharmacy setting.
➡ Shredding documents, papers, labels containing patient information instead of discarding in regular trash.
➡ Never yelling information related to a patient across the room. Speak to patients and other healthcare professionals in the most private area possible.
➡ Never discussing patients with any individual unless the patient has authorized you to do so. This authorization should be in written form.

When working in any pharmacy, be sure to read and understand the pharmacy's HIPAA policy.

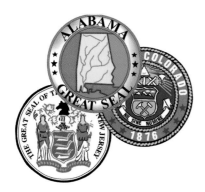

State Regulations

Community pharmacies are most closely regulated at the state level. For example, many states have mandated OBRA '90 counseling requirements for all patients, not just those on Medicaid. Also, states are increasingly requiring that technicians attain national pharmacy technician certification or they may have their own certifying process which may include registration with the state's board of pharmacy. States also regulate such things as:

➡ the ratio of pharmacists to technicians;
➡ scope of technician practice;
➡ record keeping;
➡ equipment;
➡ work areas.

ORGANIZATION

Prescription processing areas among community pharmacies may be organized differently, but they generally contain the same elements.

A number of space and equipment requirements are dictated by State regulations.

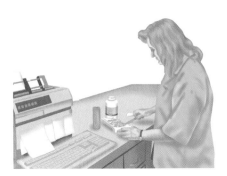

Prescription Counter

The prescription area of a pharmacy must have a counter area on which to prepare prescriptions. This counter should be kept orderly at all times.

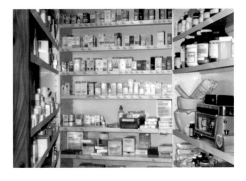

Storage

There must be adequate shelving, cabinets, or drawers for storage of medications. It is common to see several bays with shelving to hold bottles of medications. The medications may be arranged on the shelves alphabetically according to generic name or they may be arranged according to brand, or trade name.

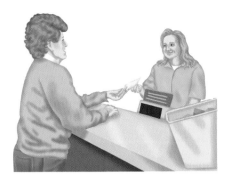

Transaction Windows

Pharmacies often have counter areas designated for intake of prescriptions being dropped off and may use the same or different counter area for dispensing the finished prescription. In accordance with HIPAA, transaction windows should be positioned so as to provide privacy for the patient. Some pharmacies are even establishing separate counseling rooms or booth areas.

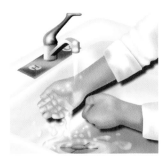

Sink

There must be an easily accessible sink that also must be kept clean at all times.

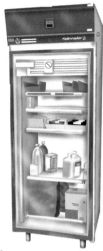

Refrigeration

There must also be a refrigerator in which to store medication that requires storage in temperatures between 2 and 8 degrees Celsius. The refrigerator must be designated for drugs only. No food products are allowed to be stored in the same refrigerator.

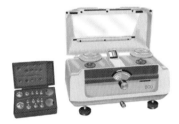

Equipment

Equipment that must be available for use in the pharmacy includes a prescription balance, a set of metric weights, a glass mortar and pestle, glass funnels, stirring rods, graduates for measuring liquids, spatulas, counting trays and or counting devices, ointment board or parchment paper for compounding creams, ointments, etc., prescription labels, and auxiliary or precautionary labels.

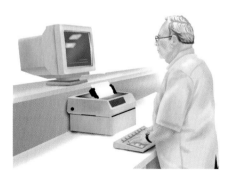

Computer System

There is an area for the computer monitor, keyboard, and printer.

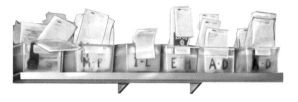

Prescription Bins or Shelves

Completed prescriptions that are not being immediately picked up are generally placed in bins or shelves alphabetized by customer.

CUSTOMER SERVICE

Customer satisfaction is the goal of customer service.

Good customer service requires presenting yourself to customers in a calm, courteous, and professional manner. It requires listening to and understanding customer requests for service and fulfilling those requests accurately or explaining to the customer's satisfaction why the request cannot be serviced.

The health of customers is a significant factor in their experience of community pharmacy service.

Customers may often feel sick or irritable and need their medication quickly. Having to wait in a line may be physically difficult or emotionally upsetting. The cost of the medication may be an additional worry. Consequently, though customer service is important in any type of retail store, it is particularly important in the community pharmacy setting.

It is important to respond to customers in a positive way at all times.

In any situation where a customer is angry, frustrated, or otherwise dissatisfied, it is especially important to give a positive response. This can be done in part by listening intently and making eye contact with the customer. Restating what the customer has said is also important, since it demonstrates that you have listened to their complaint. Use positive, not negative terms to tell the customer what you can do, not what you can't do to solve their problem.

Involve the pharmacist in all difficult situations.

If after spending some time with the customer, you have been unable to resolve the problem, you should inform the pharmacist. This should be done immediately for serious complaints regarding problems with prescriptions. Remember that employees that possess well developed interpersonal skills are good for business and will be appreciated by employers.

AT THE COUNTER

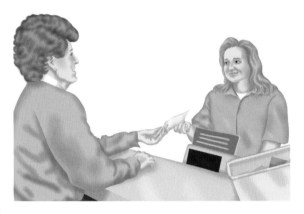

Since pharmacy technicians are generally responsible for handling the pharmacy counter, they have direct contact with customers and play a key role in assisting customers with their needs.

This involves taking in new and refill prescriptions, but also includes directing customers to requested over-the-counter products or answering other questions that do not require the pharmacist's judgment. The technician should be familiar with the layout of the store and must know where various types of products are located so that they may help customers find products quickly.

 A pharmacy technician must know when to refer a customer to the pharmacist. It is a good idea to discuss such situations with the pharmacist regularly.

ON THE TELEPHONE

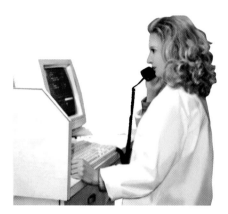

A significant part of the pharmacy technician's responsibilities includes answering the telephone. Calls must be answered in a pleasant and courteous manner, following a standard format that should be indicated by the store manager or pharmacist. Generally, this begins with stating the name of the pharmacy and your name. An example:

"Main Street Pharmacy, Joan speaking, may I help you?"

Many calls will concern the price or stock availability of prescription and over-the-counter products. Some will be to place refill requests. In that case, the same process is followed as when taking refill requests at the counter (see p. 263), except that the technician should also ask the patient when they plan to pick up the prescription.

Some calls will require the pharmacist's judgment. These should be directed immediately to the pharmacist. This applies to questions regarding medication or general health related questions. When patients raise such questions, politely ask them to hold on the line while you get the pharmacist.

INTERPERSONAL TECHNIQUES

At the Counter

Techniques for interacting with customers at the counter include:

➥ listening carefully;

➥ making eye contact;

➥ repeating what the customer has said;

➥ using positive rather than negative language to describe what you can do.

On the Phone

Techniques for interacting with customers on the telephone include:

➥ using a pleasant and courteous manner;

➥ stating the name of the pharmacy and your name;

➥ following the standard procedure indicated for your pharmacy;

➥ referring all calls that require a pharmacist's judgment to the pharmacist.

 Any time you are uncertain of whether a question requires the pharmacist's judgment, refer the question to the pharmacist.

PROCESSING PRESCRIPTIONS

A major responsibility of the pharmacy technician is to process new and refill prescriptions.

This is done using the pharmacy's computerized prescription system. Different pharmacies will use different systems. The pharmacist or another pharmacy technician will usually provide training on the system that is used. Learning to process prescriptions efficiently and accurately on the system is essential and will take some time and commitment.

PATIENT INFORMATION

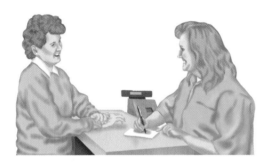

When taking in a new prescription, always ask whether the patient has ever had prescriptions filled at the pharmacy in the past. If the patient had not been to the pharmacy in the past, be sure to get the following information which will be needed for the patient profile information that must be entered into the computer:

➡ **full name of the patient**
➡ **address**
➡ **telephone number**
➡ **date of birth**
➡ **any allergies to medication.**

If a patient requests a prescription refill, **be sure to get the patient's name and the prescription number** which appears on the prescription bottle. If the prescription number is unavailable, ask for the name of the medication. Whether the patient is requesting a new or refill prescription, ask if they would like to wait or if they prefer to pick up the prescription later.

PRESCRIPTION INFORMATION

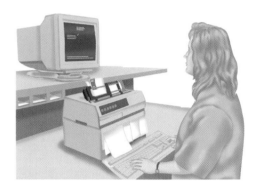

When entering a new prescription into the pharmacy prescription system, the pharmacy technician needs to enter the following information into the appropriate fields on the computer's dispensing screen:

➡ **correct drug and strength**
➡ **correct physician's name** (and physician's **DEA number** for prescriptions for controlled substances or for prescriptions being billed to a third party that requires it)
➡ **directions for use** (the signa)
➡ **quantity** (i.e. the number of tablets or the metric quantity if dispensing a liquid, cream, inhaler, etc.)
➡ **number of authorized refills**
➡ **DAW code** which indicates that a brand name or a generic product is being dispensed.
➡ **initials of the dispensing pharmacist**

ONLINE BILLING

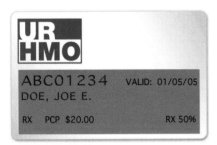

A major feature of computerized prescription systems is online billing of a prescription to a patient's insurance company or other third party. Since the majority of patients today have an insurance plan or third party coverage that will pay for the cost of their prescriptions, the technician must be familiar with all of the private and state administered prescription plans that are accepted by the pharmacy. So entering a prescription also involves entering a code identifying the plan that will be billed. This generally includes:

➡ a **group number**, which identifies the patient's employer;

➡ a **patient or policy identification number**, which is usually, but not always, the patient's social security number;

➡ a **patient code**, which indicates the specific patient covered under the plan (the primary card holder is usually 01, spouse is 02, and so on).

Once all third party billing information is entered, the technician can proceed with online billing. The third party will respond within a few moments by either stating that the claim has been paid or otherwise has been rejected. If a co-payment by the patient is required, the amount is indicated. If a rejection occurs, there will be a general message regarding why the claim has been rejected. If it is due to incorrect number entry, it can be easily corrected. Sometimes however, a call to the third party will be necessary to get the claim paid.

REFILLS

In the case of entering refill prescriptions, most pharmacy computer programs allow looking up a refill either by prescription number or through screening the patient profile for the medication. When processing a refill prescription, be sure to check that there are refills available. Most systems will indicate when no refills are available. If there are no refills, alert the pharmacist so that he or she can call the patient's physician for a new prescription. Prescriptions can be called in by a physician over the phone, but these calls should be handled by the pharmacist.

Note that when refilling prescriptions, be sure it is not too early to refill the medication. If it is more than a week early, many third parties will reject the claim. Also, refills for controlled medications should not be refilled early since they have the potential for abuse. In the case of a patient requesting an early refill of a controlled substance, involve the pharmacist right away.

SAFETY

Another important aspect of entering new and refill prescriptions has to do with screening for safety of prescription medication. Many computer software systems will flag drug interactions and allergy conflicts. When these flags occur, always alert the pharmacist so that he or she can evaluate the significance of the flag. The pharmacist may tell the pharmacy technician this is okay to proceed or will otherwise stop the process and may need to make a call to the patient's physician.

PREPARING THE PRESCRIPTION

The prescription system will print a prescription label based on the patient and prescription information that has been entered into it. Once the label is generated, it is time to prepare the prescription. This begins with locating the medication and its container.

MEASURING

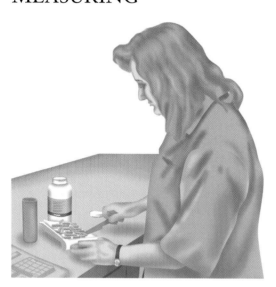

If it is a tablet or capsule, find the stock bottle on the shelf and count the correct number of pills using a **counting tray**. A counting tray is a tray that allows a pharmacist or pharmacy technician to count pills from the tray into a side container-like area. This special tray allows for the pills remaining on the tray to be easily slid back into the stock bottle. The pills that will be dispensed will slide easily into a prescription vial.

Community pharmacies that process a high volume of prescriptions may use automatic filling devices. These devices generally are cells that are each filled with a particular drug. The fastest moving drugs will be stocked in the cells. When a drug that is in one of the cells is ordered, the device quickly counts the appropriate amount of capsules or tablets into the a prescription vial. Some devices also produce the prescription label.

When necessary, solutions are measured using a graduate, and ointments are weighed using a balance.

CONTAINERS

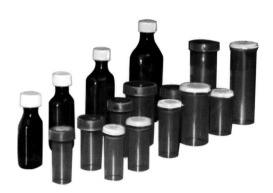

There are various size containers for tablets and capsules from which to choose an appropriate one. If preparing a liquid medication, select the appropriate size bottle and pour the correct volume of liquid into the bottle. For creams and ointments, find a tube of the correct metric quantity. If the cream or ointment is not pre-packaged in the appropriate size tube or perhaps was compounded at the pharmacy, it will be necessary to transfer the product with a spatula to an ointment jar of the correct size. It may be necessary to use a balance to weigh out the correct amount.

SAFETY CAPS

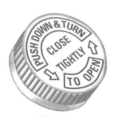

All dispensed prescription vials and bottles must have a safety cap or child resistant cap, *unless the patient requests an easy-open or non-child resistant cap.* Most computer software programs have a field in which to record the patient's preference regarding this. It is important to pay attention to which cap is indicated as some elderly or arthritic patients have extreme difficulty opening child-resistant caps.

counting tray a tray designed for counting pills.

auxiliary labels labels regarding specific warnings, foods or medications to avoid, potential side effects, and so on.

LABELS

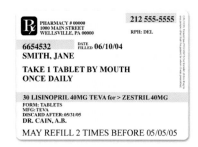

Once the desired pills or other product is put in an appropriate container, the finished prescription label is placed on the product along with any **auxiliary labels** that may be necessary. These labels identify important usage information, including specific warnings or alerts on:

- ➡ administration
- ➡ proper storage
- ➡ possible side effects
- ➡ potential food and drug interactions

Examples include "take with food", "may cause drowsiness", and others shown at right. Some computer systems automatically identify which auxiliary labels are needed. If this is not the case, ask the pharmacist which labels should be applied.

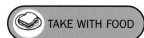
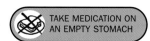
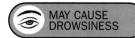
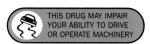
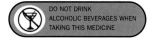
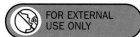
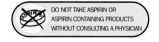
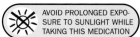

sample auxiliary labels

FINAL CHECK BY THE PHARMACIST

As a final step of the preparation process, organize the final product and all paperwork, including the original prescription, for the pharmacist's final check. Also, leave stock bottles, or other packaging next to the final product so the pharmacist can see that the correct product was used. After the pharmacist has checked the prescription, it is a responsibility of the pharmacy technician to return any products used to their proper place on the shelf, cabinet, or drawer.

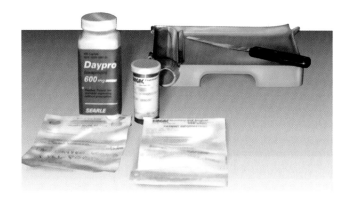

 Schedule II controlled substances must be checked and signed for by the pharmacist.

CUSTOMER PICK-UP

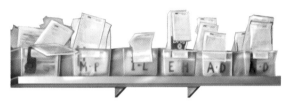

alphabetized prescription bins

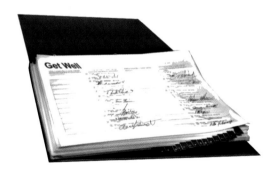

a signature log

℞ Always be sensitive to the confidential nature of prescription information. While customers may wish to hear prescription information themselves, they may not want others to.

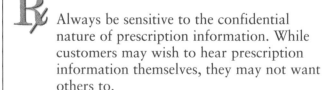

signature log a book in which patients sign for the prescriptions they receive, for legal and insurance purposes.

Picking Up the Prescription

When the customer is picking up a prescription, locate the prescription, which will usually be filed alphabetically by the last name of the patient either in bins or another storage area. For confidentiality reasons, when a prescription is located for a family member, do not ask for instance, "Would you also like to pick up your daughter's prescription while you're here?" Though this may seem helpful, it is a breach of confidentiality. Find only the prescription that was requested.

Signature Logs

Most community pharmacies will have customers sign a log which records that the prescription was picked-up. The signature log will serve as proof to a third party payer such as Medicaid or a private insurer that the prescription was dispensed to the patient. It is common for third party payers to review the signature log when conducting audits at pharmacies.

The log may serve a dual purpose of also recording that patient medication counselling was offered. The usual process is to ask the patient if they would like the pharmacist to speak with them regarding their prescription. The patient is then asked to sign that they have either accepted the offer of medication counselling, or that they have declined the offer.

For Schedule II, and sometimes also for Schedule II, IV and V, prescriptions, pharmacies may require that the person picking up the prescription show a driver's license (in addition to signing the signature log). The driver's license number will be recorded either in the log or on the back of the prescription. This identification information will help in the event that the drug is used unlawfully.

USING A CASH REGISTER

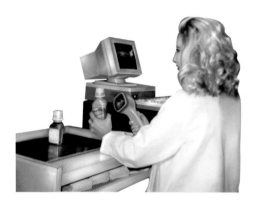

scanning a price

It is often a responsibility of the pharmacy technician to ring up prescriptions and over the counter products into the register and accept payment for them. Cash registers are integrated into the pharmacy's computerized system so prices for products can be automatically entered by using bar code scanners. Scanners can be hand-held or built into the counter. The scanner beam is targeted at the bar code and identifies the product for the register. The product's price (or discounted price if there is a prescription plan discount) is automatically entered into the register. If a mistake is made between the pricing on the product or shelf and the amount in the system, changes can be made manually, though each system is different, and technicians need to know and follow the procedures used at their pharmacy.

Operating a cash register also requires handling payments properly. When cash payment is made, it is it is important to count the payment within the customer's line of sight and to confirm the amount orally to the customer. This will avoid misunderstandings over what the customer thought they gave you. If change is necessary, the amount should be counted out loud and placed into the customer's hand. An example of such a transaction would be:

A twenty dollar bill is given as payment for a bill of $14.50.

➡ The bill should be held or placed within the customer's line of sight and the amount confirmed as "That's Twenty dollars."

➡ The amount is then entered into the register and a receipt is produced.

➡ The change is counted out as it is placed into the customer's hand, i.e. "fifty cents makes fifteen dollars, and five dollars makes twenty dollars".

➡ After the customer has received their change and is given the receipt, the twenty dollar bill is placed into the register drawer.

Following this general procedure will avoid disputes, either out of confusion or intent to deceive, over whether a larger bill was tendered or the correct change given.

The pharmacy technician must also be able to handle checks and credit cards appropriately. It is very important to follow the store policy and procedure regarding handling of these transactions. Be sure to check the identification of the customer as instructed by the store manager or pharmacist

OTHER DUTIES

The pharmacy technician should know the names and locations of the various over-the-counter products carried in the pharmacy. When asked, the technician should be able to direct customers to an OTC product. Some of the many OTC products that are available will include cough and cold preparations, laxatives and antidiarrheals, medications for the treatment of indigestion, analgesics, vitamins, first aid supplies, dental and denture care products, and infant care products.

The technician should not recommend OTC products to pharmacy customers, however.

Though OTC products may be bought freely by customers, they are not without risks. Incorrect dosages and drug-drug interactions with OTC products can produce significant adverse effects. For example, many cough and cold preparations contain ingredients that may increase blood pressure and worsen a diabetic condition. Therefore, the technician should *refer patients asking about OTC products to the pharmacist*. As always, the technician must involve the pharmacist whenever judgement is needed.

Ordering stock is another responsibility of the pharmacy technician.

As stock diminishes, it is important to reorder. The technician must know which products are used more frequently than others and reorder in appropriate quantities. For instance, popular anti-hypertensive medication should be kept well stocked, while medications that are not as popular do not need to be available in large quantities.

The pharmacy technician is also generally responsible for keeping the pharmacy clean, neat, and in proper working order.

Periodically, the counting trays, and the pharmacy counter should be wiped with alcohol. Pharmacy supplies, such as prescription bags, prescription vials and bottles, prescription labels and computer paper should be available at all times and thus, must be stocked regularly. The stock bottles of drugs on the shelves should periodically be readjusted so that they are neatly arranged with all labels facing front. At least monthly, the pharmacy technician should check all bottles for outdated expiration dates as it is unlawful to dispense outdated medications. Expired drugs must be sent back to the wholesaler or be destroyed.

RETAIL CONCEPTS

Community pharmacies do not just dispense prescriptions. They are **retail businesses** that sell over-the-counter medications and various other products. Retail businesses resell consumer ready products that they have purchased from wholesalers or manufacturers. To make a profit, the retailer sells the products at a **mark-up** from their purchase price. The mark-up is the amount of the retailer's sale price minus their purchase price. For example, if an over-the-counter medication is purchased at $5.00 a package, and the mark-up is 50%, the retailer's price to the consumer will be: $5.00 plus a $2.50 markup ($5.00 times 50%), or $7.50.

The mark-up represents the portion of sales that the retailer will clear after paying suppliers. This is what pays for the costs of doing business (building, equipment, salaries, etc.) and generates profits. So calculating the mark-up is very important to retailers. It is generally calculated by the pharmacy computer system and based on business costs and profit goals. They will differ by pharmacy and can differ by product. That is, some product lines may have lower or higher mark-ups than the standard products in the pharmacy. Each price that the technician stickers on a product includes the cost of the product and its mark-up.

Shelf Stickers

OTC products have shelf-stickers that can be scanned for inventory identification. They also indicate **unit price** information for consumers. A unit price is the price of a unit of medication (such as an ounce of a liquid cold remedy), rather than the price of the entire package. Unit prices protect the consumer from packaging and pricing that suggests that more is contained in the item than actually is.

STOCK DUTIES

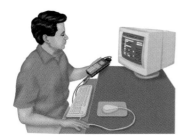

Ordering

Ordering stock in most pharmacies is done by transmitting the order to a drug wholesaler via a telephone line. Every product has a stock number which is entered, either into a computer with a modem or into a device that connects to a phone line and transmits the order to the drug wholesaler.

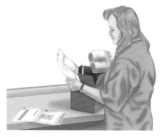

Receiving

When an order from a drug wholesaler is received, it is generally the pharmacy technician's responsibility to unpack the order and check that all items on the invoice have, in fact been received. Items must be checked to make sure the following are as ordered:

✔ **drug product**
✔ **strength**
✔ **packaging**
✔ **quantity**

In addition items must be inspected for:

✔ **damage**
✔ **expiration dates**

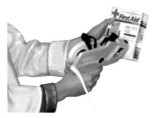

Stickering

Products are often stickered with pricing information and reorder numbers for each item. These stickers may be applied with a stickering gun or by hand. They are placed on each item. Once this process is complete, the items will need to be put on the shelves in their proper places. The invoices will also need to be filed for reference purposes.

DISEASE STATE MANAGEMENT

An important development related to community pharmacy practice is disease state management. Disease state management programs are designed to provide one-on-one pharmacist/patient consultation sessions targeted toward management of a chronic disease or condition such as diabetes. Pharmacies that offer these programs utilize a private office or area, usually located at the pharmacy, where the pharmacist can conduct consultation sessions. For example, the pharmacist can teach people with diabetes how to properly use blood glucose monitoring devices; the pharmacist may also analyze blood-glucose readings on an on-going basis and recommend medication changes to the patient's physician. Disease management programs are also offered for asthma/chronic obstructive pulmonary disease (COPD), anticoagulation, weight loss, smoking cessation and cholesterol reduction.

Fees for these services are either billed directly to the patient or to the patient's major medical insurance. The pharmacy technician may coordinate the billing, as well as schedule appointments and take patient information. As with all patient-related medical and pharmaceutical information, HIPAA regulations apply, mandating complete confidentiality.

REVIEW

KEY CONCEPTS

COMMUNITY PHARMACY

✔ In addition to prescription drugs, community pharmacies sell over-the-counter medications as well as other health and beauty products.

✔ The role of the community pharmacist in counseling and educating patients has been steadily increasing.

✔ Pharmacies in the U.S. must comply with OBRA 90 which mandates that patients be offered counseling on all new prescriptions. Pharmacies must also comply with HIPAA which mandates the protection of patients' privacy.

ORGANIZATION

✔ Pharmacies have basic space and equipment requirements that may vary slightly from state to state but generally include a prescription counter to work on, proper storage areas for drugs, designated refrigerators for drugs, equipment for compounding, a sink, computer system and areas for dispensing prescriptions.

CUSTOMER SERVICE

✔ Technicians should always respond to customers in a positive and courteous way.

✔ Telephone calls must be answered following a standard format that should be indicated by the store manager or pharmacist.

PROCESSING PRESCRIPTIONS

✔ In the case of a patient requesting an early refill of a controlled substance, involve the pharmacist right away.

PREPARING THE PRESCRIPTION

✔ Whenever the prescription system flags drug interactions and allergy conflicts, alert the pharmacist so that he or she can evaluate the significance of the flag.

✔ All dispensed prescription vials and bottles must have a safety cap or child resistant cap, unless the patient requests an easy-open or non-child resistant cap.

✔ Auxiliary labels identify important usage information, including specific warnings or alerts on: administration, proper storage, possible side effects, and potential food and drug interactions.

✔ As a final step of the preparation process, the final product and all paperwork, including the original prescription, is organized for the pharmacist's final check.

CUSTOMER PICK-UP

✔ Customer signatures in a log are required for Medicaid and most third party insurer or HMO prescriptions, along with Schedule V controlled substances, poisons, and certain other prescriptions (depending upon the state).

OTHER DUTIES

✔ OTC products may be bought freely by customers, but they are not without risks. The technician may direct customers to a product they are looking for but should involve the pharmacist when making recommendations.

✔ Ordering stock is often a responsibility of the pharmacy technician.

✔ The pharmacy technician is generally responsible for keeping the pharmacy clean, neat, and in proper working order.

SELF TEST

MATCH THE TERMS.   *answers can be checked in the glossary*

auxiliary labels

counting tray

interpersonal skills

mark-up

safety cap

shelf-stickers

signature log

transaction windows

unit price

- skills involving relationships between people.

- counter areas designated for taking prescriptions and for delivering them to patients.

- a child resistant cap

- the price of a unit of medication (such as an ounce of a liquid cold remedy).

- a tray designed for counting pills.

- specific warnings that are placed on filled prescriptions.

- a book in which patients sign for the prescriptions they receive, for legal and insurance purposes.

- the amount of the retailer's sale price minus their purchase price.

- stickers with bar codes that can be scanned for inventory identification.

CHOOSE THE BEST ANSWER.   *the answer key begins on page 347*

1. Community pharmacies that are individually owned local pharmacies are
   a. food store pharmacies.
   b. mass merchandiser pharmacies.
   c. chain pharmacies.
   d. independent pharmacies.

2. Community pharmacies, such as CVS and Eckerd, that are part of regional or national pharmacy chains are
   a. independent pharmacies.
   b. food store pharmacies.
   c. chain pharmacies.
   d. mass merchandiser pharmacies.

3. Community pharmacies that are part of regional or national food store chains such as Giant Eagle and Kroger are
   a. mass merchandiser pharmacies.
   b. food store pharmacies.
   c. chain pharmacies.
   d. independent pharmacies.

4. About 2/3 of all prescription drugs in the US are dispensed by
   a. community pharmacies.
   b. institutional pharmacies.
   c. hospital pharmacies.
   d. nursing home pharmacies.

REVIEW

5. _____ are skills involving relationships between people.
   a. Computer skills
   b. Data management skills
   c. Transaction skills
   d. Interpersonal skills

6. An easily accessible sink is an important part of a community pharmacy and must be
   a. kept clean.
   b. maintained at 2 to 8 degrees Celsius.
   c. maintained at 2 to 8 degrees Fahrenheit.
   d. portable.

7. The refrigerator in a community pharmacy may be used to store
   a. drugs only.
   b. drugs and the lunch of pharmacy personnel.
   c. drugs and sealed containers of soda pop.
   d. drugs and the pharmacist's lunch.

8. Techniques for interacting with customers at the counter include
   a. using a pleasant and courteous manner, stating the name of the pharmacy and your name, following the standard procedure indicated for your pharmacy, and referring all calls that require a pharmacist's judgment to the pharmacist.
   b. listening carefully, making eye contact, repeating what the customer has said, and using positive language to describe what you can do.

9. Patient information that must be entered into the computer includes
   a. only the name of the patient.
   b. full name of patient, address, telephone number, date of birth, and any medication allergies.
   c. diagnosis made by the technician.
   d. diagnosis made by the pharmacist.

10. Information that a pharmacy technician may enter into the computer for a new prescription includes
   a. correct drug and strength, correct physician's name, directions for use, quantity, number of refills, DAW code, and initials of the dispensing pharmacist.
   b. patient's name and prescription number.

11. When reviewing a prescription for a C-II substance, which of these is not required:
   a. NDC number
   b. patient street address
   c. DEA number
   d. DAW information

12. The group number in third party billing information usually identifies the
   a. employer.
   b. gender.
   c. family member.
   d. Social Security number of the insured.

13. When the prescription system warns of a potential interaction:
   a. tell the patient
   b. get the correct auxiliary label
   c. include it on the sig
   d. inform the pharmacist

14. All dispensed prescriptions must have a
    _____ cap unless that patient
    specifies a _____ cap.
    a. child resistant, non-child resistant
    b. child-resistant, child-resistant
    c. non-child resistant, non-child resistant
    d. non-child resistant, child-resistant

15. Labels that are placed on the prescription
    container in addition to the prescription
    label and provide specific warnings are
    a. warning stickers.
    b. flags.
    c. warning labels.
    d. auxiliary labels.

16. The pharmacist always checks the pre-
    scription
    a. after it is filled by the technician.
    b. when the patient signs the log.
    c. after it is rung on the cash register.
    d. as it is given to the patient.

17. A(An) _____ is a book
    that patients sign for the prescriptions they
    receive.
    a. exempt narcotic book
    b. patient register book
    c. patient compliance book
    d. signature log

18. Ordering stock is a responsibility of the
    a. computer system.
    b. prescription counter.
    c. pharmacy technician.
    d. third party.

19. The _____ is generally
    responsible for keeping the pharmacy
    clean, neat, and in proper working order.
    a. staff pharmacist
    b. pharmacy manager
    c. pharmacy technician
    d. weekend pharmacist

20. The difference between the price the cus-
    tomer pays and the price the pharmacy
    pays for a product is called
    a. profit.
    b. overhead.
    c. margin.
    d. mark-up.

21. Unit price information is found on shelf
    stickers for
    a. Schedule III, IV, and V medications.
    b. Schedule II medications.
    c. OTC products.
    d. legend drugs.

22. Disease state management services are
    offered in
    a. private offices or areas.
    b. public access areas.
    c. the dispensing area of the pharmacy.
    d. waiting areas.

23. Coordinating of billing for disease state
    management services is a duty of the
    a. physician.
    b. third party.
    c. pharmacy technician.
    d. staff pharmacist.

24. Scheduling appointments for disease state
    management services is a duty of the
    a. registered nurse.
    b. pharmacy technician.
    c. physician.
    d. third party

HOSPITAL PHARMACY

Hospital pharmacy technicians work as part of a team, under the supervision of a pharmacist or supervising technician, to ensure appropriate medication therapy for hospital patients.

This mainly involves entering, processing and delivery of medication orders; ordering, packaging and storage of drugs; helping the pharmacist to monitor patients' medication therapy; and assisting in quality assurance projects. Good communication skills are essential as the pharmacy technician will be interacting via the telephone or in person with many different professionals working in the hospital.

To better understand the hospital pharmacy technician's roles and responsibilities, it is important to become familiar with the interworkings and details of the hospital.

Though they may be organized differently, hospitals generally contain the same elements. Patient rooms are divided into groups called nursing units or patient care units. Patients with similar problems are often located on the same unit which allows for specialized nursing care based on similar issues, problems, or disease states. An example of this would be an area for patients who are in labor or about to deliver a baby (OB Unit), or an intensive care unit specifically for cardiology patients (CCU).

The work station for medical personnel on a nursing unit is called the nurses' station.

This area stores various items required for care of the patients on the unit, including medications.

There are several other areas of the hospital, called ancillary areas, that also provide patient care.

Each hospital has different ancillary areas, but some common ones are radiology, the cardiac catheterization lab, and the emergency room. These areas use medications and are serviced by the pharmacy department.

Every hospital has a center responsible for distributing supplies to all areas of the facility.

This is often referred to as central supply or materials management. This department supplies the pharmacy with items required for daily operations including paper towels, soap, needles, syringes, etc. Central supply does not, however, handle storage or delivery of any prescription medications.

THE HEALTH CARE TEAM

It takes a team of many different types of health care professionals to meet the needs of patients, and individual patients generally receive care from a variety of these professionals. Most health care personnel are identified by abbreviations that indicate their discipline. Each individual profession plays a part on the multidisciplinary healthcare team. Their common objective is to care for patients and assist in their recovery.

Around the Clock Care

Since hospitals are open 24 hours a day, 7 days a week, there are a lot of shifts that must be covered. This allows for a great deal of variability in scheduling. Standard eight hour shifts in the hospital are: 7am to 3:30pm; 3:00pm to 11:30pm; and 11:00pm to 7:00am. Other combinations of work times are possible using four, six, and twelve hour shifts. At smaller hospitals, the pharmacy may not be open 24 hours a day. In these situations, a pharmacist can be contacted by phone in the case of any pharmacy or medicine related questions. The nurse manager or other authorized personnel may have access to pharmacy areas during these times for emergency medication needs. State laws mandate what is acceptable in these situations.

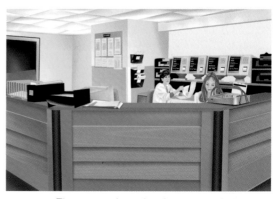

The nurses' station is a central storage and communication center for patient care in the hospital.

Medical Staff

M.D., Medical Doctor

An MD examines patients, orders and interprets lab tests, diagnoses illnesses, and prescribes and administers treatments for people suffering from injury or disease. An MD may be a general or a specialty doctor.

D.O., Doctor of Osteopathy

A osteopathic physician practices a "whole person" approach to medicine. D.O.'s may be general or specialty doctors.

P.A., Physician's Assistant

A physician's assistant coordinates care for patients under the close supervision of a MD or OD. They are allowed to prescribe certain medications.

Therapy and Other Staff

R.T., Respiratory Therapist

A respiratory therapist assists in the evaluation, treatment, and care of patients with breathing problems or illnesses.

P.T., Physical Therapist

A physical therapist provides services that help restore function, improve mobility, relieve pain, and prevent or limit permanent physical disabilities.

O.T., Occupational Therapist

An occupational therapist works with patients who have conditions that are mentally, physically, developmentally, or emotionally disabling, and helps them develop, recover, or maintain daily living and work skills.

M.S.W., Master's of Social Work

A social worker is concerned with patient social factors such as child protection, ability to pay for medications, and coping capacities of patients and their families.

R.D., Registered Dietitian

A dietitian helps assess and scientifically evaluates patients' nutritional needs and recommends appropriate modifications.

Nursing

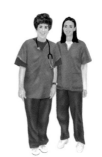

N.P., Nurse Practitioner

A nurse practitioner provides basic primary health care. The N.P. may work closely with doctors and can prescribe various medications in most states.

R.N., Registered Nurse

A nurse who provides bedside care, assists physicians in various procedures, and administers medical regimens to patients.

L.P.N., Licensed Practical Nurse

A nurse who provides basic bedside care under the supervision of an RN. An LPN may administer medication to patients.

C.N.A., Certified Nursing Assistant or L.N.A., Licensed Nursing Assistant

Nursing assistants who work under the supervision of RN's and LPN's to help provide daily care of patients but who are not allowed to administer medications.

Pharmacy

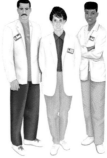

Pharm.D., Doctor of Pharmacy

A registered pharmacist with advanced training in providing pharmaceutical care.

R.Ph., Registered Pharmacist

A pharmacist who is licensed to work by the state. Duties include reviewing patient drug regimens for appropriateness, dispensing medications, and advising the medical staff on the selection of drugs.

Pharmacy Technician

Pharmacy technicians in the hospital work under the direct supervision of a pharmacist and play a vital role in the preparation, storage, and delivery of medications to patients. Technicians assist the pharmacist but are often given specific duties, such as "inventory technician." Training requirements may vary by state and hospital, but hospitals are increasingly seeking technicians that have already received certification (CPhT).

HOSPITAL PHARMACY AREAS

There are two basic organizational models for pharmacy departments within a hospital: centralized and decentralized.

In the centralized system, all pharmacy activities are conducted from one location within the hospital: the inpatient pharmacy. In a decentralized system, there are several pharmacy areas located throughout the hospital, each performing a specific function in order to provide pharmaceutical care to the entire hospital.

In the decentralized model, there is a central pharmacy which is generally responsible for the preparation and delivery of patient medication carts.

The central pharmacy also may conduct a variety of packaging functions in order to keep other areas within the department supplied with drugs they need. Medication order processing occurs at several decentralized locations throughout the hospital called pharmacy **satellites**. Satellites are responsible for providing first doses of medications, any emergency medications, and replacing missing or lost doses. Although not a primary focus of the satellite work load, a laminar flow hood may be used to prepare parenteral products as needed. There are usually several satellites located throughout the hospital, each serving a fraction of the patient care units in the hospital and each may have a specialized focus (i.e. pediatrics, oncology).

In the decentralized system, a separate area for preparation of parenteral products may be established.

This area could be a separate room or zone within the central pharmacy or exist in a separate location in the hospital. These areas, called sterile product areas, frequently contain specialized **clean rooms** for the preparation of sterile products. Laminar flow hoods will be located here since this is where the majority of parenterals will be made.

CENTRALIZED

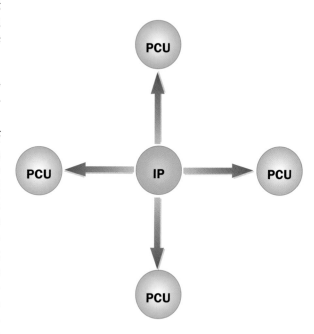

In a centralized system, all pharmacy activities are conducted at a single location, the inpatient pharmacy (IP). Medications are provided from there to the patient care units (PCU).

centralized pharmacy system a system in which all pharmacy activities in the hospital are conducted at one location, the inpatient pharmacy.

decentralized pharmacy system a system in which pharmacy activities occur in multiple locations within a hospital.

inpatient pharmacy pharmacy located in a hospital or inpatient medical facility (e.g., a nursing home) which services only those patients in the hospital/facility and ancillary areas.

outpatient pharmacy a pharmacy attached to a hospital servicing patients who have left the hospital or who are visiting doctors in a hospital outpatient clinic.

clean rooms areas designed for the preparation of sterile products.

DECENTRALIZED

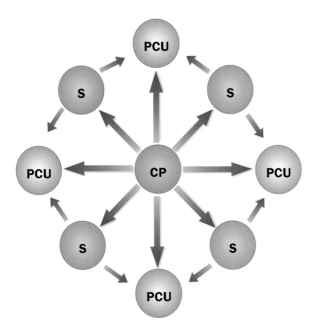

In a decentralized system, a central inpatient pharmacy (CP) is still responsible for many operations but satellite pharmacies (S) also operate at multiple locations throughout the hospital.

℞ Many larger hospitals often have a separate drug information center with important resources for answering drug-related questions. Other hospitals may set up a designated area in the pharmacy for important drug references.

A centralized area for storage of drug product may also be a part of the pharmacy department.

In larger hospitals this area requires an entire staff of its own that deals only with the order and delivery of drug products for the other pharmacy areas. Technicians often make up a large portion of this staff and may be entirely in charge of running the area. In smaller institutions, however, the functions of inventory room personnel may be only a part of the pharmacy technician's duties during their scheduled shift.

A number of hospitals have an investigational drug service which is a specialized pharmacy subsection that deals solely with clinical drug trials.

These drug studies require a great deal of paperwork and special documentation of all doses of medication taken by patients. Technicians are frequently used in this area to assist the pharmacist with the large amount of documentation required and in preparing individual patient medication supplies. The investigational drug service may provide drugs to both patients located in the hospital and those receiving study medication at home.

Quality assurance is another area in which pharmacy technicians are involved.

For example, a technician may be responsible for making sure there are no expired medications in the pharmacy, subset of the pharmacy, nursing unit floor stock or other ancillary areas such as the emergency room or cardiac catheter lab. In addition, the technician may be responsible for making sure that refrigerators and freezers are maintained at appropriate temperatures and for maintaining a daily log of the temperatures.

Hospitals frequently have doctor's offices or clinics attached to them along with an outpatient or clinic pharmacy.

These pharmacies provide prescription medications to patients visiting their doctor. They are run very similarly to a retail pharmacy, but hospital technicians may be required to staff in these areas in addition to their inpatient responsibilities. Although an outpatient or clinic pharmacy may be located within a hospital, it does not supply inpatients with medications. It only provides patients who have obtained prescriptions from their doctors at the clinic or upon leaving the hospital.

COMMUNICATION

In order to coordinate patient care, there must be communication between the various departments within the hospital.

Written and computer-generated medication orders are the routine method for letting the pharmacy know a medication is needed, but they are not the only ways pharmacy personnel interact with staff from other departments. The pharmacy technician needs to understand the variety of ways that healthcare professionals communicate with the pharmacy department.

The telephone is an important tool for communication with patient care areas and is often used to clarify orders, answer drug information questions and handle other medication-related problems (such as missing doses of a patient's medication).

The pharmacy technician is often responsible for triaging phone calls. When answering the phone the technician should identify his/herself and use good etiquette. Any drug information questions that require the pharmacist's expertise should be given to the pharmacist, but technicians should handle other phone calls related to their own job function.

Some information must be written or printed.

Fax machines and computer-generated print-outs are often used to quickly transmit written information such as drug orders from one area to another.

Two systems that allow for the mechanical transfer of written communications and drugs are the dumbwaiter and the pneumatic tube.

A dumbwaiter is like a small elevator that moves vertically, in a straight path, between different floors of the hospital. In the pneumatic tube system, compressed air tubes in the walls of the building move plastic shuttles containing medication orders and drugs to and from stations in the pharmacy and other areas of the hospital. A destination is programmed into the tube station and in minutes the shuttle arrives at the desired location. A pneumatic tube system is more advantageous than a dumbwaiter since it can move horizontally as well as vertically and, in some advanced systems, between buildings. Although the pneumatic tube has replaced the dumbwaiter in many instances, it may not be used with unstable medications, those that are too large for the tubes, and those restricted by hospital policy.

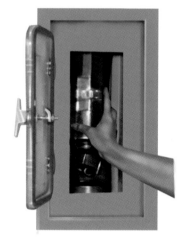

pneumatic tube and capsule

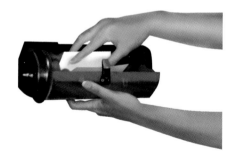

pneumatic capsule with document and medications

dumbwaiter a small elevator that carries objects (but not people) between floors of a building.

pneumatic tube a system which shuttles objects through a tube using compressed air as the force.

COMPUTER SYSTEMS

℞ For more information on sources, see chapter 12.

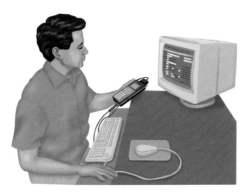

A technician using a hand held entry device for a computerized inventory system.

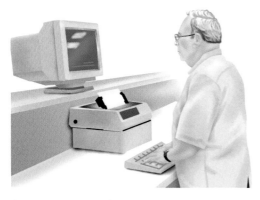

Among their many functions, hospital information systems provide quick access for the pharmacist to medication information for patients and care providers.

Most hospital information and documentation are computerized.

Information systems can integrate patient information, care and medication records, laboratory data, billing and many other types of information. However, each hospital system is customized to its own needs and therefore different. Individual systems may or may not integrate various areas of the hospital.

Hospital pharmacies rely heavily on computerized systems.

Knowledge of the hospital's pharmacy information system will be a large part of the initial training for a hospital pharmacy technician, since they must rely on it to perform many of their daily tasks including ordering pharmaceuticals, inventory control, and medication order processes.

An important responsibility for the pharmacist is to provide information on medications and their use to patients and other healthcare professionals.

Previously, much of this information was found in written form (e.g., Facts and Comparisons) or on disk. Newer hospital information systems link drug information directly with the pharmacy computer system allowing information on patients' specific medications to be viewed online.

Confidentiality and Security

The information contained on a hospital information system is *highly confidential*. In many cases (especially with patient information), it is illegal to give the information to anyone except those who are authorized to have it. As a result, access to the computer system is limited by password or other security measures. It is essential that all staff follow security and confidentiality rules.

The **Health Insurance Portability and Accountability Act (HIPAA)** is a federal privacy law enacted to safeguard a patient's protected information when it is spoken, written or transferred electronically. It includes regulations regarding privacy, confidentiality, assessing and releasing patient information, and complying with patients' rights. Technicians should never provide information patients to anyone unless specifically directed to do so by the pharmacist in charge.

ORGANIZATION OF MEDICATIONS

In most hospital pharmacies medications are organized according to a precise system.

First, medications are usually categorized and placed in defined areas of the pharmacy based on the specific route of administration such as intravenous, oral, ophthalmic, topical, etc. Intravenous medications may be further separated by vials, small volume parenterals and large volume parenterals. Oral drugs may be further divided into solid dosage forms (capsules, tablets) and liquids (suspensions, solutions) and placed in separate areas.

The second way medications are generally organized is in alphabetical order using the generic name of each drug.

This is different than most retail pharmacies which place drugs in order of brand name. Since both the generic and brand name may be on a medication label, it is important for the hospital pharmacy technician to have a good knowledge of brand vs. generic names.

Some medications require refrigeration or freezing.

It is imperative that the technician identify these items and promptly put them in the correct place so that the medications retain their stability. For example, most vaccines require refrigeration. If left at room temperature for too long, they may lose some of their effectiveness.

HOSPITAL FORMULARY

Because hospitals cannot afford to stock every medication that is available, many maintain a hospital "formulary." A **formulary** is a list of drugs that have been selected by health care professionals at the hospital based on therapeutic factors as well as cost. It is the responsibility of the Pharmacy and Therapeutics Committee to set up, add, remove and periodically evaluate medications listed on the hospital formulary. It is important, however, for anyone who orders, prepares or dispenses medications to be aware of the medications currently on the formulary. A **"closed formulary"** means that the hospital carries only formulary medications and physicians must order from this list. Of course, some exceptions apply and the pharmacy will have a section of "non-formulary" drugs. **Non-formulary** drugs may require a special form stating why the physician requires that specific medication.

formulary a list of drugs stocked at the hospital which have been selected based on therapeutic factors as well as cost.

closed-formulary a closed formulary means that a hospital carries only formulary medications and physicians must order from this list. (Some exceptions may apply.)

non-formulary drugs not on the formulary list which a physician can order; a physician may have to fill out a form stating why that specific medication is required.

The Pharmacy and Therapeutics Committee (often referred to as the P&T Committee) consists of doctors, pharmacists, nurses and other health care professionals who work as a team to review medications for the hospital formulary; evaluate medication use, adverse drug reactions, and drug-related errors in the hospital; and provide guidelines and protocols for medication use throughout the institution.

THERAPEUTIC INTERCHANGE

sample therapeutic interchange protocol

Therapeutic Interchange Protocol
H-2 Receptor Antagonists

Background:
The purpose of this protocol is to optimize patient care while considering cost containment and cost-effectiveness. This protocol defines the equivalent doses of the H-2 Receptor Antagonists. This protocol has been approved by the Pharmacy and Therapeutics Committee (P&TC) and the Medical Executive Committee (MEC).

Statement:
The P&TC will establish which H-2 receptor antagonists will be on formulary.
Pharmacists are permitted to convert orders according to the following protocol.

Protocol:
1) **Ranitidine (Zantac) is the <u>only</u> formulary agent.**
2) **Orders for nonformulary agents will be converted to the equivalent dose of ranitidine. The dosage regimens across each row are equivalent.**

Oral Conversion Table

Ranitidine (Zantac®)	Cimetidine (Tagamet®)	Famotidine (Pepcid®)	Nizatidine (Axid®)
150 mg PO BID	300 mg PO QID	20 mg PO BID	150 mg PO BID
150 mg PO BID	400 mg PO BID	20 mg PO BID	150 mg PO BID
150 mg PO BID	400 mg PO TID	20 mg PO BID	150 mg PO BID
300 mg PO HS	800 mg PO HS	40 mg PO HS	300 mg PO HS
150 mg PO QD	300 mg PO BID	20 mg PO QD	150 mg PO QD

Intravenous Conversion Table

Ranitidine (Zantac®)	Cimetidine (Tagamet®)	Famotidine (Pepcid®)
50 mg IV x 1	300 mg IV x 1	20 mg IV x 1
50 mg IV Q8H	300 mg IV Q6H	20 mg IV Q12H
50 mg IV Q12H	300 mg IV Q8H	20 mg IV Q24H
50 mg IV Q24H	300 mg IV Q12H	20 mg IV Q24H

*Nizatidine (Axid®) is not available IV.

Most hospital formularies include only a few medications in each specific class. This means that a patient who is admitted to the hospital may be taking a medication at home that is not included on the hospital formulary. In many of these cases there is another drug on the formulary that is in the same therapeutic class and works the same way but is a different drug entity (and usually of a different dose). The pharmacist is knowledgeable about therapeutic equivalence of drugs in the same class and can recommend the appropriate interchange for the doctor to order. Some hospitals have a formal therapeutic interchange program that allows the pharmacist to automatically change an order for a certain number of drugs without notifying the physician. In these cases a preset list of conditions must be fulfilled and the pharmacist must follow a strict protocol which includes entering into the computer an order for the formulary drug that was exchanged for the non-formulary drug.

UNIT DOSE SYSTEM

Oral medications are commonly provided to the nursing unit in medication carts containing 24 hour dosages for specific patients.

These carts have an individual drawer or tray for each patient on the nursing unit. Medications in the cart are packaged in individual containers holding the amount of drug required for one dose. This system is referred to as **unit dose** medication packaging. By preparing medication this way, nurses are not required to select medication from large bulk bottles, decreasing the chance of making an error.

Each individual drawer in a medication cart is filled daily to meet patient medication needs.

Technicians play a large role in this type of dispensing by either manually filling the carts or by operating equipment designed for that function. Computer generated drug profiles are prepared daily for each patient, and the appropriate amount of medications for the 24 hour period are placed manually or mechanically into each patient's tray. The trays are labeled with the patient's name and room number. The filled carts are checked by the supervising pharmacist before being delivered to the nursing units.

Some medications such as eye drops, creams and metered-dose inhalers cannot be divided into unit does increments.

In these cases, the bulk item is filled only once and used for the patient throughout the hospital admission.

At various times throughout the day adjustments in the patient trays are necessary to account for changes in medication orders.

This may require removing discontinued medications and adding new drugs where needed.

The final step in the cart filling process is the delivery of the completed medication carts to the nursing units and retrieving the used carts.

If the patient has any bulk medications the technician should transfer them to the new tray before returning to the pharmacy. All medication returned in the previous day's trays must be credited to the patient, and then the carts are prepared to go through the entire process again on the following day.

PACKAGING

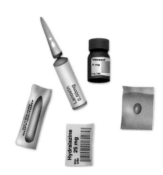

A number of different types of packages are used for unit dose medications.

Package Type	Used For
plastic blister	tablets/capsules
foil blister	tablets/capsules
paper	tablets/capsules
packet	powder
tube	ointment/cream
foil cup	oral liquid
cartridge	syringe
vial	injection

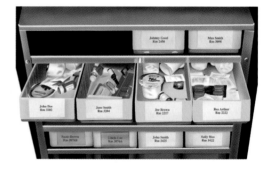

patient-specific trays

 unit dose a package containing the amount of a drug required for one dose.

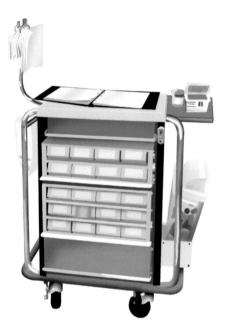

```
IBUPROFEN
600 MG
TABLET
EXP: 05/04 MFR: URL
MFR LOT#:C03803
```

a pre-pack label

a medication cart

Technicians often "pre-pack" medications that have been supplied in bulk into unit doses.

Machines that automate this process are generally used for pre-packing oral solid medications. Such systems restrict access by password or other means to authorized users and label each package with the information required by the institution. In cases where manual preparation is necessary (e.g., parenterals), technicians must follow institutional requirements exactly.

Unit dose packages are labeled with some of the same information found on multiple dose packages.

When packaged by the manufacturer, each unit dose is labeled with the name of the drug, its dosage form and strength, lot number, expiration date, and other identifying information. When pre-packed, labels must meet state and institutional requirements. Pre-packing equipment includes a label creation and application function.

Unit dose labels may contain bar codes for identification and control.

If the bar code is to be applied at the hospital, technicians may do this using a bar code printer. Bar codes enable the item to be scanned into the dispensing and inventory system at various stages up to dispensing. This reduces the chances of medication errors and improves documentation and inventory control.

Cart Filling Robots

Several machines referred to as robots have been developed to assist in the cart filling process. While this reduces the manual filling responsibilities of technicians, there is still a requirement for some medications, such as those stored in the refrigerator, to be hand filled. Additionally, there is a large amount of special packaging required to stock these robots, and technicians who would traditionally be hand filling trays often perform these duties. Cart-filling robots are very expensive and require a large amount of space within the pharmacy area; therefore, these machines are usually seen only in larger hospitals.

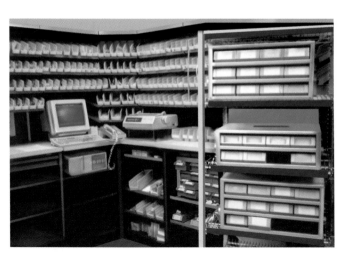

the cart filling area of a hospital pharmacy

MEDICATION ORDERS

Several different people have the ability to write medication orders in the hospital setting.

The most obvious of these is the doctor. However, both nurses and pharmacists may write orders if they are directly instructed to do so by a doctor. These are referred to as verbal orders and must be co-signed by the physician who approved them. In some hospitals, specialized healthcare providers with advanced training can write orders without the signature of a physician. These people include physician's assistants and nurse practitioners.

In the hospital, all drugs ordered for a patient are written on a medication order form and not a prescription blank as seen in a community pharmacy.

Medication order forms are an all-purpose communication tool used by the various members of the healthcare team. Orders for various procedures, laboratory tests, and x-rays may be written on the form in addition to medication orders. Several medication orders may be written on one medication order form. These forms are traditionally prepared in duplicate or triplicate so that the original remains in the medical chart and only copies are sent to other areas of the hospital for processing.

An alternative to the traditional written order is physician order entry (POE).

POE is a system in which the doctor or agent of the doctor enters orders directly into the hospital system. This helps to eliminate errors due to illegible handwriting and also expedites orders to the pharmacy, lab, radiology, etc. When a physician enters a medication order into the computer, a copy of the order is automatically printed in the pharmacy for review by a pharmacist before the medication is dispensed.

There are several different types of orders that can be written.

One is a standard medication order for patients to receive a certain drug at scheduled intervals throughout the day, sometimes called a standing order. Orders for medications that are administered only on an as needed basis are called PRN medication orders. A third type of order is for a medication that is needed right away; these are referred to as STAT orders.

MEDICATION ORDER FORMS

	PATIENT IDENTIFICATION
DOCTOR'S ORDERS	099999999 675-01
	Smith, John
	12/06/1950
	DR P Johnson

DATE	TIME	DOCTOR'S ORDERS ①	DATE/TIME INITIALS	DATE/TIME INITIALS
1/13/09	2200	Admit patient to 6th floor		
		Pneumonia, Dehydration		
		All: PCN- Rash		
		Order CBC, chem-7, blood cultures stat		
		NS @ 125ml/hr IV		
		Dr Johnson x2222		

DATE	TIME	DOCTOR'S ORDERS ②	DATE/TIME INITIALS	DATE/TIME INITIALS
2/01/09	300	Tylenol 650mg po q4-6 hrs PRN for Temp> 38°C		
		Verbal Order Dr Johnson/ Jane Doe, RN		

DATE	TIME	DOCTOR'S ORDERS ③	DATE/TIME INITIALS	DATE/TIME INITIALS
2/01/09	600	Start Clarithromycin 500mg po q12°		
		Multivitamin po qd		
		Order CXR for this am		
		Dr Johnson x2222		

sample medication order form

standing order a standard medication order for patients to receive medication at scheduled intervals (e.g., 1 tablet every 8 hours).

PRN order an order for medication to be administered only on an as needed basis (e.g., 1 tablet every 4 to 6 hours as needed for pain).

STAT order an order for medication to be administered immediately.

MEDICATION ADMINISTRATION RECORDS

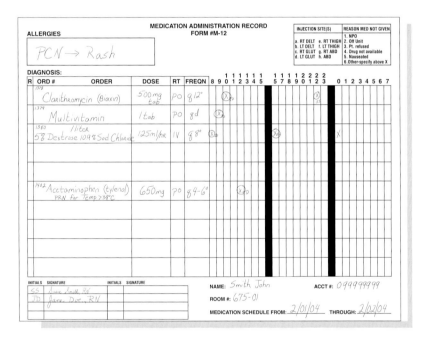

sample medication administration record

Nurses record and track medication orders on a patient specific form called the medication administration record (MAR).

This form records every medication ordered for a patient over a 24 hour period, as well as the time the medications were administered and the person who gave each dose. Whether handwritten by the nursing staff or generated by the pharmacy computer system, the accuracy of this document is crucial.

In some hospitals, nurses may chart medications directly into the computer. Alternatively, the nurse may scan the medication bar code at the patients' bedside; this information will then be processed onto a computerized MAR.

 medication administration record (MAR) a form that tracks the medications administered to a patient.

ORDER PROCESSING

There are also several ways an order can be processed.

Order entry may be performed by a nursing unit clerk, pharmacy technician, pharmacist, nurse, or physician. Before entering orders, technicians will require specialized training in the interpretation of medical orders as well as on how to use the pharmacy's computerized order-entry system.

The technician must also be aware of any specialized protocols the hospital has in place such as "restricted" medications or automatic stop orders.

In order to insure safety and appropriateness as well as contain costs, some medications may be restricted by certain services in the hospital (e.g., infectious diseases, hematology). Such restricted medications cannot be dispensed until the appropriate service approves the order. Automatic stop orders are used for certain medications or classes of medications, such as antibiotics or narcotics, which can be active for only a limited period of time after which a new medication order is required to continue. Automatic stop orders help ensure that the patient's therapy is continually reassessed and monitored.

Only a pharmacist may verify orders and check medications being sent to the nursing floors.

It is becoming more common, however, for the hospital pharmacy technician to assist the pharmacist in making sure a medication and its dose are appropriate for each individual patient. The pharmacist may ask the technician to get such information as weight, allergies or home medications from a patient's nurse or chart. The technician may also need to obtain laboratory or microbiology data from the hospital computer system.

The pharmacy technician may also screen medication orders for any that seem inappropriate.

For example, if a drug that is usually given once a day is ordered to be given four times a day, the technician alerts the pharmacist of the potential error. Although the pharmacist is required to review all orders before they are fully processed, the technician can serve as a valuable team member by flagging orders with potential problems.

MANUAL ORDER PROCESSING

✔ Medication order is written in patient chart.

✔ Copy of medication order is removed from chart.

✔ Order is picked up at nursing station or faxed or tubed to the pharmacy.

✔ Medication order is entered into the pharmacy computer system.

✔ Pharmacist reviews and verifies medication order.

✔ Medication order is filled by a pharmacy technician and checked by pharmacist.

✔ Patient-specific medication is manually delivered or tubed to nursing unit.

AUTOMATED ORDER PROCESSING

✔ Physician or agent of the physician enters medication order directly into hospital computer system which automatically communicates order to the pharmacy.

✔ Pharmacist reviews and verifies medication order.

✔ RN retrieves medication from point-of-use automated medication station.

✔ Pharmacy technician fills inventory as medication supplies fall below par.

℞ Automated order processing may include only part of the above process. Even though order processing may start with physician order entry directly into a computer, a hospital may not have point-of-use automated machines. In this case, the medication would still be manually delivered or tubed to the nursing station.

O nce the order is approved by the pharmacist, the medication order needs to be filled.

Pharmacy technicians usually prepare orders to be delivered to the nursing unit. Since many medications look similar and the same drug may come in several different doses, the technician must be vigilant in making sure the right medication and dose are being filled. Orders which require special compounding must be prepared quickly so that the patient receives his/her medication within a reasonable time. Although all medications will be checked by the pharmacist before they leave the pharmacy, it cannot be stressed enough how important it is for the technician to be accurate.

Delivery of the medication is varied depending on the hospital.

Medications may be delivered to patient care areas by pharmacy technicians, hospital delivery staff, a pneumatic tube system, or a special robot. Often these deliveries, or rounds, are done on an hourly basis.

Alternatively, some nursing stations have automated dispensing systems that contain the most common unit-dose medications used on that nursing unit.

This allows the nurse to obtain the medication much more quickly since it does not have to be delivered from the pharmacy. However, the nurse can access the medications only after a pharmacist reviews and verifies the order. Each hospital has its own policies and procedures to make sure this occurs.

The automated medication station may be used for the first dose of a new medication order or for all the doses during the length of the patient's stay in the hospital.

It is often the responsibility of the pharmacy technician to make sure these systems remain stocked. A computer-generated inventory sheet will notify the technician of the number and kind of medications which need restocking. Medications that are not stocked will need to be sent on delivery or through the pneumatic tube system.

INVENTORY CONTROL

Another responsibility that may be assigned to the hospital pharmacy technician is inventory control.

Ensuring adequate supplies of medications is the primary responsibility for staff in this area. This is especially important in the hospital setting where several of the drugs are needed in emergency situations.

Duties may include ordering medications through a special computer program that communicates with the distributor/wholesaler.

In some instances a drug company may need to be contacted directly so a special shipment can be sent directly from the manufacturer to the hospital.

When a pharmacy shipment arrives, the pharmacy technician checks the order against the invoice.

If something is on the invoice but not in the shipment, the technician should notify his/her supervisor. When all items are accounted for, the technician places the medications in the appropriate location (e.g., refrigerator, overstock area, etc.).

A primary area of concern for inventory control is narcotics, or controlled substances, which require an exact record of the location and amount of every item.

There are several systems for controlling narcotics. Some are manual and others involve electronic equipment (e.g. PYXIS). In some institutions pharmacy technicians are not allowed to handle narcotics or may require special training to do so. In contrast, some pharmacy departments assign all controlled substance management to technicians.

All patient care areas are required to have *code carts* which are used in the case of a medical emergency on the floor.

These carts contain different medications commonly used in emergency situations. Each code cart has a special lock that can be broken when the cart needs to be used. Once a lock is broken, it cannot be reused and the medication drawer must be replaced. The pharmacy is responsible for maintaining these carts. The technician refills the cart and charges the missing medications to the appropriate patient. As with all medications leaving the pharmacy, the pharmacist must first verify the work of the technician filling the carts.

 See Chapter 13 for more information on inventory systems.

INVENTORY

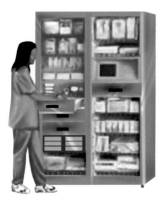

an automated Pyxis SupplyStation®

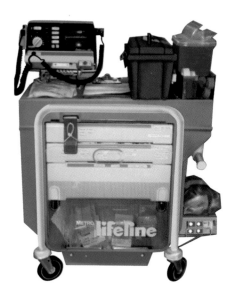

a code cart—note that the plastic yellow tie-lock must be broken to use the cart.

 code carts a locked cart of medications and other medical equipment designed for emergency use only.

floor stock- stock that does not require specific patient labeling and is stored in the nursing unit.

STERILE PRODUCTS

℞ See Chapter 8 for more information on sterile techniques and preparing parenterals.

STERILE PRODUCTS

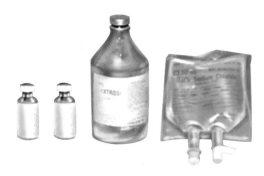

parenterals

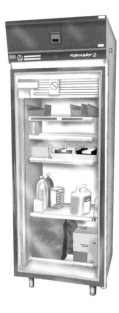

refrigerator used for storing parenterals

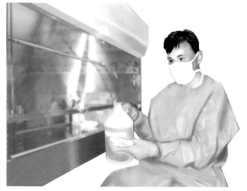

cleaning a vertical laminar flow hood

A large portion of the medication used in the hospital is administered intravenously.

The hospital pharmacy technician plays a large role in preparing these products. I.V. admixtures may include small and large volume parenterals, parenteral nutrition therapy, or chemotherapy. Preparing these products requires special safety training and the use of horizontal or vertical flow hoods. Vertical hoods offer more protection and are required for chemotherapy preparation. Most other parenterals, however, can be prepared in a horizontal hood.

A supply of some large volume parenterals may be kept on the nursing unit.

These medications are referred to as **floor stock** and do not require patient specific labeling by the pharmacy. However, a medication order is required before a nurse may administer these medications.

A daily supply of other scheduled intravenous medications will also be prepared with patient specific labels and delivered to the floor.

Since there is not enough room to store these in the medication carts, these products are stored in designated areas on the nursing unit or in the refrigerator when required.

Although IV labels are commonly computer-generated, there may be occasions when a technician must manually type out a label (such as for an ER patient).

Therefore, it is important to know what information needs to be entered on an IV label: patient name, medical record number, location of patient, name and dose of drug, amount and kind of solution used for dilution, date and time medication is to be given, expiration date, time the drug is prepared and the technician's initials.

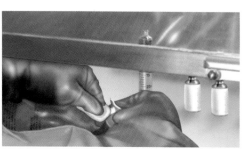

preparing parenteral admixtures in a laminar flow hood

GENERAL HOSPITAL ISSUES

Hospital employees are required to meet some conditions of employment that may not be encountered in other pharmacy settings.

First, in addition to interviewing with the pharmacy department, prospective employees are usually required to interview with the Human Resources department. This department oversees the hiring process including advertising available positions, accepting applications for employment and conducting initial interviews. They provide pharmacy with a list of potential candidates and pharmacy then conducts its own interview before making a final decision.

All hospital employees are required to undergo a physical exam and often drug testing.

In addition, employees who may be exposed to blood products, which may or may not be the case for a pharmacy technician, are encouraged to receive the hepatitis B vaccination. Many hospitals provide this vaccine, as well as flu shots, free of charge to employees.

New employees are required to attend a hospital-wide orientation.

In this session, information is given about employee benefits, rules and regulations, and safety training for various situations such as fires, exposure to blood-borne pathogens, and chemical spills. This is in addition to the training that the pharmacy department provides.

Even if a technician has previous experience working in a hospital pharmacy he or she will go through training and a probationary period.

The probationary period gives the hospital time to assess whether the employee is actually suitable and qualified for the job for which they were hired. An employee may be terminated at any time during the probationary period. At the end of the probation, the employee's status may be changed to permanent, they may be terminated, or they may be placed on an additional three month probation.

All permanent employees receive an annual or semi-annual performance review.

Technicians are rated on technical skills and interpersonal skills, as well as issues such as tardiness, dress code, and ability to complete tasks on time.

REGULATORY AGENCIES

Several different regulatory bodies oversee all aspects of hospital operations including the pharmacy department.

➡ **The Joint Commission on Accreditation of Healthcare Organizations (JCAHO)**

JCAHO surveys and accredits healthcare organizations. Healthcare Organizations must undergo this survey every 3 years. JCAHO lays out specific guidelines for every department within the hospital. Although this survey is not required, Medicare and several insurance providers now require JCAHO accreditation for reimbursement.

➡ **Health Care Financing Administration (HCFA)**

HCFA inspects and approves hospitals to provide care for Medicaid patients. Approval by this organization is required to receive reimbursement for any of these patients.

➡ **The Department of Public Health (DPH)**

The DPH is a state run organization that oversees hospitals including the pharmacy department. Hospitals undergo inspections by the DPH in order to assure compliance with laws concerning hospital practice.

➡ **The State Board of Pharmacy (BOP)**

The BOP is the agency that registers pharmacists and technicians. While their authority does not allow them to govern hospital pharmacy departments, they do regulate the registration of the pharmacists and technicians that work in this setting.

SAFETY

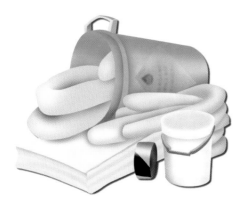

hazardous substance spill kit

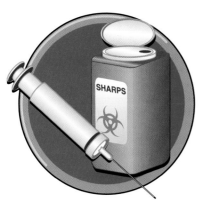

sharps container

During safety training employees learn "universal precautions" and how to handle hazardous substance spills.

Universal precautions are practices and guidelines that reduce the probability of exposure to bloodborne pathogens and that explain what to do if an exposure occurs. These precautions include the use of protective barriers (gloves, gowns, masks, and protective eyewear) and how to prevent injuries from needlesticks. Even employees who may not have direct contact with blood products must be trained in these universal precautions.

Proper waste disposal is extremely important.

Red bags are usually used for items containing blood or other body linens. Soiled linen, scrubs, and items such as cleaning rags are cleaned rather than disposed in red bags. Needles or other items that may cut or puncture the skin should always be thrown away in designated "sharps" containers.

In cases of hazardous substance spills (e.g., cytotoxic drugs, harmful chemicals), special procedures are required which involve identifying the hazardous substance, containing the spill, and disposing of the waste.

The technician should know where the Material Safety Data Sheets (MSDS) are stored since these will explain how to proceed should a spill occur. Security may need to be notified if the spill is large or if there are problems containing it. Once the situation is under control, the employee should fill out an incident report and immediately give it to the supervisor.

Chemotherapy and cytoxic drugs must be prepared in a biological safety cabinet or vertical flow hood and then placed in a bag that identifies them as hazardous or cytotoxic substances.

Special kits are used if a spill occurs at any time during processing.

The Policy and Procedure Manual

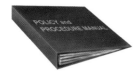

All departments within the hospital are required to maintain a policy and procedures manual by regulating agencies.

This document contains information about every aspect of the job from dress code to disciplinary actions and step by step directions on how to perform various tasks that will be required of technicians. *It is absolutely essential that technicians know what they must and must not do in their job as outlined in their institution's policy and procedure manual.*

LONG-TERM CARE

Long-term care facilities provide care for people unable to care for themselves because of mental or physical impairment.

Patients may be of any age and include chronically ill elderly, impaired children, and permanently disabled adults whose families can no longer care for their needs. Nursing homes make up the majority of long-term care facilities, but others include psychiatric institutions, chronic disease and rehabilitation facilities. The amount of time a patient may need long-term care can extend from months to years or even a lifetime.

Because of limited resources, most long-term care facilities will contract out dispensing and clinical pharmacy services.

This means that they will pay for another company to take care of the majority of patient medicines. The licensed professional pharmacy or practice that provides medications and/or clinical services to long-term care facilities and their residents is called a long-term care pharmacy organization. Although a pharmacist or pharmacy technician does not have to physically be present at the facility during all hours, pharmacy services must be made available 24 hours a day (i.e., by phone pager).

Pharmacists perform two types of functions for long-term care: distributive and consultant.

The distributive pharmacist is responsible for making sure the patients are receiving the correct medicines that were ordered. This job is mainly done outside of the long-term care facility itself.

The consultant pharmacist is responsible for developing and maintaining an individualized pharmaceutical plan for every long-term care resident.

This is done by reviewing patient charts, assessing how a patient may receive optimal benefits from their medicines, and monitoring for drug-related problems. They interact with doctors, nurses, and other health professionals. An individual consultant pharmacist is usually responsible for several different nursing homes or other facilities and so may only visit each on certain weekly or monthly intervals. It is important to make the distinction between these types of responsibilities because the pharmacy technician working for a long-term care pharmacy organization may be assisting in these different tasks.

ENVIRONMENT

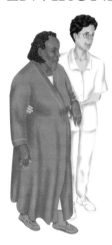

Nursing Homes

Most long-term care facilities are nursing homes that provide daily nursing care. Patients in this setting are generally referred to as **residents.**

Residents' Rights

Because residents of nursing homes were often victimized by people who were supposed to provide their care, federal and state laws were enacted in the U.S. designed to ensure residents' basic quality of life. These laws guarantee residents' rights to the following:

➡ safe and adequate care in a decent environment.
➡ privacy and confidentiality.
➡ personal property and clothing.
➡ personal privacy.
➡ freedom from abuse.

distributive pharmacist makes sure long-term care patients receive the correct medications ordered.

consultant pharmacist develops and maintains an individual pharmaceutical plan for each long-term care patient.

Training

The orientation process at a long-term care pharmacy organization is comparable to the hospital setting. There is an initial orientation and training regarding performance of assigned functions and special requirements in the long-term care setting. Also, there is a written job description of the functions the pharmacy technicians may perform in accordance with specific regulations in the state. It is important to be aware of what the pharmacy technician is able to do or not do according to the law.

Changing Responsibilities

In addition to typical duties such as preparing, packaging, stocking, and delivering medications, new opportunities are emerging for pharmacy technicians in the long-term care environment. These include working closer with the consultant pharmacist to assist in the collection of data for patient assessment, compiling quality improvement data, maintaining computerized information between dispensing and consultant pharmacists, performing reviews of drug use in individual long-term care facilities, and preparing pharmacy reports.

Automated Dispensing Systems

When a medication is needed suddenly, the time it takes for delivery from an outside supplier can present problems. Because of this, many nursing homes are turning to point-of-use automated dispensing systems. The medication order is communicated by computer to a central pharmacy system which then sends a confirmation of the order to the unit at the point of use. As soon as the unit receives this confirmation, a nurse can get the medication from the unit.

Many of the duties of pharmacy technicians in the long-term care pharmacy organization are similar to those in the hospital. These include filling medication carts, packaging prescriptions, mixing intravenous solutions, ordering medication stock, maintaining **automated dispensing systems** and emergency medication carts, and crediting returned medications. As in the hospital environment, the technician works under supervision of the pharmacist and must understand the limitations set forth by law.

In some facilities, the medication cart may be filled with enough medications to last for a week.

This is different from the hospital setting as there is much less medication and patients' drug therapies are not changed as frequently. However, if a patient receives a new medication order, there must be a system in place to make sure the appropriate drugs are received. To handle this, the pharmacy organization in charge of the facility may make arrangements with an alternative pharmacy or use an automated dispensing system. Copies of new medication orders may be faxed to an alternative pharmacy that will deliver the appropriate drugs. Some facilities may have a limited drug inventory stored in a secured location where only authorized personnel may obtain access, and pharmacy technicians may be required to keep track of inventory in these locations.

Emergency kits, or code carts, similar to those in hospitals are also located in long-term care facilities for emergency situations.

As in hospitals, if these emergency kits are opened, the appropriate patient must be charged for the medications used and the cart must be refilled. The technician is responsible for these duties and the pharmacist makes a final check before the cart is re-sealed. A pharmacy technician working with the pharmacist may also be responsible for the inventory of controlled substances stored in the long-term care facility.

automated dispensing system a system in which medications are dispensed from an automated unit at the point of use upon confirmation of an order communicated by computer from a central system.

REVIEW

KEY CONCEPTS

HOSPITAL PHARMACY

✔ Patient rooms are divided into groups called nursing units or patient care units; patients with similar problems often located on the same unit.

HOSPITAL PHARMACY AREAS

✔ In the centralized pharmacy system, all pharmacy activities are conducted from one location within the hospital -- the inpatient pharmacy. In a decentralized system, there are several pharmacy areas (satellites) located throughout the hospital, each serving a fraction of the patient care areas.

COMMUNICATION

✔ There are several ways the pharmacy communicates with other areas of the hospital including telephones, fax machines, computerized printouts, pneumatic tubes, and in person.

COMPUTER SYSTEMS

✔ Hospital information systems can integrate and store patient information such as medical records, lab data, and billing records.

ORGANIZATION OF MEDICATIONS

✔ Since hospitals cannot stock every medication available, most have a hospital formulary which is a subset of medications the pharmacy keeps on its shelves and from which doctors can order.

UNIT DOSES

✔ Medications in the cart are packaged in individual containers holding the amount of drug required for one dose, called a unit dose.

MEDICATION ORDERS

✔ In the hospital, all drugs ordered for a patient are written on a medication order form or are electronically entered through a physician order entry system.

ORDER PROCESSING

✔ Although technicians have an increasing role in order processing, only a pharmacist may verify orders in the computer system and check medications before they are sent to the nursing floors.

INVENTORY CONTROL

✔ A primary area of concern for inventory control is narcotics, or controlled substances, which require an exact record of the location of every item to the exact tablet or unit.

STERILE PRODUCTS

✔ A large portion of the medication used in the hospital is administered intravenously.

GENERAL HOSPITAL ISSUES

✔ All departments within the hospital are required to maintain a policy and procedures manual by regulating agencies.

✔ The Joint Commission on Accreditation of Healthcare Organizations (JCAHO) surveys and accredits healthcare organizations. Organizations undergo this survey every 3 years.

✔ Needles or other items that may cut or puncture the skin should always be thrown away in designated "sharps" containers.

LONG-TERM CARE

✔ Because of limited resources, most long-term care facilities will contract out dispensing and clinical pharmacy services.

SELF TEST

MATCH THE TERMS.   *answers can be checked in the glossary*

automated dispensing system

clean rooms

code cart

consultant pharmacist

distributive pharmacist

medication administration record

PRN order

satellites

standing order

STAT order

formulary

- a standard medication order for patients to receive medication at scheduled intervals.
- an order for medication to be administered only on an as needed basis.
- an order for medication to be administered immediately.
- a form that tracks the medications administered to a patient.
- a locked cart of medications designed for emergency use only.
- pharmacy locations in a decentralized systems that operate outside the central pharmacy.
- areas designed for the preparation of sterile products.
- makes sure long-term care patients receive the correct medications ordered.
- develops and maintains an individual pharmaceutical plan for each long-term care patient.
- a system in which medications are dispensed from an automated unit at the point of use upon confirmation of an order communicated by computer from a central system.
- a list of drugs stocked at the hospital

CHOOSE THE BEST ANSWER.   *the answer key begins on page 347*

1. The work station for medical personnel on a nursing unit is called
   a. satellite.
   b. the nurses' station.
   c. MARS.
   d. decentralized.

2. Ancillary areas in a hospital serviced by the pharmacy include
   a. gift shop, cafeteria.
   b. central supply, materials management.
   c. cafeteria, central supply.
   d. radiology, cardiac catheterization lab, emergency room.

3. The person in the medical staff who examines patients, diagnoses illnesses, and orders and interprets lab tests is a(an)
   a. Pharm.D.
   b. R.N.
   c. M.D.
   d. R.Ph.

4. The therapist who works with patients to help them develop, recover, or maintain daily living and work skills is a(an)
   a. O.T.
   b. R.T.
   c. P.A.
   d. P.T.

REVIEW

5. A healthcare worker that evaluates patients' nutritional needs and recommends appropriate modifications is a(an)
   a. R.N.
   b. P.T.
   c. R.T.
   d. R.D.

6. A registered nurse that has additional training and can provide some basic primary care is a(an)
   a. L.P.N.
   b. N.P.
   c. M.S.W.
   d. R.N.

7. A nurse who may administer medication to patients is a(an)
   a. R.T.
   b. R.D.
   c. R.N.
   d. O.T.

8. In a decentralized pharmacy system, pharmacy activities are conducted in
   a. clean rooms.
   b. satellites throughout the hospital.
   c. a single location in the hospital.
   d. doctors' offices.

9. A pharmacy located in a hospital that services patients within the hospital and ancillary areas only is called a(an)
   a. inpatient pharmacy.
   b. outpatient pharmacy.
   c. clinic pharmacy.
   d. nursing unit.

10. HIPAA is a federal law that is meant to protect a patient's private information when it is
    a. spoken.
    b. written.
    c. electronically transferred.
    d. all of the above

11. If a hospital has a closed formulary, the physician should
    a. order any medication s/he wants.
    b. order medications on the hospital formulary only.
    c. order non-formulary medications only.
    d. none of the above.

12. A pharmacy technician may be responsible for all of the following EXCEPT:
    a. restocking automated medication stations.
    b. triaging telephone calls.
    c. recommending a therapeutic interchange.
    d. preparing small and large volume parenterals

13. A unit dose is a(an)
    a. package that contains all non-controlled medications for a given day.
    b. package that contains all medications for a given day.
    c. controlled substance.
    d. package that contains the amount of medication for one dose.

14. Medications that have been supplied in bulk are generally pre-packaged in unit dose by
    a. pharmacy technicians.
    b. L.P.N.s.
    c. O.T.s.
    d. R.T.s.

15. Medication carts commonly provide _____ hours of medication for specific patients.
   a. 6
   b. 12
   c. 48
   d. 24

16. Orders for drugs that are administered at scheduled intervals throughout the day are
   a. PRN orders.
   b. STAT orders.
   c. parenterals.
   d. standing orders.

17. Which of the following allows a patient to receive medications on an "as needed" basis?
   a. STAT order
   b. standing order
   c. parenteral
   d. PRN order

18. Nurses track medication administration on a(an)
   a. PCU.
   b. PRN.
   c. STAT.
   d. MAR.

19. Automated dispensing systems
   a. contain unit dose medications.
   b. are often restocked by pharmacy technicians.
   c. allow nurses to obtain a medication quickly.
   d. all of the above

20. Stock (such as large volume parenterals) stored on a nursing unit that does not require patient specific labeling is called
   a. clean stock.
   b. normal stock.
   c. daily stock.
   d. floor stock.

21. Which of the following agencies is responsible for approving hospitals for Medicaid reimbursement?
   a. JCAHO
   b. HCFA
   c. DPH
   d. BOP

22. The commission that surveys and accredits healthcare organizations is
   a. DPH.
   b. ASHP.
   c. JCAHO.
   d. BOP.

23. Needles and other items that may cut or puncture the skin should be thrown away in:
   a. MSDS.
   b. designated "sharps" containers.
   c. red garbage bags.
   d. regular garbage cans.

24. The person who develops and maintains an individual pharmaceutical plan for each patient in a long-term care facility is a
   a. consultant pharmacist.
   b. community pharmacist.
   c. distributive pharmacist.
   d. pharmacy technician.

MAIL ORDER PHARMACY

While chain community pharmacies are by far the largest segment of the retail pharmacy market, mail order pharmacy is the fastest growing segment.

A mail order pharmacy sends medications to patients through mail or other delivery services. They have staffs of pharmacists, registered nurses, and technicians and can offer all the services of a community pharmacy, including compounding.

Because mail order medications involve a delivery time of at least 24-48 hours, they are used in situations where the need for the medication is known in advance.

This is true of chronic conditions like diabetes, high blood pressure, or depression, where the need for medication can be predicted and the supply can be easily maintained by mail delivery. This type of medication is called a maintenance medication, because it is used to maintain the patient with a chronic condition. By comparison, if a patient has an acute condition, such as a sudden infection, they would go to their community pharmacy to obtain the prescribed medication immediately after diagnosis.

Because they use the mail, mail order pharmacies can serve broad geographic areas.

In the U.S., for example, they can provide services to all states. This means that they can operate at a high volume. In addition to high volume discounts, this provides mail order pharmacies with economies of scale. These and other factors allow them to sell their medications at lower costs than community pharmacies. For this reason, mail order pharmacies are increasingly popular with third party insurers, a major source of their growth.

acute condition a sudden condition requiring immediate treatment.

chronic condition a continuing condition that requires ongoing treatment for a prolonged period.

maintenance medication a medication that is required on a continuing basis for the treatment of a chronic condition.

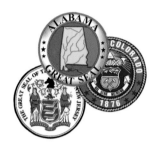

Regulation and Licensing

Though mail order pharmacies must follow federal and state requirements in processing prescriptions, they are not necessarily licensed in each state to which they send medications. As a condition for doing business there, some states now require that mail order pharmacies employ pharmacists licensed to practice in that state. However, not all do.

On-line Drugstores

On-line drugstores are a type of mail order pharmacy that use the Internet to advertise and take orders for drugs which are then mailed to the customer. Some on-line drugstores also use traditional mail order marketing methods and like mail order pharmacies they have a a full staff of pharmacists, technicians and doctors employed to ensure proper filling of prescriptions as well as provide patient counseling regarding medications.

Because of the lower cost of drugs in Canada and US cross-border regulations which allow Canadian pharmacies to fill individual prescriptions from US consumers for small amounts of drugs, the Canadian on-line drugstore industry has grown rapidly, and has been the subject of much consumer and political debate. Whether this growth trend will continue depends in part on the extent to which the US eases cross-border regulations: if the US eases them enough to allow drug wholesalers and large retailers to export drugs to the US, which is probably unlikely in the near future, then the on-line retailers may not be able to compete.

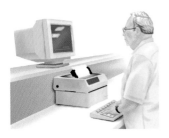

Automation and Quality Control

Mail order pharmacies are generally large scale operations that are highly automated. They use assembly line processing in which each step in the prescription fill process is completed or managed by a person who specializes in that step. For example, one technician may be responsible for entering prescriptions into the system, another for running an automated dispensing machine to fill prescriptions, and another for preparing the prescription for shipping. There are also steps for pharmacists to review the prescription before and after filling. Bar-coding of each prescription is used so that the prescription may be checked continually throughout the process against the information in the system. This ensures a high level of quality control. In fact, the increasing ability of automated systems to deliver a high quality product is one of the key contributing factors in the growth of mail order pharmacy.

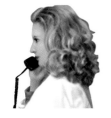

Counseling and Information

Mail order pharmacies have help desk or customer service numbers that patients can call when in need of counseling. Since calls may be related to medications, billing or other issues, these areas can be staffed with a mix of pharmacists, nurses, and technicians. As in the community pharmacy, technicians may not answer any questions related to medications, but of course can answer questions regarding forms, claims, and other non-medication issues.

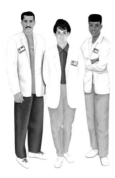

Mail Order and Community Pharmacy

Much of the growth of mail order pharmacy has come at the expense of community pharmacy, which has historically served all patients, including those with chronic conditions. The large scale and sophistication of mail order pharmacies gives them many advantages (price being an extremely important one) which will undoubtedly help them to continue growing. At the same time, the personal availability of the pharmacist and the face-to-face interaction between pharmacist and patient in the community pharmacy are advantages that are likely to ensure the continuation of their vital role in the health of their communities. Both areas offer excellent career opportunities to pharmacy technicians.

HOME INFUSION

Home care provides health care in a patient's home that might otherwise be provided in an institutional setting or physician's office. The primary providers of such care are home care agencies. Care is supervised by a registered nurse who works with a physician, pharmacist, and others to administer a care plan that involves the patient or another care giver. The primary advantage of home care over institutional care is a better quality of life, though in many cases it may also be less expensive.

The fastest growing area of home health care is home infusion.

Advances in infusion pump technology have made the infusion process more accurate and easier to administer and have been a major factor in the growth of home infusion. Pumps are available for specific therapies or multiple therapies. There are ambulatory pumps that can be worn by patients and allow freedom of movement compared to being restricted to an infusion pump attached to an administration pole.

Pumps are chosen for therapy based on various factors.

These include the type of therapy or therapies, the ambulatory status of the patient, the involvement of caregivers, and so on. The supervising nurse and the pharmacist consult on the patient's care plan and choose the appropriate pump.

One of the fundamental activities of home care is patient education.

That is, the patient is educated about their therapy: how to self-administer, monitor, report problems, and so on. The supervising nurse is the primary person responsible for personally educating the patient or their care giver about therapy. However, the pharmacist is responsible for providing medication information to the supervising nurse and the patient or care-giver. Patients or care givers are generally required by law to sign a form indicating that they have received the appropriate information.

 home care agencies home nursing care businesses that provide a range of health care services, including infusion.

Primary Providers

The primary providers of home infusion services are:

➡ **Home Care Agencies:** These are essentially home nursing care businesses that provide a range of home health care services, which can include infusion.

➡ **Home Infusion Pharmacies:** These are pharmacies with a specialized ability to deliver home infusion services. They prepare admixtures, provide infusion pumps, and are involved in various aspects of the patient's care plan.

➡ **Hospitals:** Many hospitals offer home infusion therapies as a way to ensure continued therapy outside the hospital after patients are released.

Primary Home Infusion Therapies

The primary therapies provided by home infusion services are:

➡ **Antibiotic Therapy:** Antibiotic therapy is a common home infusion service used in treating AIDS related and other infections.

➡ **Parenteral Nutrition:** Parenteral nutrition is often required for patients with various intestinal disorders or AIDS.

➡ **Pain Management:** This generally applies to the infusion of narcotics for patients with painful terminal illnesses or other types of severe chronic pain.

➡ **Chemotherapy:** In certain situations, chemotherapy is provided in the home, generally in conjunction with an oncology program at a hospital or clinic.

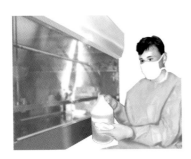

Compounding

The same rules apply to preparing parenteral admixtures in the home infusion setting as in the hospital. Compounding such admixtures requires the use of clean rooms, special equipment such as laminar flow hoods, and the use of aseptic practices. As with other parenteral admixtures, stability of the admixture for its intended use is a primary issue and storage a major concern. A complicating factor is that storage cannot be monitored as closely in a patient's home as an institutional setting. This results in short stability time limits that along with storage conditions require special attention. It also sometimes results in the on site preparation of certain therapies by the patient or care giver. In addition, automated devices that mix parenteral nutrition formulations at the time of administration are sometimes used.

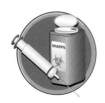

Hazardous Waste

Chemotherapy, the treatment of AIDS patients, and other infusion therapies involve the transportation, storage, and disposal of hazardous materials and is a primary area of concern. Home infusion personnel, patients and care givers must comply with all regulations governing such material. Compliance is a fundamental responsibility of home infusion personnel and is monitored by various regulatory agencies.

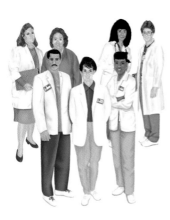

Home Care Team

The team that provides home health care includes the following:

Physician: The patient's physician orders the infusion therapy.

Registered Nurse: The nurse is responsible for coordinating and monitoring the care plan and the home care team, and for educating the patient.

Pharmacist: The pharmacist works with the supervising nurse to develop a pharmaceutical care plan which includes selection of the infusion device, identification of potential adverse reactions and interventions, and monitoring practices.

Pharmacy Technician: The technician works under the pharmacist's supervision and may be involved with compounding, labeling, delivery, and other non-consulting activities.

Home Care Aide: Aides are non-professional staff employed by the home care agency who work under the supervision of the registered nurse. They assist in various aspects of a patient's care, but generally not in medication therapy.

REVIEW

KEY CONCEPTS

MAIL ORDER PHARMACY

✔ Mail order pharmacy is used for maintenance therapy with chronic conditions that include depression, gastrointestinal disorders, heart disease, hypertension and diabetes.

✔ Mail order pharmacies must follow federal and state requirements in processing prescriptions, but are not necessarily licensed in each state to which they send medications.

✔ Mail order pharmacies are generally large scale operations that are highly automated. They use assembly line processing in which each step in the prescription fill process is completed or managed by a person who specializes in that step.

✔ Pharmacists review mail order prescriptions before and after filling.

HOME INFUSION

✔ Home care is supervised by a registered nurse who works with a physician, pharmacist, and others to administer a care plan that involves the patient or another care giver.

✔ The fastest growing area of home health care is home infusion.

✔ Infusion pumps are available for specific therapies or multiple therapies, and include ambulatory pumps that can be worn by patients.

✔ In home infusion, the patient or their care giver is educated about their therapy: how to self-administer, monitor, report problems, and so on.

✔ The primary therapies provided by home infusion services are: antibiotic therapy, parenteral nutrition, pain management and chemotherapy.

✔ The same rules apply to preparing parenteral admixtures in the home infusion setting as in the hospital.

SELF TEST

MATCH THE TERMS.   *answers can be checked in the glossary*

acute condition

antibiotic therapy

chronic condition

home care agencies

maintenance medication

pain management

parenteral nutrition

• a continuing condition that requires ongoing treatment for a prolonged period.

• a medication that is required on a continuing basis for the treatment of a chronic condition.

• a sudden condition requiring immediate treatment.

• a common home infusion service used in treating AIDS related and other infections.

• businesses that provide a range of home nursing care services, including infusion.

• infusion of nutrition solutions for patients with various intestinal disorders or AIDS.

• generally the infusion of narcotics for patients with painful terminal illnesses or other types of severe chronic pain.

CHOOSE THE BEST ANSWER. *the answer key begins on page 347*

1. Mail order pharmacies are used for maintenance medications for chronic conditions. Which of the following conditions would NOT be likely to require maintenance medication?
   a. root canal
   b. HIV/AIDS
   c. depression
   d. hypertension

2. The delivery time for mail order medications is at least
   a. 24 to 48 hours.
   b. 2 weeks.
   c. 4 weeks.
   d. 6 weeks.

3. A sudden condition requiring immediate treatment is a(an)
   a. chronic condition.
   b. PRN condition.
   c. acute condition.
   d. maintenance condition.

4. A continuing condition that requires ongoing treatment for a prolonged period is called a(an)
   a. chronic condition.
   b. acute condition.
   c. infectious condition.
   d. maintenance condition.

5. Mail order pharmacies must follow _____ requirements
   a. only state
   b. federal and state
   c. international
   d. only federal

6. The type of order processing used by mail order pharmacies in which each step in the prescription fill process is completed or managed by a person who specializes in that step is called
   a. extemporaneous processing.
   b. assembly line processing.
   c. bin fill processing.
   d. automated processing.

7. The fastest growing area of home health care is
   a. CCU.
   b. ICU.
   c. home infusion.
   d. ambulatory care.

8. The primary advantage of home care over institutional care is
   a. better quality of life.
   b. more nursing staff.
   c. more sterile environment.
   d. easier for physician to see many patients in one day.

9. Home infusion pharmacies are involved in
   a. dispensing unit doses of tablets and capsules.
   b. providing maintenance medications.
   c. mail order pharmacy.
   d. preparing admixtures and providing infusion pumps.

10. Many hospitals offer home infusion therapies.
   a. True
   b. False

REVIEW

11. The type of infusion therapy used to treat infections is called
    a. antibiotic therapy
    b. PO
    c. admixture therapy
    d. TPNs

12. The type of infusion therapy associated with patients with digestive disorders or AIDS is called
    a. admixture therapy.
    b. PO.
    c. NPO.
    d. parenteral nutrition therapy.

13. The type of infusion therapy generally associated with an oncology program at a hospital or clinic is called
    a) chemotherapy
    b) antibiotic therapy
    c) PO
    d) NPO

14. Compounding parenteral admixtures for home infusion requires all of the following EXCEPT:
    a. aseptic practices.
    b. laminar flow hoods.
    c. ointment tiles.
    d. use of clean rooms.

15. Which member of the home care team orders the infusion therapy?
    a. R.Ph.
    b. physician
    c. Pharm.D.
    d. pharmacy technician

16. Which member of the home care team coordinates and monitors the care plan?
    a. home care aide
    b. registered nurse
    c. R.Ph.
    d. Pharm.D.

17. Which member of the home care team works with the supervising nurse to select the appropriate infusion device?
    a. home care aide
    b. physician
    c. pharmacy technician
    d. pharmacist

18. Which member of the home care team may be involved with compounding, labeling, delivery, and other non-consulting activities?
    a. R.Ph.
    b. home care aide
    c. pharmacy technician
    d. Pharm.D.

19. Which member of the home care team works under the supervision of the registered nurse?
    a. home care aide
    b. pharmacy technician
    c. R.Ph.
    d. Pharm.D.

20. Which member of the home care team is not involved in medication therapy?
    a. pharmacy technician
    b. nurse
    c. home care aide
    d. physician

ANSWERS TO SELF TESTS

Chapter 1
1. b
2. a
3. c
4. b
5. a
6. b
7. a
8. c
9. a
10. a
11. b
12. c
13. d
14. c
15. d
16. c
17. a
18. c
19. b
20. d
21. d
22. c

Chapter 2
1. d
2. b
3. c
4. c
5. d
6. d
7. b
8. b
9. a
10. c
11. c
12. d
13. d
14. a
15. a
16. d
17. b
18. b
19. b
20. c
21. c

22. d
23. c

Chapter 3
1. a
2. b
3. b
4. d
5. b
6. c
7. b
8. c
9. d
10. b
11. d
12. a
13. a
14. b
15. d
16. a
17. a
18. b
19. a
20. c
21. a
22. d

Chapter 4
Matching Exercise
1. d
2. g
3. p
4. n
5. w
6. a
7. h
8. o
9. y
10. f
11. j
12. v
13. r
14. k
15. q
16. m
17. x

18. b
19. u
20. e
21. l
22. i
23. c
24. s
25. t

Multiple Choice
1. a
2. b
3. b
4. b
5. d
6. b
7. a
8. d
9. b
10. a
11. d
12. d
13. a
14. d
15. a
16. c
17. c
18. b
19. d
20. d
21. a
22. c
23. b
24. d
25. c
26. a
27. b
28. b

Chapter 5
Matching Exercise
1. h
2. b
3. d
4. c
5. e

6. a
7. g
8. f
9. i
10. l
11. m
12. n
13. j
14. k

Multiple Choice
1. b
2. c
3. c
4. a
5. c
6. b
7. d
8. c
9. d
10. b
11. c
12. c
13. b
14. a
15. b
16. d
17. c
18. a
19. a
20. a

Chapter 6
Roman Numerals
1. XVIII
2. LXIV
3. LXXII
4. CXXVI
5. C
6. VII
7. XXVIII
8. 33
9. 110
10. 1,100
11. 1.5
12. 19

13. 24
14. 14 capsules
15. 9 drops
16. 48 tablets
17. 21 tablets

Numerators,
*   Denominators,*
*   and Reciprocals*
1. 0.33
2. 0.5
3. 0.25
4. 0.3
5. 0.1
6. 5/1
7. 3/2
8. 5/2
9. 9/2
10. 15/1

Adding and
*   Subtracting*
*   Fractions*
1. 2/4 = 1/2
2. 8/8 = 1
3. 1/5
4. 4/8 = 1/2
5. 5/5 = 1
6. 4/8 = 1/2
7. 9/20
8. 7/15
9. 7/16
10. 3/8

Multiplying and
*   Dividing*
*   Fractions*
1. 1/16
2. 3/24 = 1/8
3. 2/9
4. 15/64
5. 2/3
6. 4/12 = 1/3
7. 10/5 = 2
8. 24/24 = 1

ANSWERS TO SELF TESTS

Adding Decimals
1. 1.3
2. 7.4
3. 4.34
4. 23.798
5. 72.31
6. 4.6926
7. 276.096
8. 359.3404
9. 230.4465
10. 5288.5529

Subtracting Decimals
1. -0.16
2. 8.63
3. 14.29
4. 0.9726
5. 71.965
6. 14.592
7. 251.1229
8. 20.6699
9. 459.8842
10. 368.32

Multiplying Decimals
1. 0.35
2. 0.32
3. 0.09
4. 0.15
5. 22.2
6. 0.159
7. 0.144
8. 0.0264
9. 581.0248
10. 382.6764

Metrics
1. mcg
2. l or L
3. ml or mL
4. g (gm)
5. mg
6. kg
7. 1,000
8. 1,000
9. 129.6

10. 1,000
11. 0.001
12. 0.001

Conversions
1. 7,000
2. 3,200
3. 0.0648
4. 30
5. 300
6. 7,000
7. 437.447
8. 1.1
9. 2
10. 1
11. 32
12. 0.25

Ratio and Proportion
1. 2 ml
2. 8 ml
3. 75 ml
4. 2.08 ml/mn
5. 4.8 mL

Percents
1. 60%
2. 80%
3. 12%
4. .5
5. .125
6. .99
7. 358
8. 52.5 g
9. 14 s
10. 50 ml
11. 70 ml
12. 20 ml
13. 0.12%

TPN Solutions
1. 73.5 ml Amin. 8.5%
2. 37.5 ml dext 50%
3. 2 ml KCl
4. 0.45 ml Ca Gl.

5. 5 ml Ped MVI
6. qsad 131.55 ml sterile water

Usual and Customary
1. $45.76
2. $18.40
3. $11.50
4. $328.38
5. $27.05

Discounts
1. $8.54
2. $17.49
3. $37.24
4. $94.90
5. $122.09
6. $8.09
7. $16.64
8. $35.37
9. $8.91
10. $162.50

Gross Profit and Net Profit
1. gross $24.46 net $18.46
2. gross $17.18 net $11.18
3. gross $19.90 net $13.90
4. gross $29.31 net $23.31
5. gross $23.63 net $17.63
6. gross $31.39 net $25.39
7. gross $54.06 net $48.06
8. gross $6.71 net $0.71
9. gross $25.59 net $19.59
10. gross $22.63 net $16.63

Self-Test

Conversion Exercise
1. 500,000 mg
2. 10,000 g
3. 0.25 L
4. 0.325 g
5. 0.12 mg
6. 224.4 lb
7. 3560 g
8. 0.473 L
9. 6.59 kg
10. 30,000,000 mg

Self-Test Problems
1. 7.8°
2. 3 mL
3. 2.5 mL
4. 143 mL dext 70% and 357 mL sterile water

Self-Test Multiple Choice
1. b
2. c
3. c
4. d
5. d
6. a
7. a
8. b
9. b

Chapter 7
1. d
2. d
3. d
4. d
5. a
6. c
7. b
8. b
9. d
10. d
11. a
12. d

13. b
14. b
15. a
16. a
17. b
18. c
19. b
20. b
21. c
22. a
23. d
24. c
25. b

Chapter 8
1. a
2. d
3. a
4. c
5. b
6. b
7. c
8. b
9. d
10. a
11. c
12. c
13. b
14. d
15. a
16. a
17. c
18. a
19. c
20. c
21. d
22. c
23. d
24. c
25. b

Chapter 9
1. b
2. a
3. c
4. b
5. d
6. b

ANSWERS TO SELF TESTS

7. d
8. b
9. b
10. c
11. d
12. a
13. a
14. b
15. b
16. d
17. d
18. c
19. c
20. d
21. a
22. a
23. a

Chapter 10
1. c
2. c
3. d
4. d
5. a
6. d
7. c
8. c
9. b
10. d
11. d
12. d
13. a
14. a
15. c
16. d
17. c
18. a
19. b
20. b
21. d
22. d
23. b

Chapter 11
1. d

2. d
3. c
4. a
5. d
6. a
7. c
8. b
9. b
10. a
11. c
12. a
13. a
14. b
15. d
16. c
17. c
18. c
19. a
20. c
21. b
22. d
23. a
24. d
25. b

Chapter 12
1. c
2. c
3. a
4. c
5. c
6. b
7. b
8. b
9. d
10. d
11. c
12. d
13. c
14. a
15. b
16. b
17. b
18. b
19. a

20. b
21. c
22. b
23. a

Chapter 13
1. b
2. a
3. a
4. a
5. c
6. c
7. a
8. a
9. a
10. b
11. c
12. a
13. b
14. c
15. b
16. a
17. d
18. a
19. c
20. d
21. a
22. d

Chapter 14
1. a
2. a
3. c
4. b
5. d
6. a
7. b
8. b
9. b
10. a
11. b
12. a
13. a
14. d
15. d

16. b
17. c
18. a
19. a
20. c
21. c
22. d
23. d

Chapter 15
1. d
2. c
3. b
4. a
5. d
6. a
7. a
8. b
9. b
10. a
11. a
12. a
13. d
14. a
15. d
16. a
17. d
18. c
19. c
20. d
21. c
22. a
23. c
24. b

Chapter 16
1. b
2. d
3. c
4. a
5. d
6. b
7. c
8. b
9. a

10. d
11. b
12. c
13. d
14. a
15. d
16. d
17. d
18. d
19. d
20. d
21. b
22. c
23. b
24. a

Chapter 17
1. a
2. a
3. c
4. a
5. b
6. b
7. c
8. a
9. d
10. a
11. a
12. d
13. a
14. c
15. b
16. b
17. d
18. c
19. a
20. c

DRUG NAMES & CLASSES

When a drug compound is first synthesized or isolated, it is known by its atomic composition: the types and numbers of atoms contained in it. For example, the compound $C_{14}H_{19}Cl_2NO_2$ has 14 carbon atoms, 19 hydrogen atoms, 2 chlorine atoms, 1 nitrogen atom, and 2 oxygen atoms. Besides being awkward to pronounce, this kind of identification does not really describe the structure of the molecule.

A drug's name begins with a chemical name that describes its structure and its components.

These names identify a specific compound, but they are long and complicated and not useful for general communication. As a result, highly specific chemical names are shortened to less descriptive but more easily pronounceable ones.

While a potential drug is under development, the developer gives it a code number or a "suggested nonproprietary name."

Once a suggested nonproprietary name is officially approved, it becomes the generic name of the drug compound. Many pharmaceutical companies will assign code numbers to their compounds in the earliest development stages, and then a suggested nonproprietary name if the compound shows promise of being effective as a drug. At that point, the sponsor will apply for a proprietary or trademark name from both the U.S. Patent Office and foreign agencies. If approved, the proprietary name will have the ® symbol next to it when used in interstate commerce.

When a drug is under patent protection, it has one nonproprietary name and one proprietary or brand name, but the proprietary name belongs to the sponsor.

When a drug goes off-patent, other companies may market the same compound under their own brand names. For example, ampicillin is a generic drug that has been off patent for many years. It is available as Polycillin®, Principen®, D-Amp®, Omnipen®, or Totacillin®. Each name is a brand name used by a different company. But Viagra® (which has the generic name sildenafil) is available only under one brand name because the compound is still under patent protection. The point to remember is that there is only one nonproprietary (generic) name for a drug, but it may be sold under many different brand names once its patent protection has expired.

WHAT'S IN A NAME

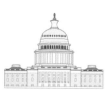

USAN

The United States Adopted Names Council (USAN) designates nonproprietary names for drugs. This council was organized in the early 1960s at the joint recommendation of the American Medical Association and the United States Pharmacopeial (USP) Convention. Other organizations, the American Pharmaceutical Association (now the American Pharmacists Association) and the FDA, were included in the Council during the latter part of the 1960s. There are publications that list "official" nonproprietary and proprietary names, as well as drug code designations, empirical names, chemical names, and show the molecular structures. The USP Dictionary of USAN and International Drug Names is such a reference.

Applying for a name

To apply for a name, the sponsoring company initiates a request for a name. The USAN and the sponsor will arrive at a "Proposed USAN" that is suitable to both. This proposed name is then submitted for consideration to US and foreign drug regulatory agencies. When approved by these different agencies, the name becomes the "official" name of the drug. The USAN guidelines for the recommendation of names include that the name should:

➡ be short and distinctive in sound and spelling and not be such that it is easily confused with existing names

➡ indicate the general pharmacological or therapeutic class into which the substance falls or the general chemical nature of the substance if the latter is associated with the specific pharmacological activity

➡ embody the syllable or syllables characteristic of a related group of compounds.

STEMS & CLASSES

Following are the USAN approved stems and the drug classes associated with them.

Stem	Drug Class
-alol	Combined alpha and beta blockers
-andr-	Androgens
-anserin	Serotonin 5-HT$_2$ receptor antagonists
-arabine	Antineoplastics (arabinofuranosyl derivatives)
-ase	Enzymes
-azepam	Antianxiety agents (diazepam type)
-azosin	Antihypertensives (prazosin type)
-bactam	Beta-lactamase inhibitors
-bamate	Tranquilizers/antiepileptics
-barb	Barbituric acid derivatives
-butazone	Anti-inflammatory analgesics (phenylbutazone type)
-caine	Local anesthetics
-cef	Cephalosporins
-cillin	Penicillins
-conazole	Anti-fungals (miconazole type)
-cort-	Cortisone derivatives
-curium	Neuromuscular blocking agents
-cycline	Antibiotics (tetracycline type)
-dralazine	Antihypertensives (hydrazine-phthalazines)
-erg-	Ergot alkaloid derivatives
estr-	Estrogens
-fibrate	Antihyperlipidemics
-flurane	Inhalation anesthetics
-gest-	Progestins
-irudin	Anticoagulants (hirudin type)
-leukin	Interleukin-2 derivatives
-lukast	Leukotriene antagonists
-mab	Monoclonal antibodies
-mantadine	Antivirals
-monam	Monobactam antibiotics
-mustine	Antineoplastics
-mycin	Antibiotics
-olol	Beta-blockers (propranolol type)
-olone	Steroids
-oxacin	Antibiotics (quinolone derivatives)
-pamide	Diuretics (sulfamoylbenzoic acid derivatives)

Drug classes are group names for drugs that have similar activities or are used for the same type of diseases and disorders. The assignment of a drug to a drug class is proposed when the sponsor makes an application to the USAN Council for an adopted name. The USAN Council and the sponsor then agree to a pharmacological or therapeutic classification. Unlike the generic and brand names, this classification is not an "official" one, however, and the drug may be listed in different classifications by different sources. For example, drugs classified one way in this chapter may appear in other classifications in other reference works.

There are common stems or syllables that are used to identify the different drug classes.

The USAN Council approves the stems and syllables and recommends using them in making new nonproprietary names. There are always new stems and syllables being approved by the Council, so the list is ever changing. On this page is a list of some common stems and syllables and the drug class associated with them.

Stem	Drug Class
-pamil	Coronary vasodilators
-parin	Heparin derivatives
-peridol	Antipsychotics (haloperidol type)
-poetin	Erythropoietins
-pramine	Antidepressants (imipramine type)
-pred	Prednisone derivatives
-pril	Antihypertensives (ACE inhibitors)
-profen	Anti-inflammatory/analgesic agents (ibuprofen type)
-rubicin	Antineoplastic antibiotics (daunorubicin type)
-sartan	Angiotensin II receptor antagonists
-sertron	Serotonin 5-HT$_3$ receptor antagonists
-sulfa	Antibiotics (sulfonamide derivatives)
-terol	Bronchodilators (phenethylamine derivatives)
-thiazide	Diuretics (thiazide derivatives)
-tiazem	Calcium channel blockers (diltiazem derivatives)
-tocin	Oxytocin derivatives
-trexate	Antimetabolites (folic acid derivatives)
-triptyline	Antidepressants
-vastatin	Antihyperlipidemics (HMG-CoA inhibitors)

CLASSIFICATION SCHEMES

There are various systems for classifying drugs: by disorder, body system affected, type of receptor acted on, type of action, etc. This text uses common classifications, but it is important to recognize that there is no standard classification system used in medicine.

A number of classifications are based on whether they influence the parasympathetic or sympathetic nervous system.

Most organs in the body are influenced by both the parasympathetic and sympathetic nervous systems. These systems generally stimulate opposing responses, which balances their effects and results in a normal state of **homeostasis**. Drugs that act on the parasympathetic system are called **cholinergic** because acetylcholine is the **neurotransmitter** of this system. Drugs that act on the sympathetic nervous system are called **adrenergic,** because the neurotransmitters for this system (norepinepherine and epinepherine) are secreted from the adrenal glands.

Many classifications are also named for the type of interaction with the receptor.

Agonist or **antagonist** interaction is the primary basis for classification (i.e., cholinergic antagonist, etc.), but drugs may be classified based on specific receptor characteristics. For example, adrenergic receptor responses may be categorized as alpha (α) and beta (β).

Classification schemes have grown significantly as different types of receptors have been discovered.

Each new type of receptor has been found to be responsible for a specific pharmacological effect. As drugs designed to interact with these receptors are developed the complexity of classifications increases.

There are also other factors that complicate classifications schemes.

One factor for drugs that affect the autonomic nervous system is the use of prefixes or suffixes such as **blocker**, **-lytic**, or **anti-** to mean antagonist, and **mimetic** to mean agonist. Another factor is the presence of neurotransmitters other than acetylcholine, norepinephrine, and epinephrine. These include serotonin, dopamine, histamine, gamma-amino butyric acid (GABA), etc. Each has subtypes, and each has agonists and antagonists that act by a variety of mechanisms.

CLASSIFICATIONS

Classification schemes for drugs can be highly complex. They can also vary greatly and any combination of terms or nomenclature schemes might be used. The classifications used in this text should provide insight into how and why the drugs in them are used, but are not the only way to classify these drugs.

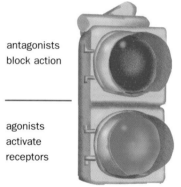

antagonists block action

_____

agonists activate receptors

 blocker another term for an antagonist drug, because antagonists block the action of neurotransmitters.

homeostasis the state of equilibrium of the body.

mimetic another term for an agonist, because agonists imitate or "mimic" the action of the neurotransmitter.

neurotransmitter substances that carry the impulses from one neuron to another.

The primary classifications used in this text are:

Analgesics
    Salicylates
    NSAIDs
    Acetaminophen
    Opiate Type
Anesthetics
    Local
    General
Anti-infectives
    Antibiotic (Antimicrobial)
    Antiviral
    Antifungal
    Antimycobacterial
    Antiprotozoal
    Antihelminthic
Antineoplastic Agents
    Antimetabolites
    Alkylating Agents
    Plant Alkaloids
    Hormonal
Cardiovascular Agents
    Antianginal
    Antiarrhythmic
    Antihypertensive
    Vasopressors
    Antihyperlipidemic
    Thrombolytic
    Anticoagulant
Dermatologicals
Electrolytes
Gastrointestinal Agents
    Enzymes
    Antidiarrheals
    Antiemetics
    Antacid / Antiulcer
    Laxatives and Stool Softeners

Hematological Agents
    Coagulation Enhancers
    Hematopoietic Agents
    Hemostatic Agents
Hormones & Modifiers
    Adrenal
    Antidiabetic
    Thyroid & Parathyroid
    Estrogen
    Contraceptive
    Androgen
    Pituitary
Immunobiologic Agents
    Vaccines
    Immune Globulins
Musculoskeletal Agents
Neurological Agents
    Antiparkinsonian
    Antialzheimer's
    Antiepileptic
    Antimigraine
Ophthalmic Agents
    Antiglaucoma agents
    Other Ophthalmics
Psychotropic Agents
    Antianxiety
    Antidepressants
    Antipsychotics
    Hypnotics
    Drug Dependency
Respiratory Agents
    Antihistamines
    Decongestants
    Antitussives
    Mucolytics
    Expectorants
    Bronchodilators
    Anti-inflammatory

LOOKALIKE / SOUNDALIKE

It is important to recognize that a number of drugs have similar sounding or looking names, but very different properties.

Besides similarity, one of the primary problems with accuracy in drug name identification is that prescriptions are still largely written by hand. However, it is also true that there are many ways drug names may be miscommunicated (by mispronunciation, typos, etc.). Therefore, the identification of a drug should be verified as many ways as possible.

Accuracy in handling and using drugs is essential.

Confusing one drug with another can lead to terrible, sometimes fatal consequences. It is critical to make certain that you have the name correct when involved in any aspect of the prescription process. At right is a list of drugs that can be mistaken for one another either by their sound or how they appear when written. There are many others, but this should illustrate the need for accuracy in drug names.

IDENTIFYING DRUG NAMES

At right is a list of drug names that might be easily misread, mispronounced, or otherwise mistaken for each other. Note that this is only a sample and that there are many other drugs with similar looking or sounding names.

Identifying Forms

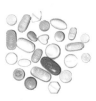

Frequent handling of a drug will help you to remember its physical characteristics (size, shape, color, markings, etc.), and this can be a valuable skill in the safe handling of drugs. It should be noted, however, that the most important step in identifying drugs is identifying the correct name. All drug information from the manufacturer to the prescriber, pharmacist, and ultimately the user is based upon communicating the correct name of the drug.exhibit text

Acetazolamide	Acetohexamide	Hydralazine	Hydroxyzine
Alfentanil	Fentanyl, Sufentanil	Hydrochlorothiazide	Hydroflumethiazide
Amitriptyline	Aminophylline	Hydrocortisone	Hydrocodone
Atenolol	Albuterol	Kanamycin	Garamycin, Gentamicin
Azathioprine	Azatadine		
Baclofen	Bactroban, Beclovent	Lisinopril	Fosinopril
Bupropion	Buspirone	Magnesium Sulfate	Manganese Sulfate
Calcitonin	Calcitriol	Methicillin	Mezlocillin
Captopril	Capitrol	Metolazone	Metaxalone
Cefamandole	Cefmetazole	Metoprolol	Metaproterenol
Cefonicid	Cefobid	Nifedipine	Nicardipine
Cefotaxime	Ceftizoxime	Oxymorphone	Oxymetholone
Cefoxitin	Cefotaxime	Pancuronium	Pipecuronium
Ceftizoxime	Ceftazidime	Pentobarbital	Phenobarbital
Cephalexin	Cephalothin	Phenytoin	Mephenytoin
Chlorpropamide	Chlorpromazine	Pramoxine	Pralidoxime
Clomiphene	Clomipramine	Prazosin	Prednisone
Clonazepam	Clofazimine	Prednisone	Prednisolone
Clorazepate	Clofibrate	Primidone	Prednisone
Clotrimazole	Co-trimoxazole	Proparacaine	Propoxyphene
Cyclosporine	Cycloserine	Quazepam	Oxazepam
Dapsone	Daypro	Reserpine	Risperidone
Dexamethasone	Desoximetasone	Ribavirin	Riboflavin
Digoxin	Digitoxin	Ritodrine	Ranitidine
Diphenhydramine	Dimenhydrinate	Sucralfate	Salsalate
Dopamine	Dobutamine	Sulfadiazine	Sulfasalazine
Doxazosin	Doxorubicin	Sulfamethizole	Sulfamethoxazole
Doxepin	Doxapram, Doxidan	Terbutaline	Tolbutamide
Dronabinol	Droperidol	Terconazole	Tioconazole
Dyclonine	Dicyclomine	Testoderm	Estraderm
Encainide	Flecainide	Thyrar	Thyrolar
Enflurane	Isoflurane	Thyrolar	Theolair
Etidronate	Etretinate	Timolol	Atenolol
Flunisolide	Fluocinonide	Tolazamide	Tolbutamide
Glyburide	Glipizide	Torsemide	Furosemide
Guanadrel	Gonadorelin	Tretinoin	Trientine
Guanethidine	Guanidine	Triamterene	Trimipramine
Guanfacine	Guaifenesin, Guanidine	Vincristine	Vinblastine
Halcinonide	Halcion	Zofran	Zoloft

ANALGESICS

Analgesic drugs create a state in which the pain from a painful medical condition is not felt.

Once pain has signaled the presence of a medical condition, its usefulness is generally complete and in most cases it can be safely blocked with the use of an analgesic.

There are several types of analgesics.

Two groups are used for mild to moderate pain, the non-steroidal anti-inflammatory drugs (NSAIDs) and the salicylates. Acetaminophen is also a popular agent for treating mild to moderate pain that some consider an NSAID but others do not.

Opiate-type narcotic analgesics are used for severe pain.

The naturally occurring opiates (morphine and codeine) and the synthetic opioids such as meperidine and propoxyphene are called "narcotic analgesics" and have a high abuse potential. In this section, we'll explore the types of analgesics and identify and describe common drug examples of each group.

 analgesia a state in which pain is not felt even though a painful condition exists.

anti-pyretic reduces fever.

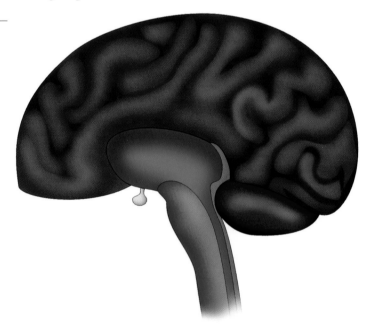

The Transmission of Pain

Nerve fibers carry pain impulses from the body's receptor sites through the spinal cord and up to the thalamus and cerebral cortex. The cerebral cortex is the ridge-like neural tissue that covers the brain's hemispheres. Analgesics are thought to depress the thalamus and interfere with the transmission of pain impulses. In addition, the brain's interpretation of pain may be altered with the use of these drugs.

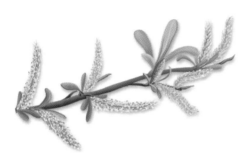

the white willow, a source of salicylic acid

Salicylates

➡ Relieve mild to moderate pain.

➡ Anti-inflammatory.

➡ Anti-pyretic.

Acetaminophen

➡ Relieves mild to moderate pain.

➡ Anti-pyretic.

NSAIDs

➡ More potent than salicylates.

➡ Relieve mild to moderate pain.

➡ Anti-inflammatory.

➡ Anti-pyretic.

Opiate-type

➡ For severe pain.

➡ Addicting.

Opiate-type Drugs & the Brain

Three specific receptors in the brain have been identified to react to opiate and opioid drugs:

➡ Mu (μ): produces euphoria, respiratory depression and physical dependence.

➡ Kappa (κ): produces analgesia,

➡ Sigma (σ): produces dysphoria and hallucinations.

An extract of willow bark, salicylic acid has been used to relieve pain for thousands of years.

Hippocrates and other ancient physicians used plants such as gaultheria and the poplar tree to obtain natural salicylates. Today, non-addicting analgesic products such as aspirin (acetylsalicylic acid) and methyl salicylate are widely used. Salicylates, acting both centrally and peripherally, are found effective as mild to moderate pain relievers, anti-inflammatory medications and fever reducers (antipyretics).

The action of non-steroidal anti-inflammatory drugs (NSAIDs) is both analgesic and anti-inflammatory.

They are generally more potent than the salicylates and serve to relieve mild to moderate pain, reduce fever and treat rheumatic symptoms. At higher doses, NSAIDs inhibit the synthesis of **prostaglandins**, a chief contributor to the inflammation process. As a result, inflammation is slowed or reduced. The effect of lower doses is analgesic. The selection and dosing of these drugs is very patient specific as one NSAID may be more effective than another for any given patient. NSAIDs may also have an antipyretic quality by which they reduce fever. The temperature regulating brain center is the hypothalamus and it is believed that some NSAIDs affect select areas of the hypothalamus to increase vasodilation, sweating, and encourage excess heat loss. Common drugs in this category include ibuprofen and naproxen.

Taken from the poppy plant, Papaver Somniferum, opium was also used in ancient times to relieve pain.

Opiate-type and opioid narcotics of today have been found to affect the CNS by reducing the awareness and perception of pain. They mimic the actions of the body's natural narcotic-like substances called endorphins. The narcotic analgesics do not eradicate the pain, but rather alter the patient's perception of it. Therefore, these drugs are thought to be most helpful if given before the severe pain is present. Common naturally occurring opiate-type drugs include morphine and codeine, while common opioid drugs include meperidine and propoxyphene.

ANESTHETIC AGENTS

Anesthetics cause an absence of sensation or pain.

They are classified into two groups: local and general.

Local anesthetics block pain conduction from peripheral nerves to the central nervous system without causing a loss of consciousness.

They do this by allowing the nerve's membrane to stabilize in a resting position and not respond to painful stimuli. Cocaine is credited by some sources as the first recognized local anesthetic, but it has a limited use today (i.e., topical application in eye and nasal surgery) and is a Schedule II substance.

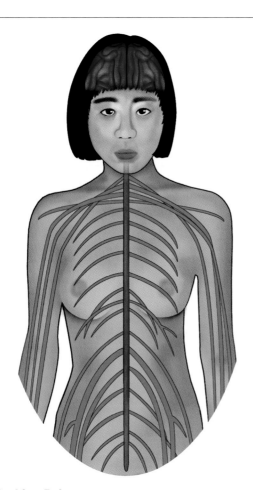

Blocking Pain

Pain is conducted from its local site through the Peripheral Nervous System (blue) to the Central Nervous System (red). Local anesthetics block pain conduction to the CNS, but do not affect the CNS, so the patient remains conscious. General anesthetics block pain sensation by depressing the CNS, causing unconsciousness.

LOCAL ANESTHETICS

Indications

Common indications for local anesthetics include:

➡ dental work or discomfort (topical or injection);

➡ birth pain (spinal, epidural or caudal IV);

➡ sunburn, hemorrhoids and skin irritations (topical).

Groups

Local anesthetics can be grouped by chemical structure as follows:

➡ **Esters** – metabolized by enzymes found in the blood or skin, short to moderate duration of effectiveness. Examples include: procaine, benzocaine, butamben, and tetracaine.

➡ **Amides** – metabolized in the liver and therefore longer acting. Examples include: lidocaine, procainamide, bupivacaine, and dibucaine.

➡ **Others** - those agents suitable for patients with allergies to esthers or amides. Examples are dyclonine and pramoxine.

ABCD *surgical anesthesia* the stage of anesthesia in which surgery can be safely conducted.

medullary paralysis an overdose of anesthesia that paralyzes the respiratory and heart centers of the medulla, leading to death.

GENERAL ANESTHESIA

The Four Stages

There are four stages of general anesthesia:

Stage I – Analgesia

Euphoria with loss of pain and consciousness.

Stage II – Excitement

Increase in sympathetic nervous system effects such as blood pressure, heart and respiratory rate.

Stage III – Surgical Anesthesia

The stage in which surgery can safely be conducted. There are four levels of surgical anesthesia, with the higher numbered levels producing deeper anesthesia and more serious systemic effects.

Stage IV – Medullary Paralysis

An overdose of anesthesia can compromise the respiratory and heart centers of the brain's medulla and cause death.

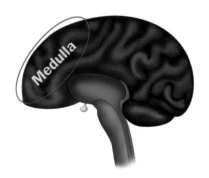

General anesthetics depress the CNS (central nervous system) to the level of unconsciousness.

The first general anesthetic, nitrous oxide (laughing gas), was developed about 150 years ago. The vapors ethyl ether and chloroform followed soon after. However, these products were found to have many safety concerns and less hazardous agents have been subsequently developed.

General anesthetics are generally classified according to their route of administration: *inhalation* or *intravenous* (*IV*).

IV anesthesia often produces a more pleasant, smoother and quicker onset than the inhaled anesthetics. A combination of various agents is widely used to avoid undesired side effects and produce the best effects of general anesthesia.

General anesthesia is administered by a medical doctor called an anesthesiologist.

The desired level of general anesthesia can be controlled by balancing the amount of anesthesia the patient receives with the amount their lungs eliminate through exhalation. In ceasing the administration of anesthesia, the process will reverse and the level of anesthesia lighten.

In addition to the anesthetic drug choice, adjunctive drugs such as analgesics, atropine-like drugs, and anti-infectives may also be used.

This is to prevent certain negative side effects (those that occur from too much of one anesthetic), potentiate other desired effects (such as pain relief and reduced amount of anesthesia), cause the drying of secretions (preventing aspiration during surgery), or act to prevent infections (post-op). The safety, comfort, and general well being of the patient are of utmost concern when an anesthesiologist chooses the anesthetic or combination of anesthetics that are the most appropriately indicated for a particular case.

Inhalation Anesthetics

Examples of inhalation anesthetics include:

➡ nitrous oxide,

➡ ether,

➡ halothane, and

➡ desflurane.

Intravenous Anesthetics

IV anesthetics include:

➡ midazolam,

➡ diazepam,

➡ fentanyl, and

➡ alfentanil.

ANTI-INFECTIVES

Anti-infectives treat disease produced by microorganisms such as bacteria, viruses, fungi, protozoa, and parasitic worms.

Historically, natural chemicals from the earth such as mercury and molds have been used to treat infections, but it wasn't until Paul Ehrlich synthesized hundreds of chemicals in the 1930's, that a chemotherapeutic approach was widely used. There are now a large number of naturally occurring, semi-synthetic and synthetic drugs and vaccines available for treatments of infectious diseases.

In this section, *antibiotics (antimicrobials)*, *antivirals* and *antifungals* will be discussed and explored.

Other forms of anti-infectives include: ***antimycobacterials*** (agents that treat tuberculosis, leprosy and the MAC complex in AIDS); ***antiprotozoals*** (agents that treat malaria, vaginitis and sleeping sickness); and ***antihelminthics*** (agents that treat parasitic worms in the GI tract). Metronidazole, a stand alone miscellaneous antibacterial and antiprotozoal agent, is also included in the drug chart.

ANTIBIOTICS

Early discovery of antibiotics comes from Sir Alexander Fleming and his work isolating the naturally occurring **penicillin**. In the latter 1930's, a team from Oxford reinvestigated this research and developed potent extracts which were important in fighting infections during WWII. Since this time, synthetic penicllins (e.g., ampicillin) and the first semisynthetic penicillin, carbenicillin, have been introduced.

Other forms of antibiotics include:

➡ **cephalosporins** (cefazolin, cefoxitin, ceftibuten, cefepime, etc.)

➡ **tetracyclines** (tetracycline, doxycycline, etc.);

➡ **sulfonamides** (sulfasoxazole, sulfamylon, etc.).

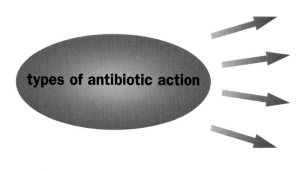

types of antibiotic action

damages the bacterial cell wall
(e.g., penicillins and cephalosporins)

modifies protein synthesis
(e.g., erythromycin and tetracycline)

modifies energy metabolism.
(e.g., sulfonamides)

modifies DNA synthesis.
(e.g., ofloxacin and ciprofloxacin)

ANTI-INFECTIVES

Antibiotic (Antimicrobial)

The terms antibiotic or antimicrobial refer to chemicals of bacterial microorganisms which suppress the growth of other microorganisms. Antimicrobials can be expanded to include both synthetic and naturally occurring antibiotics. Antimicrobials can be either **bacteriostatic** (inhibiting bacterial growth) or **bactericidal** (bacteria killing). These agents act by modifying protein synthesis, energy metabolism, DNA metabolism, and by damaging the bacteria's cell wall.

Antiviral

Antivirals inhibit the replication of viruses (**virustatic**). The viral microorganism will invade the host cell and proliferate using the cell's DNA and RNA. To effectively treat viral infections, the drug needs to stop the viral replication without destroying the patient's healthy cells. Mutations and resistance are common setbacks with this therapy. Antimicrobials are not effective with viral infections, but may be used in cases of accompanying secondary bacterial infection. **Protease inhibitors** (i.e. saquinavir, indinavir and nelfinavir) have been successful in blocking the enzyme responsible for viral replication. Other antiviral agents include: zidovudine and acyclovir.

Antifungal

Antifungals are used to treat fungal infections. Fungi are plant-like microorganisms commonly found in molds and yeast. The drugs chosen to treat these mycosis or mycotic infections are usually **fungicidal**. The fungal cell is destroyed as the drug prevents cell permeability and nutrition. Common fungal infections include: candidiasis (vaginal yeast infection), ringworm, and athlete's foot. Nystatin and fluconazole are popular antifungal drugs.

 antibiotic (antimicrobial) drug that destroys microorganisms.

antiviral drug that attacks a virus.

antifungal drug that destroys fungi or inhibits its growth.

antimycobacterial drug that attacks mycobacteria, the organisms that cause tuberculosis and leprosy.

antiprotozoal drug that destroys protozoa.

antihelminthic drug that destroys worms.

bactericidal bacteria killing.

bacteriostatic bacteria inhibiting.

virustatic drug that inhibits the growth of viruses.

ANTINEOPLASTICS

Antineoplastics inhibit the new growth of cancer cells or *neoplasms*.

Typically, cancer cells are abnormal in structure and growth rate. They offer no useful function, have unusual genetic content, and often reproduce quickly and uncontrollably. Antineoplastics present a **chemotherapeutic** approach to the treatment of cancer and together with surgery, radiation and perhaps alternative medicine, comprise an often hopeful and successful treatment protocol.

The term *malignancy* is used to denote the presence of a life-threatening cancerous group of cells or tumor.

If this original (primary) cell group spreads to other areas, often via the lymphatic or circulatory systems, it is said to have **metastasized**. Treatment to **remission** (state of cancer inactivity) or cure is more successful if little or no metastasis has occurred. However, current chemotherapeutic research and development is offering encouragement for cancers in later stages of growth.

The side effects caused by many of these drugs are often uncomfortable and serious.

They include immunosuppression (compromising one's immune system), anemia (decreased count of red blood cells), alopecia (hair loss), GI ulceration, and dehydration/weight loss caused by nausea and vomiting.

normal cell mitosis

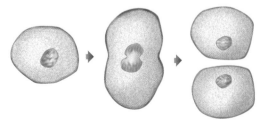

ABCD *lymphocyte* a type of white blood cell that releases antibodies that destroy disease cells.

metastasis when cancer cells spread beyond their original site.

neoplasm a new and abnormal tissue growth, often referring to cancer cells.

remission a state in which cancer cells are inactive.

The Lymphatic System

The lymphatic system is the center of the body's **immune system**. It collects plasma water from the blood vessels, filters it for impurities through the **lymph nodes**, and returns the **lymph** fluid back to the general circulation. Carried in the lymph are **lymphocytes**, a type of white blood cell that releases **antibodies** that attack and destroy **antigens** like bacteria and disease cells (including cancer). This is the body's **immune response** to antigens. **T-cells** and **B-cells** are the primary lymphocytes. Maintenance of the body's lymphocyte supply is largely performed by the bone marrow.

Antineoplastic drugs are targeted at cells with fast growth rates, which not only includes cancer cells but bone marrow as well. As a result, a serious side effect of antineoplastics is that they depress the immune system (**immunosuppression)**, leaving chemotherapy patients prone to infections.

Controlling Cell Growth

Normal cell growth (shown at left) is highly structured and steady, but cancer cells often reproduce quickly and uncontrollably. Antineoplastic drugs act on various stages of the cell replication process to stop the growth of cancerous cells.

Since cancer cells can mutate in many ways, different chemicals are used to stop their growth. This results in the "cocktail" approach to chemotherapy, in which a number of drugs are administered to a patient. Of course, these cocktails also affect normal cells, so they are administered in cycles that allow patients to recover from their adverse effects before the next round of administration.

Antimetabolites

Classified in accordance with the substances they interfere with, these antineoplastic drugs inhibit cell growth and replication by mimicking natural metabolites and taking their place within the cells. These fake metabolites inhibit the synthesis of important cellular enzymes, including DNA.

Alkyating Agents

These drugs interfere with mitosis or cell division by binding with DNA and preventing cellular replication. The early alkylating drugs were developed in World War I to introduce chemical warfare. Known as nitrogen mustard gases, these chemicals possessed properties which inhibited cellular growth and sperm counts while depressing bone marrow and damaging intestinal mucosa. Although these agents will adversely affect all cells, those that are growing at a more rapid rate (presumably cancerous) will be more affected. Nitrosureas, a more recent type of alkylating agent, are lipid soluble and pass easily into the brain where they are effective in treating brain cancers.

The rosy periwinkle of Madagascar is the source of the antineoplastic vincristine.

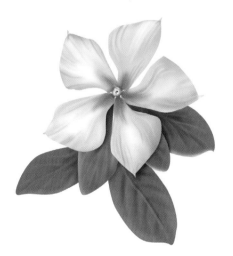

D ue to the toxicity of many antineoplastics, normal healthy cells are destroyed along with the cancerous cells.

Rapidly replicating cells such as those of the GI tract, bone marrow, and hair follicles are most often affected by selected antineoplastics, causing nausea/vomiting, bone marrow suppression, and hair loss.

Current widely used antineoplastic drugs include *alkylating agents* (nitrogen mustards), *antimetabolites,* and *plant alkaloids.*

They are usually given in cycles (e.g., 3-4 weeks between treatments), allowing rest and recovery periods for the patient. In theory, during the healthy cells recovery, neoplastic cells are entering a rapid division phase and are destroyed in greater numbers when chemotherapy is again begun. Drug resistance to a particular antineoplastic agent may occur, however, so a combination of these drugs may be given at one time to assure effectiveness. This "cocktail," as it is sometimes called, offers drugs of different actions and structure to address whatever type of cancerous cell group is suspected to be present.

Hormones, antibiotics, and radioactive isotopes are also classified as antineoplastic agents, generally for specific site treatment.

For example, if a tumor is found to be hormone dependent, surgical removal of the affected organ is often indicated (e.g., prostate, breast, or uterus), thus eliminating the chance for hormonal support. In addition, the synthetic antiestrogen agent, tamoxifen, is often used for the treatment of breast cancer in post-menopausal women. Certain antibiotics such as bleomycin and doxorubicin will be ordered to treat skin cancers, lymphomas, and leukemias. The radioactive isotopes, such as gold (AU198) and iodine (I131), are also generally organ specific, but are radioactive and special caution is needed during their use.

Plant Alkaloids

Derived from natural products or semisynthetically produced using natural products, some of these drugs inhibit the enzyme topoisomerase.

Topoisomerase is required for molecular cell growth or mitosis and therefore certain plant alkaloids interfere with cellular DNA replication. Other mechanisms of growth inhibition are not clearly understood.

CARDIOVASCULAR AGENTS

Some of the most widely used medications available are used to treat diseases and conditions of the cardiovascular system.

Cardiovascular agents include **antianginals, antiarrhythmics, antihypertensives, vasopressors, antihyperlipidemics, thrombolytics** and **anticoagulants**. They are used in treating myocardial infarction (heart attack), angina, cerebral vascular accident (CVA) or stroke, hyper/hypotension (high/low blood pressure), congestive heart failure (CHF), coronary artery disease (CAD), arrhythmias, high cholesterol, unwanted blood clots, and arteriosclerosis.

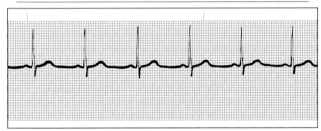

An EKG strip for a normal heart rhythm — variations from this pattern indicate an arrhythmia. The type of arrhythmia can be determined by the nature of the variation.

Arrhythmias

Normally, the electrical system of the heart causes it to contract (or beat) in a regular and organized rhythm that can be graphed by an **electrocardiogram** (**EKG** or **ECG**). An arrhythmia is an abnormal heart rhythm that can interfere with the heart's ability to pump in an effective, organized manner. Arrhythmias range from minor to life-threatening. They are classified by degree of seriousness, site of origin (where the electrical impulse causing the rhythm came from), and rate or speed. Familiar arrhythmias include:

➡ tachycardia;

➡ bradycardia;

➡ premature or ectopic beats;

➡ flutter and fibrillation.

THE HEART

Conduction

The heart is a pump that uses complex chemical and electrical processes to function. Chemically charged particles (ions) stimulate heart muscle to contract and relax systematically, pumping blood through the cardiovascular system. This contraction and relaxation is referred to as the **cardiac cycle**.

The **SA node** is the fastest generating electrical impulse area of the heart and it sets the pace. The atria and ventricles follow the conduction signal while the **AV node** together with the fine fibers (**Purkinje Fibers**) at the base of the heart transmit the impulse.

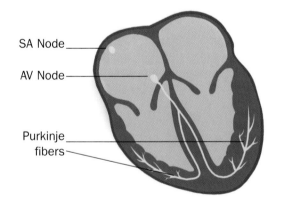

SA Node

AV Node

Purkinje fibers

arrhythmia an abnormal heart rhythm.
cardiac cycle the contraction and relaxation of the heart that pumps blood through the cardiovascular system.
diastolic pressure the minimum blood pressure when the heart relaxes; the second number in a blood pressure reading.
electrocardiogram (EKG or ECG) a graph of the heart's rhythms.

embolism, embolus a clot that has traveled in the bloodstream to a point where it obstructs flow.
myocardium heart muscle.
systolic pressure the maximum blood pressure when the heart contracts; the first number in a blood pressure reading.
thrombus a blood clot.

The Heart and Circulation

The heart is a muscular organ which powers blood circulation for the entire body. Divided into four chambers, the right and left **atria** (top chambers) and the right and left **ventricles** (bottom chambers), the heart receives deoxygenated blood into the right side (referred to as **pulmonary circulation**) and oxygenated blood into the left side (referred to as **systemic circulation**).

The right ventricle pumps blood to the lungs where it will mix with oxygen. The left ventricle pumps oxygenated blood to the body. The **myocardium** (heart muscle) is supplied fresh oxygen-rich blood by the **coronary arteries**, which branch from the **aorta** and circle back to the heart.

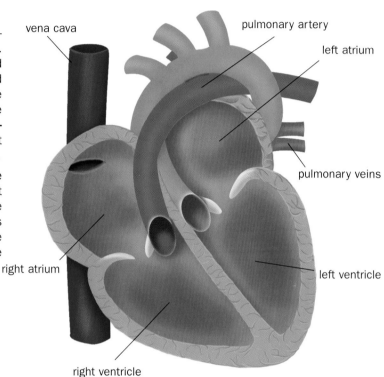

vena cava
pulmonary artery
left atrium
pulmonary veins
right atrium
left ventricle
right ventricle

Blood Clotting

Clotting is an essential function of blood that prevents excessive blood loss from injuries. Though **clotting factors** are the primary influence on clotting, adequate **platelets** and healthy blood vessel walls are also important. Too much clotting can be dangerous, however. If a clot (**thrombus**) is formed in the bloodstream, it can be carried to a location where it blocks a blood vessel and blood flow. Such blockages are called **embolisms**, and they can cause strokes and death.

Blood Pressure

Blood pressure is the outward pressure of the blood against the arteries as it is pumped through the body by the heart. Current literature recommends a blood pressure no higher than 135/85 for 40% of a normal healthy adult's day. The first number is the **systolic** value that represents the maximum pressure as the heart contracts to pump blood out. The second number is the **diastolic** value that represents the minimum pressure in the artery as the heart relaxes.

CARDIOVASCULAR AGENTS

CLASSES

Antianginals

Antianginals are used to treat cardiac related chest pain (angina) resulting from ischemic heart disease.

Patients with this condition suffer a lack of oxygen and blood flow to the myocardium. Nitrates, beta-blockers, and calcium channel blockers are examples of antianginals.

Antiarrhythmics

Antiarrhythmics are used to treat irregular heart rhythms.

They regulate the conduction activity of the heart by inhibiting abnormal pacemaker cells or recurring abnormal impulses and restoring a normal rhythm. Antiarrhythmics include beta blockers and drugs that block sodium channels, potassium ion channels, and calcium channels.

Antihypertensives

Antihypertensives are used to reduce a sustained elevation in blood pressure.

Factors affecting blood pressure include stress, blood volume, arterial narrowing, age, gender and general condition of health. Common antihypertensives include beta-blockers to reduce cardiac output, diuretics to decrease fluid volume, ACE inhibitors to reduce salt and water retention and inhibit vascular constriction, and calcium channel blockers to relax blood vessels.

Vasopressors

Vasopressors act to increase blood pressure.

If a patient is in a state of shock due to decreased blood volume, inadequate cardiac output or severe infection, fluids may be introduced to provide adequate blood volume. In addition to fluid replacement, vasopressors may be used to help supply blood to the brain and kidney.

Antihyperlipidemics

Antihyperlipidemics are used to lower high levels of cholesterol that can lead to blocked blood vessels.

Cholesterol is a **lipid** normally present in the body that is essential for healthy cell function. Proteins and carbohydrates, as well as fat are responsible for natural cholesterol production. Cholesterol levels are measured as **total cholesterol, LDL (low-density lipoprotein)**, and **HDL (high-density lipoprotein)**. Excess amounts of LDL can lead to blocked blood vessels and cardiovascular problems. HMG-CoA Reductase inhibitors are used to treat high LDL levels.

Thrombolytics / Anticoagulants

Thrombolytics are used to dissolve blood clots and anticoagulants are used to prevent their formation.

Thrombolytics can be dangerous since blood clotting can be disturbed, resulting in profuse bleeding and even bleeding to death. However, in cases of impending myocardial infarction or stroke, a travelling blood clot (**embolus**) can be dissolved and the stroke prevented. There has been much success with this group of drugs in recent years. A common thrombolytic agent is alteplase. Common anticoagulants include warfarin and heparin.

Beta blockers	Drugs that reduce the oxygen demands of the heart muscle.
Calcium channel blockers	Drugs that relax the heart by reducing heart conduction.
Diuretics	Drugs that decrease blood pressure by decreasing blood volume. They decrease volume by increasing the elimination of salts and water through urination.
ACE inhibitors	The "-pril" drugs, they relax the blood vessels. Note: the "-sartan" drugs are considered a subgroup of ACE inhibitors.
Vasodilators	Drugs that relax and expand the blood vessels.

DERMATOLOGICALS

The skin is the body's protective barrier.

It is the largest of the body's organs and protects the other organs against microorganisms, trauma, extreme temperature and other harmful elements. It is comprised of several layers: the epidermis (top layer), dermis (middle layer), and subcutaneous tissue (bottom layer). Within these layers, structures such as hair follicles and shafts, sebaceous and sweat glands, veins, arteries, and sensory nerves are found.

Dermatological refers to a drug used to treat a condition or disease related to the skin.

Pathological medical conditions and diseases which occur on or in the skin can be caused by inflammation, infection, growth rate changes, trauma, or structural dysfunction. Examples of skin conditions are: burns, cuts, rashes, dandruff, eczema, and skin cancer.

THE SKIN

The skin, also called the **Integumentary System,** is generally 3-5 millimeters thick, though it is thicker in the palms of the hands and soles of the feet and thinner in the eyelids and genitals. The outer layer of the epidermis (called the **stratum corneum**) is constantly replenished with new cells from underneath. The turnover time from cell development to shedding (**sloughing**) is about 21 days.

Skin Conditions

The following are examples of skin reactions that selected dermatologicals address:

➡ trauma (burns, cuts, abrasions, bruises).

➡ fluid accumulation (edema, cellulitis, blisters).

➡ discoloration and pigmentation, rashes, freckles, drug or allergy related photosensitivity,

➡ hyper or hypo melanin (skin pigment).

➡ dry skin or scaling (dandruff).

➡ cancers (basal cell, squamous cell or melanoma).

➡ non-malignant growths (keratoses).

In addition, the following common skin diseases are often treated with both prescription and non-prescription medications:

➡ eczema.

➡ psoriasis.

➡ acne.

➡ fungal infections (athlete's foot, ringworm).

➡ viral infections (herpes simplex).

➡ general dermatitis, hives or other allergic reactions caused by food, plants, insects, or sunburn.

dermatological a product used to treat a skin condition.

integumentary system the skin.

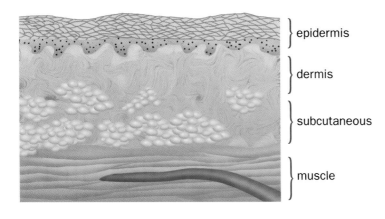

epidermis

dermis

subcutaneous

muscle

Other Structures

Contained within the skin are accessory structures: hair follicles, sweat glands, sebaceous glands, and nails.

Note also that the subcutaneous layer is not always considered a part of the skin but simply loose connective tissue that separates the skin from the underlying organs. It is, however, so closely interconnected that it is generally described with the integumentary system.

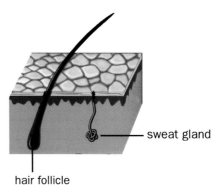

sweat gland

hair follicle

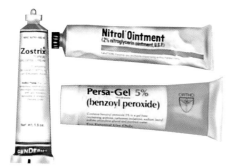

Dermatological Agents

Steroids, antihistamines, and inti-infectives are commonly used to treat skin disorders. Examples of commonly prescribed dermatological agents include:

➡ hydrocortisone cream

➡ diphenhydramine

➡ silver sulfadiazine cream

➡ doxycycline hyclate

➡ ofloxacin

Note: The drying agent zinc oxide is often seen in a combination product with the local anesthetic camphor, moisture absorbing agent kaolin, and an anti-infective such as triclosan when treating diaper rash.

ELECTROLYTIC AGENTS

Maintaining the proper balance of body fluids is essential to health and body function.

Water is the primary element in the body, accounting for more than half of body weight. It is found inside cells (**intracellular fluid**) and outside them (**extracellular fluid**) in plasma and tissue (**interstitial**) fluid.

Electrolytes are water soluble minerals that are contained in our body fluids as salts.

They form electrically charged particles called **ions**, which attract water. They have both positive and negative charges and are responsible for fluid movement into and out of cells. Changes in the body's normal electrolyte count affect fluid movement and balance and consequently various body functions.

Examples of common electrolytes include sodium (Na^+), potassium (K^+), calcium (Ca^{++}), chloride (Cl^-) and magnesium (Mg^{++}).

The plus and minus signs indicate their electrical charges. Functions these electrolytes affect include blood pressure, blood coagulation, muscle contractions, myocardial conduction, energy levels and enzyme production. Electrolytic therapy is aimed at restoring normal sodium, potassium, calcium and magnesium balances.

anions a negatively charged ion.

cations a positively charged ion.

dissociation when a compound breaks down and separates into smaller components.

electrolytes a substance that in solution forms ions that conduct an electrical current.

extracellular fluids the fluid outside the body's individual cells found in plasma and tissue fluid.

intracellular fluids cell fluid.

interstitial fluid tissue fluid.

ions electrically charged particles.

Opposites Attract

Water molecules (H_2O) are **polarized**. That is, they have positively and negatively charged sides. For this reason, many compounds **dissociate** (come apart) in water to form ions and the ions in turn **associate** with the water molecules.

The dissociation of sodium chloride (NaCl) into Na^+ and Cl^- ions followed by their association with water molecules is depicted at right. H_2O is attracted at its negative pole to the positive sodium ion and at its positive pole to the negative chloride ion.

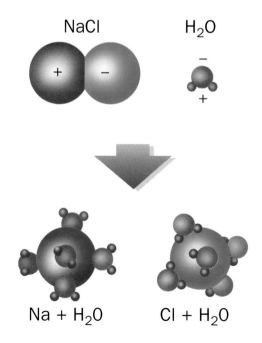

IMMUNOBIOLOGIC AGENTS

VACCINES

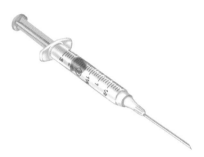

A vaccine is a suspension containing infectious agents used to boost the body's immune system response.

Two forms of vaccines presently exist: one allows **passive immunity** by giving an individual the antibody. This form generally offers a shorter period of protection. The other form stimulates the patient's immune system to produce an antibody, referred to as **active immunity**. This is the longer lasting type of immunity.

The **Smallpox Vaccine** was successfully introduced in Europe in the late 1700's by Dr. Edward Jenner. Since that time, other vaccines such as **DPT** (diptheria, pertussis and tetanus), **MMR** (measles, mumps and rubella), **Polio Typhoid**, **Rabies**, **Hepatitis A and B**, and **BCG** (an antitubercular agent) have been developed and utilized.

Today, most children are required to receive a series of these vaccines prior to attending school and this has resulted in a dramatic reduction in these diseases. Certain childhood diseases such as measles, mumps, and chicken pox, once contracted, should not reoccur due to active immunity created with the antibody formation. **Haemophilus Influenzae Type B** (Hib), a different Hepatitis series and the new **Chicken Pox** vaccine are examples of more recently developed vaccines.

Both *passive* and *active immunity* offer the body a defense against pathogens.

Passive immunity is developed by the introduction of preformed antibodies into the body. This provides immediate passive immunity. Active immunity occurs when the body is exposed to a pathogen, develops the disease, and manufactures antibodies against a future invasion. **Acquired active immunity** occurs when the body is purposefully injected with a weakened or even dead pathogen, but still produces antibodies against reoccurring exposures.

One negative aspect of passive immunity is that the life of some of the antibodies is shorter than the life of antibodies found with active immunity.

Another concern is the possibility of allergic reaction that may occur in some individuals. Further, hypersensitization may follow the receipt of passive immunity and render the host more prone to allergic response with each subsequent exposure. Severe anaphylactic reactions are possible.

***Immunobiologic agents* contain antibodies that have been produced by other humans or animals.**

These antibodies are recovered through high tech purification processes and made available commercially through **vaccines, toxoids** (e.g., DPT), and **immune globulins.**

Animal Antibodies

Pathogens for which passive immunity from animals may be used include:

➡ Diphtheria (using Antitoxin, USP)
➡ Rabies (using Antirabies serum)
➡ Botulism
➡ Black Widow Spider Venom

Human Antibodies

Human passive immunity is often used in the treatment of:

➡ Measles (using Measles Immune Globulin, USP)
➡ Pertussis (using Pertussis Immune Globulin, USP)
➡ Mumps (using Mumps Immune Globulin, USP)
➡ Tetanus (using Tetanus Immune Globulin, USP)
➡ Hepatitis A and B.

Note: Diphtheria, Tetanus, Hepatitis B, Measles, Mumps and Rabies may also be treated with agents producing active immunity.

GASTROINTESTINAL AGENTS

Gastrointestinal agents are used to treat disorders of the stomach and/or the intestines.

The drugs that address and treat various stomach and intestinal disorders include enzymes, antidiarrheals, antiemetics (anti-vomiting), antiulcer agents, laxatives, and stool softeners.

The GI organs are intimately related to the digestive system as a whole.

The other alimentary tract organs (mouth and esophagus), the accessory organs of digestion (salivary, gastric, and intestinal glands, liver, gall bladder, and pancreas), and the organs of elimination (rectum and anus) are often affected by direct GI disorders. For example, it is not uncommon for a colon cancer to metastasize not only to the stomach, but to the pancreas, liver, and rectum as well. As a result, although specific site antineoplastic drugs and treatments are available, agents may be used that treat more than one site and cell type at a time. **Gastric reflux** is another example. Gastric hyperacidity will often travel toward the chest and throat area via the esophagus. Antacid drugs that inhibit acidity of the stomach will provide for rest and healing of the esophagus when this happens.

THE DIGESTIVE SYSTEM

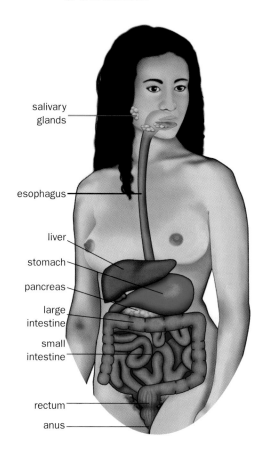

The stomach lies in the upper left quadrant of the abdomen between the lower end of the esophagus and the beginning of the small intestine (duodenum). This organ serves to store and chemically break down food using hydrochloric acid and pepsinogen. **Chyme** is the semi-liquid form of food as it enters the duodenum. **Peristalsis** is the wave-like motion which moves the food products along the intestinal tract.

Together, the small intestine and the large intestine make up about 28 feet of bowel (intestine). Most food absorption takes place in the small intestine. The large intestine absorbs water and connects to the rectum and anus for stool evacuation.

The GI organs are large in mass compared to other systems' organs and play a major role in normal body function. As a result, dysfunction, abnormality or other pathologic medical conditions of the GI tract may require serious and immediate drug therapy as well as other forms of medical or surgical intervention. Similar to other organ systems, preventive care and early detection of pathology is suggested and encouraged.

chyme the semi-liquid form of food as it enters the intestinal tract.

peristalsis the wave like motion of the intestines that moves food through them.

Enzymes

Pepsin is a normally present gastric enzyme that breaks down proteins. However, in the absence of pepsin, it is still possible for the digestive system to break down protein molecules into amino acids using **proteolytic enzymes** from the pancreas that are found in the small intestine. These enzymes are capable of attacking starches and fats. If a patient's condition warrants treatment using **enzyme therapy** (as with cystic fibrosis and chronic pancreatitis), products that contain pancreatin, an agent prepared from hog pancreas, or pancrelipase may be indicated. **Malabsorption** conditions such as **steatorrhea**, where fat is inadequately digested and is excreted in large amounts in feces, may be treated with pancrelipase.

Antidiarrheals

Diarrhea is a condition of frequent watery stools which results from microorganism invasion, drug or stress reaction, and/or other circumstances causing a decrease in intestinal absorption of water, an increased secretion of electrolytes into the intestines or an excessive amount of mucus production. **Antiperistalsis drugs** slow the movement of the intestinal contents to allow for greater water and electrolyte absorption. Loperamide is a common antiperistalsis agent and diphenoxylate plus atropine is another popular antidiarrheal agent. Bismuth subsalicylate (Pepto-Bismol) is a **secretion inhibitor** that acts to prevent organisms from attaching to the intestinal mucosa and may deactivate certain toxins as well. In cases of infectious diarrhea, antibiotics such as metronidazole and vancomycin may also be indicated and ordered in conjunction with other therapies. Note: Some antibiotics can kill normal bacterial flora or facilitate regrowth of resistant microorganisms, and so lead to diarrhea.

GASTROINTESTINAL AGENTS

Antiemetics

This class of drugs treats the condition of nausea and vomiting. There are many causes for this condition which is usually a symptom or side effect as opposed to being the actual condition itself: food or drug reaction or allergy, pregnancy, anxiety, exhaustion, dehydration, and a large number of diseases or illnesses such as cancer, or a microorganism related infectious process such as a middle ear infection. Often, antiemetics are ordered concurrently with other drug therapies used to treat the underlying condition. Vomiting is a reflex that occurs from a variety of stimuli. The treatment is to reduce the hyperactivity of stimuli receptors and lower the impulse rate. Also, decreasing the sensitivity to emetic chemicals found in the blood will inhibit the vomiting reflex. Dehydration and electrolyte imbalance are of major concern with prolonged vomiting.

Antacid/Antiulcer Agents

Antacids, generally composed of inorganic salts such as calcium carbonate, aluminum hydroxide, and magnesium hydroxide are popular antiulcer agents that act to neutralize existing acid, as opposed to inhibiting its production. Antacids are most indicated at the onset of hypergastric activity, are pain relieving yet short acting, and not strong enough for a diagnosed ulcer condition. Caution should be exercised to not rely on anatacids alone or for a prolonged time. If ulcer symptoms persist, the physician should be notified. Maalox is an example of a common antacid.

Cimetidine is a **histamine receptor antagonist.** It inhibits the secretion of gastric acid by blocking the effects of histamine. This type of agent was first approved for use in 1977 and revolutionized standard antacid therapy. Cimetidine has a history of drug interactions, however, and improved histamine antagonists (ranitidine, famotidine, and nizatidine) have since been developed.

Peptic ulcer is caused by hypergastric acidity that erodes tissue in localized areas of the stomach and intestines. While these lesions are normally benign, they may produce symptoms that are mild and of minor discomfort or they may be more serious and extend to underlying layers of connective tissue and smooth muscle. In these cases, blood vessels can be affected and bleeding can occur. A special dietary regime (i.e., frequent, small, bland, non-acid containing meals) together with selected drug therapy is commonly recommended for treatment of this condition.

Gastric Reflux

Gastric Reflux is a more serious gastric acid condition that is often treated with a strong antacid.

374

Laxatives and Stool Softeners

Enemas

Enemas may be placed into this category since they are indicated in cases of constipation, pre-medical treatment, and to ease the stress of bowel movements. Fleets, sodium biphosphate and sodium phosphate, is a popular saline enema.

These agents are commonly prescribed to treat **constipation**, the condition of dehydrated stool in which bowel movements are infrequent, hard, and often painful and difficult. Aside from changing a patient's diet, fluid intake and activity level, drug therapy may be suggested. Laxatives promote defecation without stress or pain and are often suggested for use prior to certain medical procedures related to the bowel (e.g., colonoscopy, barium enema), for constipation, and for patients who have hemorrhoids, recent hernia surgery, or a heart attack.

There are several types of laxatives available: **bulk forming,** that swell as they mix with intestinal contents; **stimulant,** that irritate the lining and nerves of the intestine; **saline,** that rapidly promote watery stool by drawing water into the intestine; and **osmotic,** that increase the stool's water content using osmosis. The osmotic laxative is often used as a **retention enema,** although it can be powerful and cause cramping. Lactulose (Chronulac® Syrup) is an example of a commonly prescribed saline laxative.

Docusate sodium (Colace®) is a commonly ordered **stool softener,** or emollient laxative. It promotes the mixing of fatty and watery intestinal substances to soften the stool's contents and ease the evacuation of feces.

HEMATOLOGICAL AGENTS

Blood coagulation or clotting is a complex process in which the protein *fibrinogen* is transformed to an insoluble fiber called *fibrin.* The enzyme thrombin, which comes from prothrombin, acts on fibrinogen in the blood to cause the transformation. Prothrombin and fibrinogen are *clotting factors* or coagulation factors. Other clotting factors, adequate platelets, and healthy blood vessel walls are also essential components to balanced coagulation.

Each stage of clot development can be affected by clotting factors as well as drugs.

For example, patients with hemophilia A have a genetic deficiency in factor VIII (*most clotting factors are denoted by Roman Numerals*) and can be successfully treated with concentrates of Antihemophilic Factor (AHF) that are commercially available. Factor VIII concentrate or cryoprecipitate and desmopressin acetate are other agents that will act to shorten bleeding time. Von Willebrand's disease, a very common congenital coagulation disorder, is also caused by a deficiency in factor VIII. Factor IX concentrates (Christmas factor) are available for patients with hemophilia B, a condition marked by a deficiency in clotting factor IX.

Phytonadione, or Vitamin K$_1$, is a drug that stimulates the liver to produce several clotting factors and mimics the action of Vitamin K (a natural clotting promoter).

Patients who may develop Vitamin K deficiency and require coagulation enhancer therapy include "at risk" infants whose liver and intestines are not fully developed, users of antibiotics that "sterilize" the intestines and prevent vitamin K synthesis, and those with malabsorption disorders such as Whipple's Disease and obstructive jaundice. In addition, patients with liver disease may suffer with bleeding disorders since the liver is responsible for the synthesizing of many clotting factors.

---

 clotting factors factors in the blood coagulation process.

fibrinogen Factor I.

fibrin the fiber that serves as the structure for clot formation.

Clotting

The main stages of natural clot formation and dissolution are:

Thromboplastin is formed from blood and tissue (**platelet aggregation** at injury site).

Thrombin is formed from prothrombin and thromboplastin.

The fiber fibrin is formed from thrombin acting on fibrinogen (clot formation).

Fibrinolysin breaks down fibrin (clot breakdown).

 Aside from drug therapy, patients with excessive bleeding may receive whole blood and blood products such as packed cells, platelets, and plasma to treat this serious situation.

Hematopoietics **are drugs that treat various forms of anemias by stimulating or helping to stimulate blood cell growth.**

Anemias are generally characterized by a decrease in hemoglobin or red blood cells which leads to a series of other disorders manifested by oxygen deficiency. The classifications of anemias include cell shape and structure, cause, and the pathophysiology or disease tract the particular anemia will take.

Most commonly, anemias develop in the elderly from iron deficiency, as a result of genetic predisposition (e.g., Sickle Cell anemia), or due to vitamin B$_{12}$ deficiency (*pernicious anemia*).

An additional type of anemia is associated with chronic disease. Correction of the underlying illness will improve this anemia. Anemias may also occur as a result of cancer or other diseases and treatments that cause bone marrow suppression and decrease of erythropoietin (which stimulates red blood cell production). In addition, a decrease in the granulocyte colony stimulating factor (G-CSF) and granulocyte macrophage colony stimulating factor (GM-CSF), excessive blood loss, infections, and inflammatory processes contribute to anemia. Common drug therapies for anemias include ferrous sulfate for iron-deficiency anemia and cyanocobalmin for vitamin B$_{12}$ deficiency anemia.

***Hemostatic* drugs are used to treat or prevent excessive bleeding.**

Patients who have hemophilia or thrombocytic purpura may receive hemostatic medications. They suffer from a lack of platelets and/or blood clotting factors found in the first stage of clotting. Systemic hemostatic agents include aminocaproic acid, tranexamic acid, and aprotinin. Their indications range from preventing hemorrhages during dental procedures to prevention of blood loss in cardiopulmonary bypass surgery. Their primary action is to inhibit the activation of plasminogen. ***Topical hemostatics*** are used for minor bleeding of small blood vessels when sutures are not appropriate. Examples of topical hemostatics include thrombin powder, microfibrillar collagen hemostat, and oxidized cellulose.

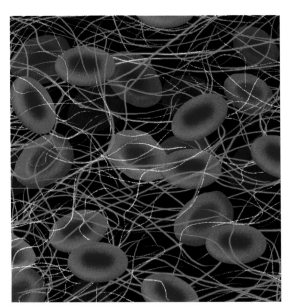

Strands of fibrin interweave and trap red blood cells to form a blood clot.

ABCD *anemia* a decrease in hemoglobin or red blood cells.

hematopoietics drugs used to treat anemia.

hemostatic drugs drugs that prevent excessive bleeding.

topical hemostatics drugs used for minor bleeding when sutures are not appropriate.

HORMONES & MODIFIERS

Hormones are secretions of the *endocrine system's* ductless glands.

These substances control or influence a selected organ or set of organs to produce an effect. If a patient does not naturally produce enough or produces too much of a particular hormone, selected drugs can be given to stimulate or inhibit hormone secretion. These hormones and **hormone modifiers** can either be extracted from animals or reproduced synthetically.

The *pituitary gland* is also known as the "master gland" because it regulates the activities of the entire endocrine system.

This pea-sized organ is located deep within the cranium, at the base of the brain. In turn, another major system, the nervous system, greatly controls the pituitary gland and together these two systems are responsible for a large number of our body's regulatory processes.

The *thyroid gland* is located in front of the trachea and secretes hormones that affect metabolism, growth, and central nervous system development.

Thyroxine (T_4) and triiodothyronine (T_3) are thyroid hormones. Their normal secretion is dependent on appropriate amounts of iodine and **TSH (thyroid stimulating hormone)** in the circulating blood. **Hyperthyroidism** is a disorder of overproduction of thyroid hormones that increases the metabolism. Symptoms include increased nervousness and heart rate. Treatment includes surgery and antithyroid medications. **Hypothyroidism** is a disorder of underproduction of thyroid hormone, resulting in a lower metabolism. Symptoms include tiredness, low blood pressure, slow heart rate, and weight gain. Treatment includes thyroid hormone and increased dietary intake of iodine.

corticosteroid hormonal steroid substances produced by the cortex of the adrenal gland.

endocrine system the system of hormone secreting glands.

hormone a chemical secretion that influences or controls an organ or organs in the body.

hyperthyroidism overproduction of thyroid hormone.

hypothyroidism underproduction of thyroid hormone.

THE ENDOCRINE SYSTEM

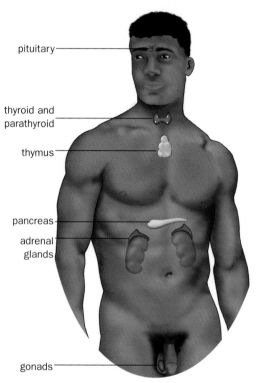

pituitary

thyroid and parathyroid

thymus

pancreas

adrenal glands

gonads

Note: the gonads of males are called **testes** and of females, **ovaries**.

Pituitary Gland
➡ Regulation of Endocrine system and growth.

Thyroid and Parathyroid
➡ Metabolic and calcium regulation.

Thymus
➡ Lymphatic regulation.

Pancreas
➡ Blood sugar regulation.

Adrenal Glands
➡ Metabolism and energy regulation.

Gonads
➡ Sexual characteristics.

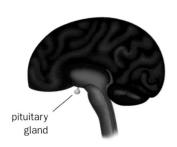

pituitary gland

Pituitary Gland

Divided into posterior and anterior lobes, this organ controls metabolism, growth, water loss and retention, electrolyte balance, and the reproductive cycle. An example of a hormone secreted by the posterior lobe is ADH or antidiuretic hormone. Also known as **vasopressin**, this hormone acts to help the kidneys conserve water and prevent dehydration. Diabetes Insipidus is caused by a deficiency in this hormone and marked by excretion of large amounts of urine (polyuria) and excessive thirst (polydipsia).

Oxytocin is another posterior lobe hormone. It helps stimulate uterine contraction and promote birth or inhibit uterine bleeding post birth.

FSH or follicle stimulating hormone is an anterior lobe hormone called a **gonadatropin** (stimulator of reproductive organ function). It acts to stimulate the egg follicle to produce eggs. Clomiphene is a popular synthetic nonsteroidal agent used to induce ovulation and establish fertility in otherwise unfertile women.

Adrenal Glands

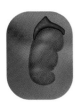

The adrenal glands sit atop the kidneys. They secrete corticosteroids and epinepherine, which influence many aspects of metabolism and energy regulation.

PTH (parathyroid hormone) **and calcitonin are the hormones secreted by the parathryroid glands.**

These hormones regulate the body's serum calcium and phosphorus levels which are integral to normal muscle contraction, bone formation, blood coagulation, milk production in the lactating mother, and nerve impulse conduction. These four small round organs are located behind the thyroid gland and reduction of their function can cause low calcium levels, convulsions, and possible death. Calcitonin-salmon is a common parathyroid gland synthetic hormone.

Located above each kidney, the *adrenal glands* consist of an outer section, the *cortex*, and an inner section, the *medulla*.

The cortex secretes **corticosteroids** which regulate the body's ability to handle stress, resist infection, affect glucose, fat, protein and carbohydrate metabolism and maintain salt and water balance. The adrenal medulla secretes the neurotransmitter **epinephrine** which acts as a stimulator to the sympathetic nervous system. This hormone, referred to as a **catecholamine**, is generally released during stress or activities of "fight or flight." Epinephrine will generally cause a rise in blood pressure, strength and rate of heart beat, blood glucose, metabolic rate, a relaxation of bronchi muscles, coronary and uterine muscles, and dilation of the eye's pupil. Epinephrine is commercially available and used often in serious or medical emergency situations.

Corticosteroids

Hydrocortisone and **cortisone** are two adrenal cortex corticosteroids that act to control anti-inflammatory response and the immune response system. In the 1940's cortisone was recognized as having anti-inflammatory properties. Since then, many synthetic corticosteroids such as prednisone and trimcinolone have been developed and indicated for a number of inflammatory diseases (e.g., arthritis and Crohn's).

The corticosteroid aldosterone helps maintain an adequate supply of serum sodium which accommodates sufficient extracellular fluid or blood volume. A severe deficiency in aldosterone could lead to low blood pressure and circulatory collapse.

HORMONES & MODIFIERS

The pancreas secretes the hormones *insulin* and *glucagon*.

The pancreas is an irregularly shaped organ located between the adrenal glands and behind the stomach. A specialized cluster of pancreatic beta cells called the **Islands (or Islets) of Langerhans** produce insulin, a hormone that controls the body's use of glucose, its normal source of energy. The alpha cells of the pancreas secrete the hormone glucagon which helps convert amino acids (by products of protein digestion) to glucose and raise the level of **serum glucose** (blood sugar). As the serum glucose level increases in a healthy individual, insulin secretion is stimulated. Glucagon and insulin ideally work together to strike a delicate balance and maintain **homeostasis**. Glucagon is available commercially and given to release glucose into the blood stream for severely hypoglycemic patients.

Without adequate insulin levels, serum glucose is not reabsorbed into the intestine, and it spills into the urine for excretion.

Instead of using glucose as it should, the body uses fat and protein as energy sources. This condition, **diabetes mellitus**, is marked by frequent urination, excessive thirst, elevated blood glucose levels, and positive urine glucose and acetone levels. In the early 1920's, Canadian researchers noted a link between the absence of a pancreas and diabetic symptoms. A young boy was subsequently treated with insulin and the diabetic symptoms abated. Insulin, in a variety of types, is given to treat diabetes mellitus, and several oral diabetic agents are also available (e.g., glyburide). Note that insulin does not cure diabetes. It is merely a treatment for it.

 insulin a hormone that controls the body's use of glucose.

glucagon a hormone that helps convert amino acids to glucose.

diabetes mellitus a condition in which the body does not produce enough insulin or is unable to use it efficiently.

serum glucose blood sugar.

Islands (or Islets) of Langerhans specialized cells of the pancreas that secrete insulin.

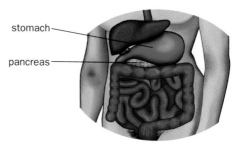

The pancreas is located behind the stomach.

stomach
pancreas

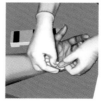

Glucose Monitoring

Patients with diabetes mellitus routinely monitor their blood glucose levels with a **glucometer**. This involves taking a small blood sample, usually from a fingertip, and inserting the sample into the glucometer for analysis. Newer systems that read glucose levels through the skin and do not require blood specimens are being developed.

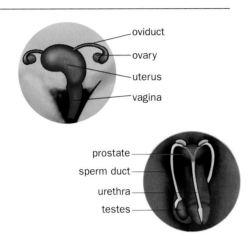

oviduct
ovary
uterus
vagina

prostate
sperm duct
urethra
testes

The *ovaries* are almond shaped organs found on either side of the uterus within the female pelvis.

Under control of the anterior pituitary gland, the ovaries are responsible for the production of ova (eggs) as well as the secretion of the hormones **estrogen** and **progesterone**. These hormones are essential for primary and secondary sex characteristic development, menstruation, healthy pregnancies (gestation), and milk production (lactation).

The *testes* secretes the male hormone testosterone.

Male hormones are called **androgens**. The development and maintenance of the male reproductive tract includes enhancement of secondary sexual characteristics, muscle development, sex organ growth, and body fat distribution. In addition, testosterone also contributes to the building of tissues and prevention of their breakdown. Commercially available testosterone products are often indicated in cases of male hypogonadism or in females for certain breast cancers or engorgement. Fluoxymesterone is a common example of this androgen.

Estrogen

First produced in large quantities at puberty, women secrete estrogens until menopause. Due to their adjunctive role in calcium and phosphorus conservation, many women receive replacement estrogen therapy in their post menopausal years. Women who experience a lack of these hormones during their child bearing years and/or post menopause, may receive them as natural and synthetic products. Synthetic estrogen may also be indicated in cases of breast engorgement, to stunt female growth in height, and for men with prostate cancer. Estrogens are generally contraindicated in cases of breast and/or genital cancer history or if there has been unexplained uterine bleeding.

Progesterone

Progesterone, which is naturally responsible for placenta development and prevention of ovulation, may be indicated in cases of amenorrhea (absence of menstruation), endometreosis (sloughing off of uterine tissue with subsequent attachment to other pelvic organs), dysfunctional uterine bleeding, and for oral contraceptive use.

Oral Contraceptives

There are three types of oral contraceptives:

➡ **monophasic**,

➡ **biphasic**, and

➡ **triphasic**.

Monophasic contraceptives offer a fixed dose of estrogen and progestin (progesterone) while the biphasic and triphasic types deliver the hormones more as they would be naturally secreted by the ovaries. Ortho Novum®, depending on its estrogen/progestin mix, is an example of an oral contraceptive available as any one of the three above mentioned types.

androgens male sex characteristic hormones.

estrogen female sex characteristic hormone that is involved in calcium and phosphorus conservation.

progesterone a female sex characteristic hormone that is involved in ovulation prevention.

testosterone the primary androgen.

MUSCULOSKELETAL AGENTS

Rheumatoid arthritis is a chronic and often progressive inflammatory condition linked to the dysfunction of the immune system. Antibodies called **rheumatoid factors** contribute to the course of the disease. Inflammation caused by the release of histamine and prostaglandins leads to swelling, feelings of warmth, and pain in joints (especially in the hands, wrists, feet, hips, knees, and ankles). As the disease progresses, a decrease in range of motion and an increase in bony fusion and muscle deformity may occur. Patients often show fatigue, low-grade fever, stiffness, and joint pain, especially in the morning.

There is no known cure or method of prevention for rheumatoid arthritis.

Treatment may include drug therapy, physical therapy, occupational therapy, weight reduction, rest, and the use of adaptive or assistive devices. Drug therapy primarily consists of NSAIDs that inhibit prostaglandins synthesis and reduce inflammation. They are also the first line drug of choice due to their analgesic properties. However, as the condition progresses, **disease modifying antirheumatic drugs (DMARD's)** such as methotrexate (see chapter 13, Antineoplastics) as well as gold preparations such as gold sodium thiomate (aqueous) and aurothioglucose (suspended in oil) are indicated.

Gout **is an inflammatory condition in which an excess uric acid and urate crystals accumulate in** *synovial fluids* **of the joints.**

This leads to joint swelling, redness, warmth, and pain. The cause of the gout may be dietary or due to a metabolism dysfunction. A patient may experience an acute attack of gouty arthritis with severe pain, fever, swelling of joints, and inflammation. Stress, diet (e.g., foods high in iodine such as shellfish), alcohol, and infection can precipitate an attack. A first line drug used to treat gouty arthritis would be colchicine. **Uricosuric** drugs (e.g., probenecid) increase elimination of uric acid and **xanthine oxidase inhibitors** (e.g., allopurinol) interfere with uric acid synthesis.

gout a painful inflammatory condition in which excess uric acid accumulates in the joints.

rheumatoid arthritis a chronic and often progressive inflammatory condition with symptoms that include swelling, feelings of warmth, and joint pain.

MUSCULAR SYSTEM

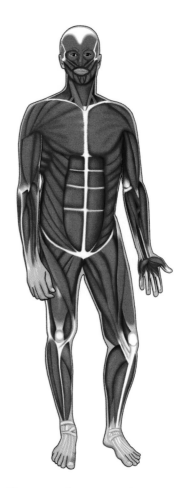

The muscular system is a complex system of connecting and overlapping muscles that completely cover the body. There are **cardiac muscles** in the heart and **smooth muscles** in the arteries and digestive tract, but most muscles are **skeletal muscles** attached to the skeleton by **tendons**. These muscles are made up of long muscle fibers that expand and contract to push and pull bones and cause body movement.

SKELETAL SYSTEM

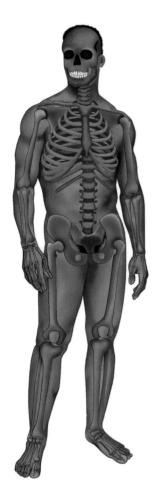

The skeletal system works with the muscular system to provide precise and powerful movement. The system's 206 bones are called **axial** (brain and spinal column) or **appendicular** (arms, legs, and connecting bones). They are held together at **joints** by connective tissue called **ligaments** and **cartilage**. Joints range from rigid to those allowing full motion. The **hinge joints** of the knee, elbow and ankle allow motion along a single axis. The **ball-and-socket joints** of the hips and shoulders allow a much broader range of movement.

Osteoarthritis is marked by weight-bearing bone deterioration, decreasing range of motion, and increasing pain, deformity, and disability.

Water content changes in the bone cartilage weakens the bones, causes cartilage damage and prevents repair. Inflammation may occur. Deep aching and local pain is experienced but can initially be relieved by rest. However, as the disease progresses, pain becomes chronic. Deformity also occurs in the later stages and bony enlargements (**osteophytes**) develop on the fingers and toes.

Drug therapy, physical therapy, adaptive or assistive devices, patient education, and possibly surgery are part of a comprehensive treatment approach.

Drug therapy primarily consists of analgesics, NSAID's, and corticosteroids. Since the majority of patients are elderly, drug treatment is directed at pain relief and is traditionally more conservative than aggressive.

Muscle spasms are painful occurrences that can be infrequent, chronic, or acute, depending on their origin and the patient's underlying medical condition.

Trauma, overwork, or a disorder such as connective tissue irritation can cause painful muscle contractions and involuntary spasms. Severe **spasticity** is usually linked to central nervous system disorders. Traditionally, treatment of muscle spasms is directed at muscle relaxation, pain relief, ability to exercise the muscle, and prevention of motion loss. Centrally acting **antispasmodics** (e.g., diazepam) eliminate contracture and cramps without affecting normal muscle activity. The sedative action of agents such as carisoprodol, chlorzoxazone, and chlorphenesin helps relieve acute musculoskeletal pain while cyclobenzapine decreases muscle tone and reduces spasm.

---

osteoarthritis a disorder characterized by weight-bearing bone deterioration, decreasing range of motion, pain, and deformity.

uricosuric drugs drugs used to treat gout that increase the elmination of uric acid.

NEUROLOGICAL AGENTS

Since nerve cells do not contact other neurons and the muscles they affect directly, nerve impulses are communicated by chemical transmission.

These chemical mediators are **neurotransmitters** or **neurohormones**. They cross the **synapses** (the junctions between nerve cells) and allow transmission of impulses from one neuron to another. Two common peripheral nerve neurotransmitters are **acetylcholine** and **norepinephrine**.

Several common neurological disorders are affected by abnormalities in neurotransmitter release and/or response.

This includes the following disorders: Parkinson's Disease, Alzheimer's Disease, epilepsy, and migraine headaches.

NERVOUS SYSTEM

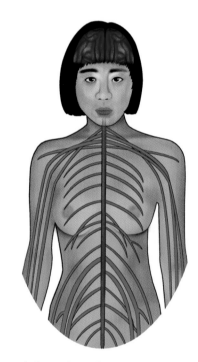

The Nervous System

The nervous system is divided into two main subsystems: the **central nervous system (CNS)** and the **peripheral nervous system.** The central nervous system consists of the brain and spinal cord. The peripheral nervous system carries information throughout the body and links the body's systems together. It is made up of the **somatic nervous system** and the **autonomic nervous system.**

The somatic nervous system is associated with voluntary movements of the musculoskeletal system and sensations (heat, cold, pressure and pain). The autonomic nervous system is responsible for automatic movements (breathing, digestion, etc.).

The autonomic nervous system is divided into the **sympathetic** and **parasympathetic** systems. The sympathetic branch works with the adrenal

gland's medulla and regulates energy in times of stress such as danger, emotional tensions and severe illness. The parasympathetic branch influences bodily functions to slow down and conserve energy. The sympathetic and parasympathetic nervous systems effect a delicate balance and maintain homeostasis on a daily basis within the human body. Drugs referred to as mimics act upon these systems to affect this balance and force a reaction.

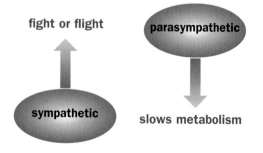

A Delicate Balance

The balance between the sympathetic and parasympathetic systems is illustrated in the "fight or flight" response. In the event of being threatened and frightened, the sympathetic system reacts to increase heart rate, deep breathing, and blood pressure (increases circulation of oxygen), dilate pupils (provides extra light for vision), increase liver glycogen breakdown (supplies glucose and oxygen to muscles for energy), and halt peristalsis. The parasympathetic system will restart digestive and peristaltic actions, constrict the pupils, slow the heart and respiratory rates, and lower blood pressure when the threat is removed.

DISORDERS

THERAPIES

Parkinson's Disease

Parkinson's Disease is a progressive neuromuscular condition that usually affects patients above 50 years of age and is characterized by flat emotionless expression, bent posture, shuffling and unsteady gait, fine tremors, and difficulty chewing and swallowing. Early symptoms may include muscle aches, numbness, coldness, and loss of sensation or tingling. It is associated with low levels of the neurotransmitter **dopamine** in the brain and increased levels of acetylcholine. Brain tumors, arteriosclerosis, severe infectious processes, and excessive use of some antipsychotic drugs may also cause this disease.

Drug therapy will not stop the progress of this disease. Instead, an increased quality of life, decreased side effects, and minimization of disabilities are the goals of chemical treatment. Levodopa, carbidopa and levodopa together, amantadine, and selegiline hydrochloride are commonly prescribed antiparkinsonian drugs. In addition, dopamine agonists (e.g., pergolide and bromocriptine) are indicated when patients are experiencing a decrease in L-dopa's responsiveness. Anticholinergics are used for the treatment of tremors and decreased muscle tone.

Alzheimer's Disease

Alzheimer's, a progressive **dementia** often classified as a psychiatric disorder, has been linked to neurotransmitter abnormalities. It primarily affects the elderly. Loss of memory is often one of the first signs of this condition, with speech impairment, frustration, depression and decreased socialization soon occurring. These symptoms are generally followed by an inability to conduct the activities of daily living as well as a loss of spatial relationships. Ultimately, an inability to recognize familiar people and surroundings, wandering, combative aggression and incontinence occur.

Drug therapy can be divided into treatment for cognitive symptoms most closely associated with dementias and noncognitive symptoms such as depression. Tacrine and donepezil are examples of cognitive symptom agents while secondary amine tricyclic antidepressants (e.g., nortriptyline and desipramine) and SSRI's (e.g., paroxetine and sertraline) are indicated for symptoms such as depression in the Alzheimer patient.

Epilepsy

Epilepsy is a neurologic disorder associated with neuron transmission instability and characterized by recurrent seizure activity. Though there are other causes for seizures (trauma, fever, stress, etc.), the excess excitability seen in seizures may be linked to an imbalance of dopamine and acetylcholine release coupled with factors such as improper pH balance or an inadequate supply of glucose, oxygen, potassium, calcium or amino acids.

Common antiepileptic drugs include phenytoin and phenobarbital. Other drugs include valproic acid and carbamazepine. With anticonvulsant agents, the diagnosis needs to be conclusive and the most appropriate drug for the specific seizure type is chosen.

Migraine Headaches

There are two common theories on the causes of migraine headaches: the *vascular* and *nerve theories*. The vascular theory is that arterial vasoconstriction causes loss of oxygen and inflammation that stimulates sensory nerves in the head and results in possible auras and pain. An aura is an unusual sensation that can include hallucination. Stress, intense lights, colors, and sounds, and sleep deprivation are all considered stimulants of vasoconstriction. The nerve theory is that inflammation of nerve endings in the brain by inflammatory neurotransmitters (i.e., prostaglandins) causes pain.

Aspirin is considered the drug of choice (with caution used when treating children), and NSAID's are especially useful if the patient is female and menstruating. Other drug therapies include: ergotamine, sumatriptan, and midrin. Prophylactic treatment may include: beta-blockers, antidepressants, calcium channel blockers and anticonvulsants.

OPHTHALMIC AGENTS

Ophthalmic agents are used to treat various conditions or disorders of the eye.

Disorders include **glaucoma**, infection, pain, and inflammation, but agents may also be used for eye examinations and in preparation for surgery. Ophthalmic agents are generally applied topically as drops or ointments.

Due to the special requirements for ophthalmic formulations, there are often many ingredients in a product besides the active ingredient.

Preservatives, antioxidants, buffers, and wetting agents that control such factors as pH, sterility, and proper isotonic percentages are often included.

Glaucoma represents several disorders characterized by abnormally high pressure within the eye that leads to optic nerve damage and progressive loss of vision.

The onset of glaucoma can be a slow process that may not be apparent to the patient and may only be detected during an eye examination. Early detection is essential for successful treatment and prevention of vision loss.

Although infection and inflammation can increase *intraocular pressure* temporarily, the common cause of glaucoma is a structural defect in the eye.

This form is called **primary glaucoma** and is divided into two types: **narrow or closed angle** and **wide or open angle**. Narrow angle glaucoma is corrected with surgery. Open angle glaucoma can be successfully treated with antiglaucoma drugs such as cholinergic receptor agonists, acetylcholinesterase inhibitors, carbonic anhydrase inhibitors, beta-adrenergic receptor antagonists, and adrenergic receptor agonists.

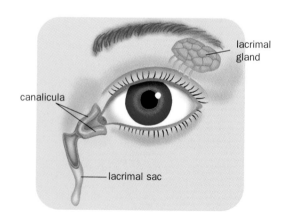

THE EYE

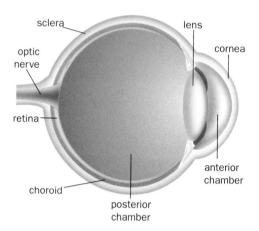

The eyeball has three layers:

- → the outer layer contains the **sclera** (white part) and the **cornea** (clear);
- → the middle vascular layer called the **choroid** contains the **iris** and **pupil**;
- → the inner layer contains the **retina,** responsible for visual reception.

Both the anterior and posterior optic chambers are filled with a liquid called **aqueous humor**. The **lens** is located behind the **iris**. Ocular muscles control the movement of the eyeball and accommodate focusing. The thickness of the lens helps determine the distance at which one can see an object. Behind the lens, a jelly-like substance called the **vitreous body** helps maintain the shape of the eyeball.

Similar to a camera, the pupil allows light to enter. The lens focuses the light, and the retina receives the image. A complex chemical reaction within the retina processes the picture. The optic nerve then carries the image to the visual area of the brain.

Accessory structures to the eyeball include eyelids, ocular muscles, conjunctiva, eyelashes, and lacrimal glands.

Conjunctivitis ("pink eye") is a common eye infection resulting from conjuctival irritation due to infectious organism or allergy.

Conjunctivitis infections are highly contagious. Symptoms are redness of the conjunctiva and pus-like crusty exudate that often leads to the eyelid closing. Antibiotics such as gentamicin, bacitracin, neomycin, sodium sulfacetamide, norfloxacin, and ciprofloxacin are indicated if the infection is bacterial. For viral infections such as herpes simplex and cytomegalovirus retinitis, idoxuridine, vidarabine, and trifluridine are used. If the conjunctivitis is caused by an allergy, histamine blocking agents such as levocabastine, olopatadine, and emedastine may be ordered.

Inflammation of the eye may be treated with both NSAID's and corticosteriods.

Agents such as medrysone, prednisolone, and loteprednol are common ophthalmic corticoseriods while flurbiprofen, suprofen, and ketorolac are NSAID's available for ophthalmic application. Note: flurbiprofen and ketorolac are often used following cataract extraction surgery.

Other drugs include *mydriatics*, anesthetics, and lubricating agents.

Mydriatics are drugs that dilate the pupil and are commonly indicated prior to eye exams. When the pupil is dilated, more light is allowed in and visualization into the eye is enhanced. Phenylephrine and hydroxyamphetamine are popular examples. For optic related pain, a topical anesthetic such as proparacaine (also known as ophthaine) or tetracaine may be prescribed. To provide lubrication to the eyes if abnormal drying is occurring, the isotonic solution Artificial Tears® is available as an over-the counter agent. Lacrisert® is a prescription lubricating drug.

Ophthalmic Administration

➡ Hands should always be washed prior to drug administration.

➡ If more than one agent is to be instilled, wait the suggested time (5 minutes between solutions, 10-15 minutes before ointments) between administrations.

➡ Do not rub eyes. Carefully instill, as per order, onto conjunctiva, one eye at a time.

➡ Do not touch the applicator to the eye at any time.

➡ Replace the applicator cap carefully and do not touch the top of the applicator.

➡ Be aware that temporary vision distortion may occur and encourage the patient accordingly.

➡ The physician should be notified if condition symptoms do not alleviate.

Note: The incidence of adverse reactions to ophthalmic agents is small. Systemic absorption may cause allergic response and steroidal side effects in some cases.

Antiglaucoma Agents

Cholinergic receptor agonists such as pilocarpine and acetylcholine were the first antiglaucoma drugs developed. More recently, **acetylcholinesterase agents** such as physostigmine and demecarium are preferred, since they are more potent, longer acting, and include both reversible and irreversible properties.

Beta-adrenergic receptor antagonists are also now used more commonly than the cholinergic receptor agonists as they are considered more effective and have fewer side effects. Examples of this type include: betaxolol, carteolol, metipranolol, and timolol.

Adrenergic receptor agonists such as epinepherine, atropine, and dipivefrin are used to lower intraocular pressure by increasing outflow of aqueous humor from the eye.

conjunctivitis inflammation of the conjunctiva (eyelid lining).

glaucoma disorders characterized by abnormally high pressure within the eye that leads to optic nerve damage and loss of vision.

intraocular inside the eye.

mydriatics drugs that dilate the pupil.

PSYCHOTROPIC AGENTS

Psychotropic agents **are drugs that affect behavior, psychiatric state, and sleep.**

They act on specialized areas of the brain to suppress or control the symptoms of common psychological disorders such as bipolar disorder, anxiety, depression, schizophrenia, and drug abuse. The primary drug types in this class are **antidepressants**, **antipsychotics**, and **antianxiety agents**. Other related psychotropic agents include **sedatives** and **hypnotics**.

THE BRAIN

The brain is an incredibly versatile and complex organ responsible for a vast number of the body's functions. To a great extent, the structures or areas of the brain are specialized by function. These specialized structures are shown below.

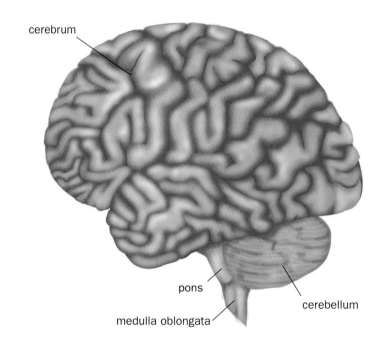

cerebrum

pons

medulla oblongata

cerebellum

Cerebrum

➡ concerned mostly with learned behavior, thought, memory, sensation and voluntary motion. It is divided into lobes: Frontal, Occipital (back) Parietal (top) and Temporal (side).

Cerebellum

➡ controls balance and muscle coordination.

Medulla Oblongata (brain stem)

➡ controls processes that affect the heart, breathing, temperature control and circulation.

Pons

➡ bridges from the medulla oblongata to the cerebellum and also works on muscle coordination.

Thalamus

➡ above the Pons, receives sensations such as heat, cold, pressure and pain.

Hypothalamus

➡ below the Thalamus, controls blood sugar levels, body temperature, emotions, appetite and sleep.

Midbrain

➡ works to control blood pressure and the Pineal Gland secretes the hormone melatonin which effects the body's biological rhythms.

Limbic System

➡ an interconnecting network of brain cells inside the brain that affects behavior, emotions, sociosexual drives, motivation, learning, and memory storage and retrieval.

Sedatives and Hypnotics

Sedatives are drugs that are intended to relax and calm. They reduce restlessness and may produce mild drowsiness. Antianxiety medications that include benzodiazepines (e.g., diazepam and chlordiazepoxide) are included in this group.

Hypnotics are often referred to as "sleeping pills" and are designed to induce and, in some cases, prolong sleep. This group includes barbiturates such as secobarbital and pentobarbital. Nonbarbiturate sedative-hypnotics include chloral hydrate and meprobamate.

DISORDERS

THERAPIES

Bipolar Disorder

Also known as **Manic-Depression**, this disorder is characterized by mood, energy, and behavior swings from periods of elation to episodes of depression. These swings are found to occur in a cyclical and recurring pattern. Theories of cause include chemical imbalance and neurotransmitter alterations in the brain. There is a high degree of family history associated with this disorder.

Although psychotherapy is included in the suggested treatment, antipsychotic drugs such as lithium combined with benzodiazepines such as lorazepam are commonly prescribed. Carbamazepine and valproic acid are often added to this therapy to treat seizure activity secondary to psychotropic agents.

Anxiety

People experiencing anxiety may appear abnormally tired or energetic, withdrawn, tremorous, tense and restless and may suffer from insomnia, phobias and panic attacks. Theories of cause include a hypersensitive sympathetic nervous system, excessive serotonin release, and an inability to chemically receive the body's natural calming agents.

In conjunction with psychotherapy and various relaxation techniques, the commonly prescribed drugs include antianxiety agents such as the benzodiazapines (diazepam, lorazepam, and alprazolam).

Depression

Depression is characterized by mood disturbances that may be mild (e.g., lack of interest or inability to experience joy) or severe (e.g., physical aggression or suicide attempts). Sleep disturbances, crying episodes, gastro-intestinal upset and heart palpitations may occur. Theories of cause include: experience of trauma (real or perceived), loss, as well as poor neurotransmitter response of norepinephrine.

While psychotherapy and even shock therapy are often prescribed treatment, antidepressants such as amitriptyline, paroxetine, and sertraline are common drug suggestions

Schizophrenia

This is characterized by extreme and inappropriate behavior and dysfunctional daily routine. Hearing "voices," experiencing delusions, becoming agitated or hostile and perhaps a lack of response at all (flat affect) are examples of schizophrenic behavior. Theories of cause include: family history and chemical imbalances, especially norephinephrine and serotonin, noted in the limbic system.

Patients experiencing schizophrenia must undergo a complete medical and psychological examination. The drug therapy selected will result from the findings. Antipsychotic agents commonly used may include: chlorpromazine, trifluoperazine, and haloperidol.

Drug Dependency

Addiction to drugs and alcohol may occur for various reasons, including chronic usage without adequate physician supervision, chemical intolerance, error in personal judgement or purposeful abuse. Family history and social situation may be contributing factors.

Treatment for dependency often encompasses an on-site treatment program designed to identify and address the patient holistically. Adjunct drug therapy may or may not be included in this. For example, disulfiram and naltrexone may be used to dissuade the alcoholic from drinking, desipramine curbs cocaine desire, and methadone is prescribed for narcotic detoxification.

RESPIRATORY AGENTS

Balancing oxygen and carbon dioxide levels correctly is essential to health.

The cells of the body use oxygen for energy and produce carbon dioxide as waste. The respiratory system is responsible for exchanging oxygen from the air with carbon dioxide from the body. High carbon dioxide levels alert the medulla of the brain to signal **inspiration** (breathing in) to the **diaphragm** and **intercostal muscles** of the rib cage. It is their action that drives normal respiration. There are two phases of respiration: the **mechanical phase** which involves the diaphragm and the rib cage and allows air to enter the lungs, and the **physiologic phase** in which oxygen and carbon dioxide are exchanged between the lungs and the blood cells. Dysfunction can occur at any time during either phase.

Emotional stimuli as well as medical disorders may alter gas exchange and breathing patterns.

Abnormal breathing patterns can occur for a variety of reasons and include **dyspnea** (labored breathing), wheezing, hyperventilation, and **apnea** (absence of breathing). Common respiratory disorders include: asthma, emphysema, bronchitis, COPD, croup, pneumonia, and allergy (see below).

Drugs commonly indicated in the treatment of respiratory diseases and disorders include *antihistamines, decongestants, antitussives,* **and** *bronchodilators.*

These agents act in a variety of ways to clear the airways and restore normal respiration.

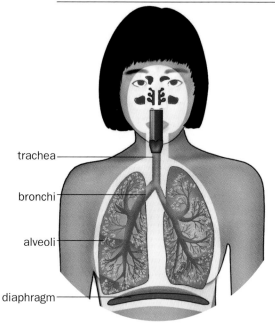

trachea —
bronchi —
alveoli —
diaphragm —

The **trachea** ("windpipe") connects the larynx or "voicebox" and the **bronchi**, the two airway branches that carry air to the lungs. The smaller bronchial tubes are called **bronchioles**, They carry the air to the **alveoli** (air sacs) of the lungs where gas exchange takes place.

Common Respiratory Disorders

➡ **Asthma**: chronic airway inflammation related to stimuli hyperresponsiveness, resulting in airflow obstruction with symptoms such as wheezing and potentially acute spasms and breathlessness.

➡ **Allergy**: allergic response to food, drugs, animals, insect bites, pollens, or dust.

➡ **Emphysema:** chronic airway obstruction due to lung hyperinflation and diminished oxygen intake, characterized by breathlessness and flushed color.

➡ **Croup** (bronchiolitis): an infection of the bronchioles occurring in young children and resulting in airway obstruction and labored breathing.

➡ **Bronchitis**: infection producing excess mucus in the bronchial tree that makes breathing difficult.

➡ **COPD** (chronic obstructive pulmonary disease): also termed COLD (lung) or COAD (airway) by some sources. Abnormal lung function that generally encompasses both emphysema and chronic bronchitis that is present at least for 3 months a year for 2 consecutive years.

➡ **Pneumonia**: infectious process of either bacterial or viral origin whereby fluid accumulates in the lungs causing inadequate or in severe cases, impossible, air exchange at the alveolar level.

AGENTS

Antihistamines

Antihistamines act to respond to the release of **histamine** or inflammation producing substance from white blood cells that occurs with an injury or allergic reaction. Antihistamine agents replace histamine at the inflammation receptor sites to reduce inflammation, swelling, and irritation. Additional properties of antihistamines include: antipruritic (anti-itching), antiemetic, and sedative. Common antihistamines listed by chemical structure are **alkylamines** (e.g., triprolidine), **piperizines** (e.g., hydroxyzine), **phenothiazines** (e.g., promethazine), **piperidines** (e.g., loratidine), **ethanolamines** (e.g.,), and **ethylenedramines** (e.g., pyrilamine).

Decongestants

Decongestants cause mucous membrane vasoconstriction, reduction of nasal passage drainage and relief of stuffiness. These products are available as both oral agents (e.g., pseudoephedrine) and nasal sprays (e.g., phenylephrine).

Antitussives

Antitussives are products which treat both productive (with phlegm) and non-productive (without phlegm) coughs. These agents are available in both narcotic and non-narcotic preparations. Dextromethorphan is the most widely used antitussive agent. Codeine sulfate is a widely used narcotic antitussive agent. **Mucolytic** drugs that act to liquefy thickened bronchial mucous and assist in clearing airways are included in this category by some sources. Acetylcysteine is a commonly indicated mucolytic agent. The **expectorant** guaifenesin is often used with antitussives. It increases the production of respiratory secretions and decreases irritation caused by dryness in the airways.

Bronchodilators

Bronchodilators are drugs which act to relieve **bronchospasm** (a narrowing of the bronchi, accompanied by wheezing and coughing, i.e, an "asthma attack," as seen in disorders such as asthma, emphysema and bronchitis). **Sympathomimetics** (e.g., proventil and metaproterenol) dilate the bronchi. **Xanthine derivatives** (e.g., amoline and theopylline) directly relax the smooth muscle of the bronchi. Both categories of bronchodilators increase the opening of the bronchi and allow more airflow to occur. Note: corticosteroids such as prednisone and anticholinergics such as Atrovent may be used to decrease respiratory airway inflammation and produce some bronchodilation in cases where bronchodilators have failed.

COMMON DRUGS

The following are common drugs listed by classification, generic names, and a limited description of their therapeutic use.

ANALGESICS

Acetylsalicylic Acid (Aspirin)	antipyretic, pain relieving, anti-inflammatory, and anticoagulant.
Methyl Salicylate	topical anti-inflammatory.
Acetaminophen	antipyretic, pain relieving.
Ibuprofen	antipyretic, pain relieving, anti-inflammatory agent.
Nabumetone	non-steroidal anti-inflammatory (NSAID) pain relieving agent.
Naproxen	NSAID, anti-inflammatory, pain relieving.
Oxaprozin	long acting anti-inflammatory, antipyretic, pain relieving agent.
Tramadol Hydrochloride	serotonin reuptake inhibitor for moderate to severe pain.
Hydrocodone Bitartate & Acetaminophen	a narcotic analgesic.
Morphine Sulfate	a narcotic analgesic.
Meperidine Hydrochloride	synthetic opioid analgesic.
Propoxyphene Hydrochloride	mild narcotic analgesic.

ANESTHETICS

Procaine	injection local anesthetic.
Tetracaine	injection local anesthetic.
Bupivacaine	injection local anesthetic.
Dibucaine	injection local anesthetic.
Nitrous Oxide	inhalation general anesthetic.
Halothane	inhalation general anesthetic.
Midazolam	injectable general anesthetic.
Fentanyl Citrate/Droperidol	injectable general anesthetic.

ANTI-INFECTIVES

Ampicillin	penicillin-like antibiotic.
Amoxicillin / Clavulanate	semi-synthetic antibiotic.
Cerufoxime Axetil	cephalosporin antibiotic.
Cefprozil Monohydrate	cephalosporin antibiotic.
Cefaclor	cephalosporin antibiotic.
Cephalexin Hydrochloride	cephalosporin antibiotic.
Levofloxacin	quinolone antibiotic.
Ciprofloxacin	quinolone antibiotic.
Azithromycin	macrolide antibiotic.

Clarithromycin	macrolide antibiotic.
Penicillin V Potassium	anti-infective antibiotic.
Amoxicillin	penicillin-like antibiotic.
Sulfisoxazole	sulfa antibiotic.
Trimethoprim / Sulfamethoxazole	sulfa antibiotic.
Tetracycline	bacteriostatic antibiotic.
Metronidazole	antibacterial and antiprotozoal agent.
Zidovudine	antiviral protease inhibitor.
Acyclovir	antiviral.
Nystatin	fungicidal, fungistatic agent.
Fluconazole	antifungal

ANTINEOPLASTICS

Cyclophosphamide	alkylating agent.
Cisplatin	alkylating agent.
Busulfan	alkylating agent.
Methotrexate	antimetabolite.
5-Fluorouracil	antimetabolite.
Mercaptopurine	antimetabolite.
Vincristine	plant alkaloid.
Paclitaxel	plant alkaloid.
Etoposide	plant alkaloid.
Tamoxifen Citrate	anti-estrogen.

CARDIOVASCULAR AGENTS

Nitroglycerin	antianginal agent.
Nifedipine	antianginal calcium channel blocker.
Verapamil Hydrochloride	antianginal calcium channel blocker.
Isosorbide Mononitrate	vasodilator.
Bretylium Tosylate	antiarrhythmic.
Lidocaine Hydrochloride	antiarrhythmic.
Diltiazem Hydrochloride	antihypertensive calcium channel blocker.
Doxazosin Mesylate	antihypertensive.
Losartan Potassium	antihypertensive.
Losartan / Hydrochlorothiazide	combination antihypertensive diuretic.
Amlodipine Besylate	antihypertensive calcium channel blocker.

COMMON DRUGS (CONT'D)

Felodipine	antihypertensive calcium channel blocker.
Metaprolol Tartrate	antihypertensive beta blocker.
Furosemide	diuretic.
Benazepril Hydrochloride	antihypertensive ACE inhibitor.
Bisoprolol / Hydrochlorothiazide	combination antihypertensive beta blocker and diuretic.
Atenolol	antihypertensive beta blocker.
Terazosin Hydrochloride	antihypertensive.
Lisinopril	antihypertensive ACE inhibitor.
Hydrochlorothiazide	diuretic.
Dobutamine Hydrochloride	diuretic.
Dopamine Hydrochloride	diuretic.
Lovastatin	antihyperlipidemic.
Atorvastatin Calcium	antihyperlipidemic.
Simvastatin	antihyperlipidemic.
Fluvastatin Sodium	antihyperlipidemic.
Pravastatin Sodium	antihyperlipidemic.
Alteplase	thrombolytic.
Warfarin Sodium	anticoagulant.
Heparin	anticoagulant.

DERMATOLOGICALS

Hydrocortisone Cream	steroidal cream
Diphenhydramine Hydrochloride	antihistamine.
Silver Sulfadiazine	topical sulfa antibiotic.
Doxycycline Hyclate	tetracycline group antibiotic.
Clotrimazole / Betamethasone	topical antifungal and steroid.
Ofloxacin	broad spectrum antibiotic.

ELECTROLYTIC AGENTS

Potassium Chloride	potassium replacement
Sodium Chloride	salt replacement
Calcium Chloride	mineral
Magnesium Chloride	mineral

GASTROINTESTINAL AGENTS

Pancrelipase	pancreatic enzyme.
Loperamide Hydrochloride	antidiarrheal.
Diphenoxylate / Atropine	antidiarrheal.

Trimethobenzamide Hydrochloride	antiemetic.
Prochlorperazine Maleate	antiemetic.
Cimetidine	antacid, antiulcer.
Famotidine	antacid, antiulcer.
Lansoprazole	antacid, antiulcer.
Nizatidine	antacid, antiulcer.
Ranatidine Hydrochloride	antacid, antiulcer.
Cisapride	antacid, antiulcer.
Omeprazole	antacid, antiulcer.
Lactulose	laxative.
Docusate Sodium	stool softener.

HEMATOLOGICAL AGENTS

Desmopressin Acetate	coagulation enhancer.
Phytonadione	coagulation enhancer.
Ferrous Sulfate	hematopoietic.
Cyanocobalamin	hematopoietic.
Aminocaproic Acid	hemostatic agent.
Thrombin Powder	hemostatic agent.

HORMONES & MODIFIERS

Fludrocortisone	adrenal agent.
Epinephrine	adrenal agent.
Glyburide	oral antidiabetic.
Glucagon	antidiabetic.
Insulin	antidiabetic.
Troglitazone	oral antidiabetic.
Glipizide	oral antihyperglycemic.
Metformin Hydrochloride	oral antidiabetic.
Glimepride	oral antihyperglycemic.
Methimazole	antithyroid agent.
Levothyroxine Sodium	synthetic thyroid hormone.
Calcitonin-Salmon	synthetic calcitonin.
Norethindrone / Ethinyl Estradiol	oral contraceptive.
Norethindrone / Mestranol	oral contraceptive.
Fluoxymesterone	androgen.
Sildenafil Citrate	erectile dysfunction agent.
Oxytocin	uterine contraction stimulant.
Clomiphene Citrate	fertility agent

COMMON DRUGS
(CONT'D)

IMMUNOBIOLOGIC AGENTS
Diptheria Antitoxin   Diphtheria agent.
Immune Globulin   Hepatitis A, Rubeola, Varicella agent.
Hepatitis B Immune Globulin   Hepatitis B agent.
Rabies Immune Globulin   Rabies agent.
Tetanus Immune Globulin   Tetanus immunization agent.

MUSCULOSKELETAL AGENTS
Gold Sodium Thiomalate   rheumatoid arthritis agent.
Colchicine   anti-inflammatory.
Allopurinol   anti-gout.
Carisoprodol   muscle pain relief agent.
Cyclobenzaprine Hydrochloride   muscle antispasmodic and pain relief.
Diazepam   antispasmodic, antianxiety.

NEUROLOGICAL AGENTS
Carbidopa / Levodopa   anti-Parkinson's agent.
Benztropine Mesylate   anti-Parkinson's agent.
Tacrine Hydrochloride   anti-Alzheimer's.
Gabapentin   antiepileptic.
Phenytoin Sodium   antiepileptic.
Phenobarbital   barbiturate antiepileptic.
Ergotamine / Caffeine   antimigraine.
Sumatriptan Succinate   antimigraine.

OPHTHALMIC AGENTS
Physostigmine Sulfate   anti-glaucoma agent.
Betaxolol Hydrochloride   anti-glaucoma agent.
Timolol Maleate   anti-glaucoma agent.
Dipivefrin Hydrochloride   anti-glaucoma agent.
Gentamicin Sulfate   antibiotic.
Dexamethasone / Tobramycin   combination steroid and antibiotic.
Prednisolone Acetate   steroid.
Ketoralac Tromethamine   NSAID.

PSYCHOTROPIC AGENTS
Carbamazepine   mood stabilizer, anticonvulsant.
Divalproex Sodium   antidepressant, antianxiety, anticonvulsant.
Diazepam   antianxiety.

Lorazepam	antianxiety, sedative.
Alprazolam	antianxiety.
Buspirone Hydrochloride	antianxiety.
Paroxetine Hydrochloride	antidepressant SSRI.
Sertraline Hydrochloride	antidepressant SSRI.
Fluoxetine Hydrochloride	antidepressant SSRI.
Amitriptyline Hydrochloride	tricyclic antidepressant, sedative, pain relief.
Trazodone Hydrochloride	antidepressant.
Bupropion Hydrochloride	antidepressant.
Olanzapine	antipsychotic.
Chlorpromazine Hydrochloride	antipsychotic.
Trifluoperazine Hydrochloride	antipsychotic.
Haloperidol	antipsychotic.
Risperidone	antipsychotic.
Zolpidem Tartrate	hypnotic.
Disulfiram	alcohol aversion agent.
Naltrexone Hydrochloride	alcohol and narcotic addiction therapy.

RESPIRATORY AGENTS

Diphenhydramine Hydrochloride	antihistamine.
Fexofenadine Hydrochloride	antihistamine.
Loratidine	long acting antihistamine.
Cetirizine Hydrochloride	antihistamine.
Pseudoephedrine Hydrochloride	decongestant.
Phenylephrine Hydrochloride	decongestant.
Codeine / Guaifenesin	antitussive.
Benzonatate	antitussive.
Dextromethorphan	antitussive.
Acetylcysteine	mucolytic.
Guaifenesin	expectorant.
Metaproterenol Sulfate	bronchodilator.
Ipratropium Bromide	bronchodilator.
Albuterol Sulfate	bronchodilator.
Salmeterol Xinofoate	bronchodilator.
Theophylline	bronchodilator.
Triamcinolone Acetonide	anti-inflammatory.
Beclomethasone Dipropionate	anti-inflammatory.
Fluticasone Propionate	anti-inflammatory.

GLOSSARY

absorption the movement of the drug from the dosage formulation to the blood.

abstracting services services that summarize information from various primary sources for quick reference.

active transport the movement of drug molecules across membranes by active means, rather than passive diffusion.

acute condition a sudden condition requiring immediate treatment.

acute viral hepatitis a virus caused systemic infection that causes inflammation of the liver.

additive a drug that is added to a parenteral solution.

additive effects the increase in effect when two drugs with similar pharmacological actions are taken.

adjuvant a drug added to a prescription to enhance the action of the primary drug ingredient.

admixture the resulting solution when a drug is added to a parenteral solution.

adverse effect an unintended side affect of a medication that is negative or in some way injurious to a patient's health.

agonist drugs that activate receptors to accelerate or slow normal cell function.

agonist-antagonist a drug with agonist activity at some receptors but antagonist activity at others.

alimentary tract the organs from the mouth to the anus. The GI tract is a portion of the alimentary tract.

aliquot a portion of a mixture.

alveolar sacs (alveoli) the small sacs of specialized tissue that transfer oxygen out of inspired air into the blood and carbon dioxide out of the blood and into the air for expiration.

ampules sealed glass containers with an elongated neck that must be snapped off.

anaphylactic shock a potentially fatal hypersensitivity reaction producing severe respiratory distress and cardiovascular collapse.

anhydrous without water molecules.

androgens male sex hormones.

anemia a deficiency of red blood cells in blood.

antagonist drugs that bind with receptors but do not activate them. They block receptor action by preventing other drugs or substances from activating them.

antibiotic a substance which harms or kills microorganisms like bacteria and fungi.

anticipatory compounding compounding in advance of expected need.

antidote a drug that antagonizes the toxic effect of another drug.

antihyperlipidemics drugs that lower cholesterol and triglyceride levels.

antitoxin a substance that acts against a toxin in the body; also, a vaccine containing antitoxins, used to fight disease.

antitussive a drug that acts against a cough.

aqueous water based.

arrest knob the knob on a balance that prevents any movement of the balance pans.

aseptic techniques methods that maintain the sterile condition of products.

automated dispensing system a system in which medications are dispensed from an automated unit at the point of use upon confirmation of an order communicated by computer from a central system.

auxiliary labels labels regarding specific warnings, foods or medications to avoid, potential side effects, and so on.

bactericidal kills bacteria.

bacteriostatic retards bacteria growth.

bevel an angled surface at the tip of a needle.

bioavailability the relative amount of an administered dose that reaches the general circulation and the rate at which this occurs.

biocompatibility not irritating or infection or abscess causing to body tissue.

bioequivalence the comparison of bioavailability between two dosage forms.

biopharmaceutics the study of the factors associated with drug products and physiological processes, and the resulting systemic concentrations of the drugs.**blocker** another term for an antagonist drug, because antagonists block the action of neurotransmitters.

body surface area a measure used for dosage that is calculated from the height and weight of a person and measured in square meters.

bronchodilators a medication that decongests the bronchial tubes.

bronchospasm a narrowing of the bronchi, accompanied by wheezing and coughing, i.e, an "asthma attack."

browser a software program that allows users to view Web sites on the World Wide Web.

buccal inside the cheek.

buffer system ingredients in a formulation designed to control the pH.

calcium channel blockers drugs that lower blood pressure by relaxing blood vessels.

calibrate to set, mark, or check the graduations of a measuring device.

carcinogenicity the ability of a substance to cause cancer.

centralized pharmacy system a system in which all pharmacy activities in the hospital are conducted at one location, the inpatient pharmacy.

cation a type of ion.

certification a legal proof or document that an individual meets certain objective standards, usually provided by a neutral professional organization.

chronic condition a continuing condition that requires ongoing treatment for a prolonged period.

cirrhosis a chronic and potentially fatal liver disease causing loss of function and increased resistance to blood flow through the liver.

clean rooms areas designed for the preparation of sterile products.

closed formulary a limited list of approved medications.

co-insurance an agreement for cost-sharing between the insurer and the insured.

co-pay the portion of the price of medication that the patient is required to pay.

code carts a locked cart of medications designed for emergency use only.

colloids particles up to a hundred times smaller than that those in suspensions that are, however, likewise suspended in a solution.

colon the large intestine.

competent being qualified and capable.

complexation when molecules of different chemicals attach to each other, as in protein binding.

compliance doing what is required.

compounding record a record of what actually happened when the formulation was compounded.

compression molding a method of making suppositories in which the ingredients are compressed in a mold.

concentration the strength of a solution as measured by the weight-to-volume or volume-to-volume of the substance being measured.

confidentiality the requirement of health care providers to keep all patient information private among the patient, the patient's insurer, and the providers directly involved in the patient's care.

conjunctiva the eyelid lining.

consultant pharmacist develops and maintains an individual pharmaceutical plan for each long-term care patient.

contraceptive device or formulation designed to prevent pregnancy.

GLOSSARY

controlled substance mark the mark (CII-CV) which indicates the control category of a drug with a potential for abuse.

conversions the change of one unit of measure into another so that both amounts are equal.

coring when a needle damages the rubber closure of a parenteral container causing fragments of the closure to fall into the container and contaminate its contents.

counting tray a tray designed for counting pills.

data information that is entered into and stored in a computer system.

database a collection of information structured so that specific information within it can easily be retrieved and used.

DEA number required on all controlled drug prescriptions; identifies the prescriber.

decentralized pharmacy system a system in which pharmacy activities occur in multiple locations within a hospital.

deductible a set amount that must be paid by the patient for each benefit period before the insurer will cover additional expenses.

degradation the change of a drug to a less effective or ineffective form

denominator the bottom or right number in a fraction which is divided into the numerator to give the fraction's value.

depot the area in the muscle where a formulation is injected during an intramuscular injection.

depth filter a filter that can filter solutions being drawn into or expelled from a syringe, but not both ways at the same time.

desiccated thyroid a dried animal thyroid.

dialysis movement of particles in a solution through permeable membranes.

diluent a solvent that dilutes a freeze-dried substance or dilutes a solution.

disintegration the breaking apart of a tablet into smaller pieces.

disposition a term sometimes used to refer to all of the ADME processes together.

dissolution when the smaller pieces of a disintegrated tablet dissolve in solution.

distributive pharmacist makes sure long-term care patients receive the correct medications ordered.

diuretics drugs that increase the elimination of salts and water through urination.

drug-diet interactions when elements of ingested nutrients interact with a drug and this affects the disposition of the drug.

dual co-pay co-pays that have two prices: one for generic and one for brand medications.

dumbwaiter a small elevator that carries objects (but not people) between floors of a building.

duration of action the time drug concentration is above the minimum effective concentration (MEC).

edema swelling from abnormal retention of fluid.

elimination the processes of metabolism and excretion.

emulsifier a stabilizing agent in emulsions.

emulsions mixture of two liquids that do not dissolve into each other; one liquid is spread through the other by mixing and using an emulsifier for stability.

endogenous produced from within the body or within a cell.

enteral a route of administration to any organ in the alimentary tract (ie.e, from the mouth to the anus).

enterohepatic cycling the transfer of drugs and their metabolites from the liver to the bile in the gall bladder and then into the intestine, and then back into circulation.

enzyme a complex protein that catalyzes chemical reactions into other substances.

enzyme induction the increase in enzyme activity that results in greater metabolism of drugs.

enzyme inhibition the decrease in enzyme activity that results in reduced metabolism of drugs.

equivalent weight a drug's molecular weight divided by its valence, a common measure of electrolyte concentration.

esterification combining an organic acid with an alcohol to form an ester.

extemporaneous compounding the on-demand preparation of a drug product according to a physician's prescription, formula, or recipe.

final filter a filter that filters solution immediately before it enters a patient's vein.

finger cots protective coverings for fingers.

first pass metabolism the substantial degradation of a drug caused by enzyme metabolism in the liver before the drug reaches the systemic circulation.

flexor movement an expansion or outward movement by muscles.

flocculating agent electrolytes used in the preparation of suspensions.

floor stock stock (such as large volume parenterals) that does not require patient specific labeling.

flow rate the rate (in ml/hour or ml/minute) at which solution is administered to the patient.

formulary a list of medications that are approved for use.

formulation record formulas and procedures (i.e., recipes) for what should happen when a formulation is compounded/

fusion molding a suppository preparation method in which the active ingredients are dispersed in a melted suppository base.**gastric emptying time** the time a drug will stay in the stomach before it is emptied into the small intestine.

gauge a measurement with needles: the higher the gauge, the smaller the lumen.

geometric dilution a technique for mixing two powders of unequal quantity.

glomerular filtration the blood filtering process of the kidneys.

gonadotropins sex gland stimulants.

gram stain a method for identifying microorganisms based on staining characteristics.

HCFA 1500 Form the standard form used by health care providers, such as physicians, to bill for services; it can also be used to bill for disease state management services.

Health Insurance Portability and Accountability Act (HIPAA) a federal act that, among other things, protects the privacy of individuals and the sharing of protected health information.

hemorrhoid painful swollen veins in the anal/rectal area, generally caused by strained bowel movements from hard stools.

HEPA filter a high efficiency particulate air filter.

heparin lock an injection device which uses heparin to keep blood from clotting in the device.

hepatic disease liver disease.

hepato a prefix meaning "of the liver."

HMOs a network of providers for which costs are covered inside but not outside of the network.

home care agencies home nursing care businesses that provide a range of health care services, including infusion.

homeostasis the state of equilibrium of the body.

hormones chemicals produced by the body that regulate body functions and processes.

hub the part of the needle that attaches to the syringe.

human genome the complete set of genetic material contained in a human cell.

hydrates absorbs water.

hydrophilic capable of associating with or absorbing water.

hydrophilic emulsifier a stabilizing agent for water based dispersion mediums.

GLOSSARY

hydrophobic water repelling; cannot associate with water.

hypersensitivity an abnormal sensitivity generally resulting in an allergic reaction.

hyperthyroidism a condition in which thyroid hormone secretions are above normal, often referred to as an overactive thyroid.

hypertonic when a solution has a greater osmolarity than that of blood.

hyperuricemia an abnormal concentration of uric acid in the blood.**hypothyroidism** a condition in which thyroid hormone secretions are below normal, often referred to as an underactive thyroid.

hypotonic when a solution has a lesser osmolarity than that of blood.

hypoxemia low oxygen levels in the blood, which can be caused by asthma.

idiosyncrasy an unexpected reaction the first time a drug is taken, generally due to genetic causes.

immiscible cannot be mixed.

induction a drug causes more metabolic enzymes to be produced, thus increasing the metabolic activity.

infusion the gradual intravenous injection of a volume of fluid into a patient.

inhibition a drug blocks the activity of metabolic enzymes in the liver.

injunction a court order preventing a specific action, such as the distribution of a potentially dangerous drug.

inotrope a drug that increases the force of cardiac contraction.

inpatient pharmacy pharmacy located in a hospital or inpatient facility which services only those patients in the hospital/facility and ancillary areas.

inspiration breathing in.

integumentary system the body covering, i.e., skin, hair, and nails.

Internet Service Provider (ISP) a company that provides access to the Internet.

interpersonal skills skills involving relationships between people.

inventory to make an accounting of items on hand; also, with people, to assess characteristics, skills, qualities, etc.

ion molecular particles that carry electric charges.

isomer a variation of a drug that has the same molecular formula but a different arrangement of the atoms in the molecule.

isotonic when a solution has an osmolarity equivalent to that of blood.

IUD an intrauterine contraceptive device that is placed in the uterus for a prolonged period of time.

labeling important associated information that is not on the label of the drug product, but is provided with the product in the form of an insert, brochure, or other document.

lacrimal canalicula the tear ducts.

lacrimal gland the gland that produces tears for the eye.

laminar flow continuous movement at a uniform rate in one direction.

legend drug any drug which requires a prescription and either of these "legends" on the label: "Caution: Federal law prohibits dispensing without a prescription," or "Rx only."

levigation triturating a powder drug with a solvent in which it is insoluble to reduce its particle size.

liability legal responsibility for costs or damages arising from misconduct or negligence..

lipoidal fat like substance.

lipophilic emulsifier a stabilizing agent for oil based dispersion mediums.

local effect when drug activity is at the site of administration.

look-alikes drug names that have similar appearance, particularly when written.

lumen the hollow center of a needle.

lymphocytes a type of white blood cells that helps the body defend itself against bacteria and diseased cells.

lyophilized freeze-dried.

maintenance medication a medication that is required on a continuing basis for the treatment of a chronic condition.

mark-up the difference between the retailer's sale price and their purchase price.

materia medica generally pharmacology, but also refers to the drugs in use (from the Latin materia, matter, and medica, medical).

Material Safety Data Sheets (MSDS) OSHA required notices for hazardous substances that provide hazard, handling, clean-up, and first aid information.

maximum allowable cost (MAC) the maximum price per tablet (or other dispensing unit) an insurer or PBM will pay for a given product.

Medicaid a federal-state program, administered by the states, providing health care for the needy.

Medicare a federal program providing health care to people with certain disabilities over age 65; it includes basic hospital insurance and voluntary medical insurance.

medication administration record (MAR) a form that tracks the medications administered to a patient.

medication order the form used to prescribe medications for patients in institutional settings.

membrane filter a filter that attaches to a syringe and filters solution through a membrane as the solution is expelled from the syringe.

meniscus the curved surface of a column of liquid.

metabolite the substance resulting from the body's transformation of an administered drug.

milliequivalent (mEq) a unit of measure for electrolytes in a solution.

mimetic another term for an agonist, because agonists imitate or "mimic" the action of the neurotransmitter.

minimum effective concentration (MEC) the blood concentration needed of a drug to produce a response.

minimum toxic concentration (MTC) the upper limit of the therapeutic window. Drug concentrations above the MTC increase the risk of undesired effects.

miscible capable of being mixed together.

modem computer hardware that enables a computer to communicate through telephone lines.

molecular weight the sum of the atomic weights of one molecule.

mucilage a wet, slimy liquid formed as an initial step in the wet gum method.

mydriatics drugs that dilate the pupil.

myocardial infarction heart attack.

myometrium the muscular wall of the uterus.

nasal cavity the cavity behind the nose and above the roof of the mouth that filters air and moves mucous and inhaled contaminants outward and away from the lungs.

nasal inhaler a device which contains a drug that is vaporized by inhalation.

nasal mucosa the cellular lining of the nose.

NDC (National Drug Code) number the number assigned by the manufacturer. The first five digits indicate the manufacturer. The next four indicate the medication, its strength, and dosage form. The last two indicate the package size.

necrosis the death of cells.

negligence failing to do something that should or must be done.

nephron the functional unit of the kidneys.

nephrotoxicity the ability of a substance to harm the kidneys.

neurotransmitter chemicals released by nerves that interact with receptors to cause an effect.

GLOSSARY

nomenclature a system of names specific to a particular field.

nomogram a chart showing relationships between measurements.

non-formulary drugs not on the formulary which the physician can order; a physician may have to fill out a form stating why that particular drug is needed.

numerator the top or left number in a fraction that indicates a portion of the denominator to be used.

OBRA '90 a federal act that is generally credited for states mandating pharmacist counseling on all new prescriptions.

obstructive jaundice an obstruction of the bile excretion process.

oil-in-water emulsion an emulsion in which oil is dispersed through a water base.

online adjudication the resolution of prescription coverage through the communication of the pharmacy computer with the third party computer.

onset of action the time MEC is reached and the response occurs.

open formulary a system that allows the pharmacy to purchase any medication that is prescribed

ophthalmic related to the eye.

Orange Book the common name for the FDA's Approved Drugs Products.

orthostatic hypertension a drop in blood pressure upon standing up.

osmotic pressure a characteristic of a solution determined by the number of dissolved particles in it.

osmosis the action in which a drug in a higher concentration solution passes through a permeable membrane to a lower concentration solution.

outpatient pharmacy a pharmacy attached to a hospital servicing patients who have left the hospital or who are visiting doctors in a hospital outpatient clinic.

panacea a cure-all (from the Greek panakeia, same meaning).

parenteral a route of administration to any organ outside of the alimentary tract (e.g., ophthalmic, dermal).

passive diffusion the movement of drugs from an area of higher concentration to lower concentration.

patient assistance programs manufacturer sponsored prescription drug programs for the needy.

pediatric having to do with the treatment of children.

percutaneous absorption the absorption of drugs through the skin, often for a systemic effect.

perpetual inventory a system that maintains a continuous record of every item in inventory so that it always shows the stock on hand.

personal digital assistant (PDA) a fully functioning computer the size of a notebook.

pH the pH scale measures the acidity or the opposite (alkalinity) of a substance. 7 is the neutral midpoint of the scale, values below which represent increasing acidity, and above which represent increasing alkalinity.

pharmaceutical alternative drug products that contain the same active ingredients, but not necessarily in the same amount or dosage form.

pharmaceutical equivalent drug products that contain identical amounts of the same active ingredients in the same dosage form.

pharmaceutical of or about drugs; also, a drug product.

pharmacogenetics a new field of study which defines the hereditary basis of individual differences in absorption, distribution, metabolism, and excretion (the ADME processes).

pharmacognosy derived from the Greek words "pharmakon" or drug and "gnosis" or knowledge; the study of physical, chemical, biochemical and biological properties of drugs as well as the search for new drugs from natural sources.

pharmacology the study of drugs—their properties, uses, application, and effects (from the Greek pharmakon: drug, and logos: word or thought).

pharmacopeia an authoritative listing of drugs and issues related to their use.

pharmacy benefits managers companies that administer drug benefit programs

piggybacks small volume solutions added to an LVP.

placebo an inactive substance given in place of a medication.

pneumatic tube a system which shuttles objects through a tube using compressed air as the force

point of sale system (POS) an inventory system in which the item is deducted from inventory as it is sold or dispensed.

policy and procedure manual documentation of required policies, procedures, and disciplinary actions in a hospital.

positional notation the position of the number carries a mathematical significance or value.

POSs a network of providers where the patient's primary care physician must be a member and costs outside the network may be partially reimbursed.

potentiation when one drug with no inherent activity of its own increases the activity of another drug that produces an effect.

PPOs a network of providers where costs outside the network may be partially reimbursed and the patient's primary care physician need not be a member.

prefix a modifying component of a term located before the other components of the term.

prescription a written order from a practitioner for the preparation and administration of a medicine or device.

prescription drug benefit cards cards that contain third party billing information for prescription drug purchases.

primary emulsion the initial emulsion to which ingredients are added to create the final product.

primary literature original reports of clinical and other types of research projects and studies.

PRN order an order for medication to be administered only on an as needed basis.

prodrug an inactive drug that becomes active after it is transformed by the body.

professional practice journals official publications of pharmacy organizations.

protein binding the attachment of a drug molecule to a plasma or tissue protein, effectively making the drug inactive, but also keeping it within the body.

protocols specific guidelines for practice

punch method a method for filling capsules by repeatedly pushing or "punching" the capsule into an amount of drug powder.

purchase order number the number assigned to each order for identification.

pyrogens chemicals produced by microorganisms that can cause pyretic (fever) reactions in patients.

qsad the quantity needed to make a prescribed amount.

Qualified Medicare Beneficiaries Medicare patients who may at times qualify for prescription drug coverage through a state administered program.

recall the action taken to remove a drug from the market and have it returned to the manufacturer.

receptor the cellular material at the site of action that interacts with the drug.

GLOSSARY

reorder points minimum and maximum stock levels which determine when a reorder is placed and for how much.

resorption absorption of bone elements into the blood.

rheumatoid arthritis a disease in which the body's immune system attacks joint tissue.

root word the base component of a term which gives a word its meaning and which may be modified by other components.

safety caps a child-resistant cap.

satellites pharmacy locations in a decentralized systems that operate outside the central pharmacy.

saturated solution a solution containing the maximum amount of drug it can contain at room temperature.

search engine software that searches the web for information related to criteria entered by the user.

secondary literature general reference works based upon primary literature sources.

selective (action) the characteristic of a drug that makes its action specific to certain receptors and the tissues they affect.

sensitivity the amount of weight that will move the balance pointer one division mark on the marker plate.

sharps needles, jagged glass or metal objects, or any items that might puncture or cut the skin.

shelf stickers stickers with bar codes that can be scanned for inventory identification.

signa the directions for use on the prescription that must be printed on the prescription label.

signature log a book in which patients sign for the prescriptions they receive, for legal and insurance purposes.

site of action the location where an administered drug produces an effect.

solution a clear liquid made up of one or more substances dissolved in a solvent.

solvent a liquid that dissolves another substance in it.

sonication exposure to high frequency sound waves.

spatulation mixing powders with a spatula.

sphygmomanometer a device used to measure blood pressure.**point of sale system (POS)** an inventory system in which the item is deducted from inventory as it is sold or dispensed.

stability the chemical and physical integrity of the dosage unit, and when appropriate, its ability to withstand microbiological contamination.

standing order a standard medication order for patients to receive medication at scheduled intervals.

STAT order an order for medication to be administered immediately.

steatorrhea a condition of excess fat in the feces.

sterile a sterile condition is one which is free of all microorganisms, both harmful and harmless.

stratum corneum the outermost cell layer of the epidermis.

sublingual under the tongue.

suffix a modifying component of a term located after the other components of the term.

supersaturated solution a solution containing a larger amount of drug than it normally contains at room temperature.

suspending agent a thickening agent used in the preparation of suspensions.

suspensions formulations in which the drug does not completely dissolve in the liquid.

synergism when two drugs with similar pharmacological actions produce greater effects than the sum of the individual effects.

synthetic with chemicals, combining simpler chemicals into more complex compounds, creating a new chemical not found in nature as a result.

syringeability the ease with which a suspension can be drawn from a container into a syringe.

Syrup USP 850 grams of sucrose and 450 ml of water per liter.

systemic effect when a drug is introduced into the circulatory system.

teratogenecity the ability of a substance to cause abnormal fetal development when given to a pregnant woman.

tertiary literature condensed works based on primary literature, such as textbooks, monographs, etc.

therapeutic serving to cure or heal.

therapeutic equivalent pharmaceutical equivalents that produce the same effects in patients.

therapeutic window a drug's blood concentration range between its minimum effective concentration and minimum toxic concentration.

topical applied for local effect, usually to the skin.

total nutrient admixture (TNA) solution a TPN solution that contains intravenous fat emulsion.

total parenteral nutrition (TPN) solution complex solutions with two base solutions (amino acids and dextrose) and additional micronutrients.

transaction window counter area designated for taking prescriptions and delivering them.

transcorneal transport drug transfer into the eye.

trituration the process of grinding particles to reduce particle size.

turnover the rate at which inventory is used, generally expressed in number of days.

tuberculosis an infectious disease which primarily affects the respiratory system.

U&C or UCR usual and customary—the maximum amount of payment for a given prescription, determined by the insurer to be a usual and customary (and reasonable) price.

unit dose packaging a package containing the amount of a drug required for one dose.

unit price the price of a unit of medication (such as an ounce of liquid cold remedy).

universal claim form a standard claim form accepted by many insurers.

URL (uniform resource locator) a web address.

valence the number of positive or negative charges on an ion.

vasoconstriction a constriction of the blood vessels.

vasodilators drugs that relax and expand the blood vessels.

variable an unknown value in a mathematical equation.

ventricular fibrillation irregular heart action seen in cardiac arrest patients.

vial a small glass or plastic container with a rubber closure sealing the contents in the container.

viscosity the thickness of a liquid.

volumetric measures volume.

water soluble the property of a substance being able to dissolve in water.

water-in-oil emulsions an emulsion in which water is dispersed through an oil base.

waters of hydration water molecules that attach to drug molecules.

wheal a raised blister-like area on the skin, as caused by an intradermal injection.

workers' compensation an employer compensation program for employees accidentally injured on the job.

World Wide Web a collection of electronic documents at Internet addresses called Web sites.

QUICK INDEX